Evaluation, Care and Management of Musculoskeletal Disorders

Evaluation, Care and Management of Musculoskeletal Disorders

Edited by Daphne Horton

hayle
medical

New York

Hayle Medical,
750 Third Avenue, 9th Floor,
New York, NY 10017, USA

Visit us on the World Wide Web at:
www.haylemedical.com

ISBN: 978-1-63241-712-1

Cataloging-in-Publication Data

Evaluation, care and management of musculoskeletal disorders / edited by Daphne Horton.
    p. cm.
Includes bibliographical references and index.
ISBN 978-1-63241-712-1
1. Musculoskeletal system--Diseases. 2. Musculoskeletal system--Diseases--Diagnosis.
3. Musculoskeletal system--Diseases--Treatment. I. Horton, Daphne.
RC925 .E83 2019
616.7--dc23

Table of Contents

Preface

The purpose of the book is to provide a glimpse into the dynamics and to present opinions and studies of some of the scientists engaged in the development of new ideas in the field from very different standpoints. This book will prove useful to students and researchers owing to its high content quality.

Musculoskeletal disorders refer to the pain, disorders and injuries in the human musculoskeletal system, including the joints, nerves, ligaments and muscles. Such disorders result from sudden exertion caused due to the lifting of heavy objects, repetition of same motions, or awkward postures. Some common musculoskeletal disorders include tension neck syndrome, tendinitis, epicondylitis and carpal tunnel syndrome. In order to diagnose musculoskeletal disorders, doctors often use lab tests, Nordic questionnaire, physical examination, X-rays and magnetic resonance imaging. Electrical muscle stimulation is used to prevent disuse muscle atrophy from occurring after musculoskeletal injuries. This book provides significant information of musculoskeletal disorders to help develop a good understanding of their evaluation, care and management. The topics included herein on musculoskeletal disorders are of utmost significance and bound to provide incredible insights to readers. The extensive content of this book provides the readers with a thorough understanding of the subject.

At the end, I would like to appreciate all the efforts made by the authors in completing their chapters professionally. I express my deepest gratitude to all of them for contributing to this book by sharing their valuable works. A special thanks to my family and friends for their constant support in this journey.

Editor

The prevalence of myofascial trigger points in neck and shoulder-related disorders

Daniel Cury Ribeiro[*] [iD], Angus Belgrave, Ana Naden, Helen Fang, Patrick Matthews and Shayla Parshottam

Abstract

Background: Neck and shoulder disorders may be linked to the presence of myofascial trigger points (MTrPs). These disorders can significantly impact a person's activities of daily living and ability to work. MTrPs can be involved with pain sensitization, contributing to acute or chronic neck and shoulder musculoskeletal disorders. The aim of this review was to synthesise evidence on the prevalence of active and latent MTrPs in subjects with neck and shoulder disorders.

Methods: We conducted an electronic search in five databases. Five independent reviewers selected observational studies assessing the prevalence of MTrPs (active or latent) in participants with neck or shoulder disorders. Two reviewers assessed risk of bias using a modified Downs and Black checklist. Subject characteristics and prevalence of active and latent MTrPs in relevant muscles was extracted from included studies.

Results: Seven articles studying different conditions met the inclusion criteria. The prevalence of MTrPs was compared and analysed. All studies had low methodologic quality due to small sample sizes, lack of control groups and blinding. Findings revealed that active and latent MTrPs were prevalent throughout all disorders, however, latent MTrPs did not consistently have a higher prevalence compared to healthy controls.

Conclusions: We found limited evidence supporting the high prevalence of active and latent MTrPs in patients with neck or shoulder disorders. Point prevalence estimates of MTrPs were based on a small number of studies with very low sample sizes and with design limitations that increased risk of bias within included studies. Future studies, with low risk of bias and large sample sizes may impact on current evidence.

Keywords: Shoulder pain, Neck pain, Trigger point, Myofascial pain, Trigger point, Rotator cuff muscle

Background

Neck and shoulder pain are common complaints that may significantly impact a person's activities of daily living and their ability to work [1]. In New Zealand, shoulder pain is the third most common musculoskeletal condition. Neck pain is the 4th highest condition in terms of years lived with disability [2]. Within New Zealand, ACC reports the 12-month prevalence estimates for neck pain in the adult population lie between 30 and 50%, and accounts for 15% of the global burden of disease [2].

Myofascial trigger points (MTrPs) are considered to be hypersensitive, tender areas over a taut band of muscle [3].

They are palpable, produce localised and referred pain to other structures with mechanical stimulation [4, 5]. MTrPs can be further differentiated as active or latent [3]. Active and latent MTrPs elicit local and referred pain, however active MTrPs also reproduce patient symptoms, whereas latent MTrPs do not [3, 4, 6]. Latent MTrPs may later become active [3, 7]. It is considered that both active and latent MTrPs can cause muscle imbalances, weakness and impaired motor recruitment, disrupting muscle function, and exposing joint to suboptimal loading [8].

The theory of trigger points causing myofascial pain syndrome is controversial with limited external validity to support it [9]. Despite that, physiotherapy interventions commonly target MTrPs [10, 11]. Active and latent MTrPs may contribute to neck and shoulder pain symptoms [12].

* Correspondence: daniel.ribeiro@otago.ac.nz
Centre for Health, Activity and Rehabilitation Research (CHARR), School of
Physiotherapy – University of Otago, PO Box 56, Dunedin 9054, New Zealand

In a study with small sample size, active MTrPs were found to present higher concentration of inflammatory mediators, neuropeptides, cytokines, and catecholamines if compared to latent MTrPs or other body regions with no MTrPs [13]. Latent MTrPs were found to impact on motor recruitment patterns [14], accelerate fatigue [15] in agonist muscles, and seem to be linked to increased muscle activity of antagonist muscles [16].

Patients with chronic, non-traumatic neck and shoulder pain were found to have higher prevalence of MTrPs when compared to healthy controls, with different distributions between muscles of two opposing anatomical structures [12]. For example, active MTrPs were prevalent in the infraspinatus and upper trapezius muscles, whilst latent MTrPs were prevalent in the teres major and anterior deltoid muscles [12]. Studies investigating shoulder impingement have reported active MTrPs in infraspinatus, subscapularis, supraspinatus, and pectoralis major muscles [17]. Together, these findings suggest that MTrPs are likely to be present in different shoulder and neck disorders, and may vary in muscle distribution and type (i.e. active or latent).

Knowledge of MTrP common locations at the neck and shoulder can help clinicians to optimally prescribe interventions to manage neck and shoulder disorders. To our knowledge no previous systematic review summarized findings from and assessed the methodological quality of studies assessing the prevalence of MTrPs in the upper quadrant (i.e. neck and shoulder disorders). A previous review focused on spinal disorders only, without assessing patients with shoulder disorders [18]. Given the link between these structures (i.e. neck, scapula and shoulder), we deemed appropriate to conduct a systematic review assessing the upper quadrant. Therefore, the objective of this study was to synthesize the current evidence on the prevalence of active and latent MTrPs in subjects with acute or chronic neck and shoulder disorders. The specific aims were to: (1) identify the prevalence of MTrPs in neck, scapular and shoulder muscles; and (2) compare the prevalence of MTrPs in subjects with diagnosed acute or chronic neck or shoulder-related disorders to healthy controls.

Methods
The protocol of this review is described in Additional file 1.

Study retrieval and screening
A comprehensive literature search of databases including CINAHL, Embase, Pubmed, Scopus and Web of Science was completed on August 12, 2017. The search strategy used is presented in Table 1. Screening of reference lists from included studies was also performed. Articles were then exported into Endnote and duplicates were removed. The retrieved articles were screened for eligibility by title, followed by full-article screening. There was no attempt to access unpublished studies or supplementary 'grey' literature.

Initially, two independent reviewers screened articles by titles, and a third reviewer was available if consensus was not achieved. Full texts of potential eligible studies were retrieved and assessed independently against the inclusion criteria by two reviewers (A.B., and P.M.). Discrepancies between reviewers regarding full text eligibility were resolved in a consensus meeting and a third reviewer (DCR) was consulted.

Eligibility criteria
The following study designs were included in this review: (1) full-text articles published in a peer-reviewed scientific journal; (2) observational, cross-sectional, or prospective studies assessing the prevalence of active and/or latent MTrPs in at least one group of adult subjects (> 18 years old) with a shoulder, scapular, or neck disorder (as diagnosed by the original study); and (3) inclusion of manual assessment of MTrPs in at least one specific neck, scapular or shoulder muscle. Articles in any languages and medical diagnoses indicating the presence of shoulder, scapular, or neck were accepted and included in this review. All study designs other than the aforementioned were excluded, unless randomised control trials included the prevalence of MTrPs as a baseline measurement.

Risk of bias within included studies
A modified Downs and Black checklist [19] was used to assess the risk of bias within included studies. This checklist is a 27 item checklist; however, 11 items were excluded as these were not applicable for this systematic review. Each study was assessed independently by 2 reviewers. Disagreements were resolved through consensus, if consensus was not reached, then a third author (D.R) was consulted. Studies scoring 50% or more were considered to have low risk of bias; whilst studies presenting with a Downs and Black score lower than 50% were considered to have a high risk of bias. For the purpose of this review, we arbitrarily selected a 50% cut-off. This threshold been used by a previous systematic review assessing observational studies [18].

Data extraction
Characteristics from each study and additional patient and control group information were extracted and recorded. The proportion of participants with active/latent MTrPs in all assessed muscles were documented from each study. When available, we extracted information regarding the duration of the condition (i.e. acute or chronic). The data was independently extracted by two reviewers, and double-checked for accuracy.

Table 1 Search strategy and key terms used

Database	Keywords	Number of Studies
CINAHL	(1) shoulder/ or glenohumeral/ or scapular/ or scapula/ or neck/ or cervical; (2) trigger point/ or trigger points; (3) prevalence; (4) disease/ or musculoskeletal diseases; (5) 1 and 2 and 3 and 4	3
Embase	(1) shoulder/ or glenohumeral/ or scapular/ or scapula/ or neck/ or cervical; (2) trigger point/ or trigger points; (3) prevalence; (4) disease/ or musculoskeletal diseases; (5) 1 and 2 and 3 and 4	2
Pubmed	(1) shoulder/ or glenohumeral/ or scapular/ or scapula/ or neck/ or cervical; (2) trigger point/ or trigger points (3) prevalence (4) "disease" [MeSH Terms]/ OR disease [All Fields]/ or disorder [All Fields]/ or condition [All Fields]/ or "musculoskeletal diseases" [MeSH Terms] (5) 1 and 2 and 3 and 4	40
Scopus	(1) shoulder/ or glenohumeral/ or scapular/ or scapula/ or neck/ or cervical; (2) trigger point/ or trigger points; (3) prevalence; (4) disease/ or musculoskeletal diseases; (5) 1 and 2 and 3 and 4	30
Web of Science	(1) shoulder/ or glenohumeral/ or *scapula*/ or neck/ or Cervical; (2) trigger* point*; (3) prevalence; (4) disease/ or musculoskeletal diseases; (5) 1 and 2 and 3 and 4	38
Total number of articles identified		113
Excluding Duplicates		84

Data analysis

As each included study analysed a different disorder, it was not possible to conduct a meta-analysis. Therefore, a narrative discussion of findings is presented.

Results

The flow of studies in the review is presented in Fig. 1. Seven articles were included in this systematic review, with a sample size of 433 participants. Four studies had a cross-sectional design, while three studies used a case-control design.

Risk of bias within included studies

The risk of bias within included studies is presented in Table 2. Overall, studies were considered as having low risk of bias. There is some risk of bias for external validity. For example, subjects were considered as not representative of the entire population in three studies, and it was not possible to determine this in two studies (Item 8, Table 2). Risk of bias for internal validity was mainly due to participants not being recruited from the same population (Item 14 – Table 2) or due to lack of clarity about the recruitment period (not clear in four studies – Item 15, Table 2). Finally, three studies did not estimate sample size a priori.

Characteristics of included studies

The included studies analysed the following disorders: chronic tension-type headache, chronic non-traumatic unilateral shoulder pain, non-specific upper quadrant pain, acute whiplash disorder, unilateral shoulder impingement syndrome and episodic migraine. For each disorder, MTrP prevalence was assessed in different muscles (e.g. upper trapezius, supraspinatus, sternocleidomastoid) (Table 3). The characteristics of the subjects included in the studies is presented in Table 4, and the

point prevalence of active MTrPs in subjects with shoulder or neck disorders is presented in Table 5.

Chronic tension-type headache

Alonso-Blanco et al. (2011) analysed the prevalence of active MTrPs in dominant and non-dominant temporalis, upper trapezius, sternocleidomastoid (SCM), and bilateral suboccipital muscles [5]. The sample contained 20 adults and 20 children with chronic tension-type headache. Results showed adults had a significantly ($p = 0.001$) higher number of active MTrPs (4, SD = -0.8) than children (3, SD = -0.7). Significant differences in the distribution of active MTrPs between adults and children were found in the dominant upper trapezius ($p < 0.001$), and the non-dominant SCM ($p = 0.032$) muscles. This study had some external validity and power bias.

Chronic non-traumatic unilateral shoulder pain

Bron et al. (2011) reported on the prevalence of MTrPs in 72 subjects with chronic non-traumatic unilateral shoulder pain [20]. This study analysed the prevalence of MTrPs on upper trapezius, middle trapezius, lower trapezius, infraspinatus, supraspinatus, subscapularis, teres minor, teres major, posterior deltoid, middle deltoid, anterior deltoid, pectoralis major, pectoralis minor, biceps, triceps, scalenes and subclavius muscles. Muscles containing active MTrPs were present in all participants, and the median number of MTrPs was 6 (range 2–16) per subject. Latent MTrPs were found in 67 participants with a median of 4 (range 0–11). Active MTrPs were most prevalent in the infraspinatus ($n = 56$) and the upper trapezius muscles ($n = 42$); whereas latent MTrPs were most prevalent in the teres major ($n = 35$), anterior deltoid ($n = 27$) and upper trapezius (n = 27) muscles. Although there was no difference found between left and right sides, this study demonstrated a high prevalence of active and latent MTrPs in muscles of patients with

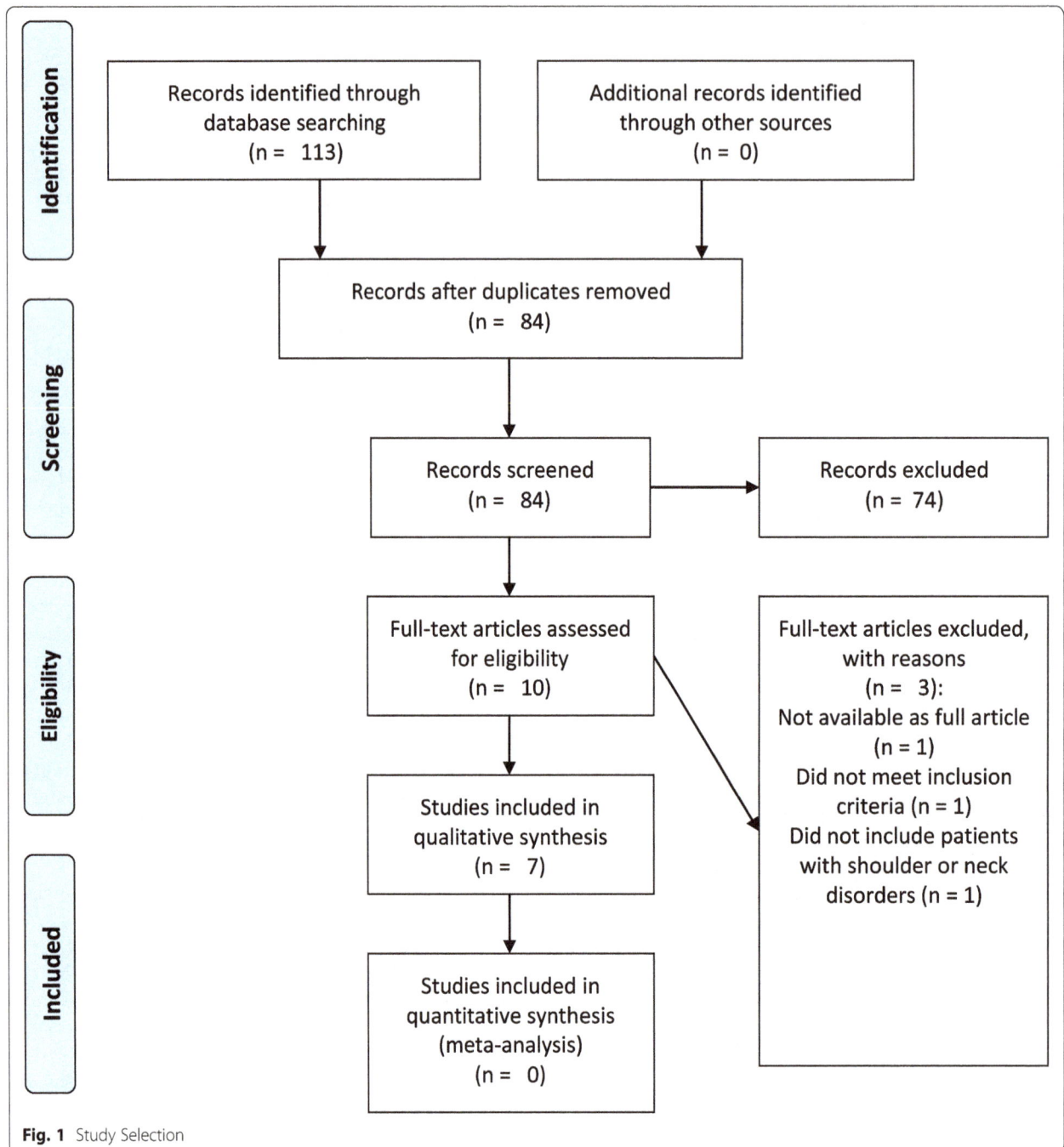

Fig. 1 Study Selection

non-traumatic shoulder pain. This study had small reporting and external validity bias.

Non-specific upper quadrant pain

Fernández-De-Las-Peñas et al. (2012) analysed the prevalence of active MTrPs in the head, neck an d arm between manual (blue collar) and office (white-collar) workers with nonspecific neck or shoulder pain [21]. There was a similar number of MTrPs in the upper quadrant musculature with the most prevalent being upper trapezius, infraspinatus, levator scapulae, and extensor carpi radialis brevis muscles for both groups. No significant difference between groups was found with regards to the distribution of active and latent MTrPs, or the total number ($p = 0.503$) of active ($p = 0.657$) and latent ($p = 0.605$) MTrPs. Manual workers demonstrated a mean of 6 (SD = 3) active MTrPs, and 10 (SD = 6) latent MTrPs compared to the 6 (SD = 4) active and 11 (SD = 5) latent MTrPs shown in office workers [21]. This study had some reporting, external and internal validity risk of bias.

Table 2 Risk of bias within included studies

Study	Reporting Bias							External Validity			Internal validity					Power	Risk of Bias
	Item 1	Item 2	Item 3	Item 4	Item 5	Item 6	Item 7	Item 8	Item 9	Item 10	Item 11	Item 12	Item 13	Item 14	Item 15	Item 16	
Alonso-Blanco et al., 2011	✓	✓	✓	✓	✓	✓	✓	✓	✗	✗	✓	✓	✓	✓	✓	✗	Low
Bron et al., 2011	✓	✓	✓	✓	✓	✓	✗	✓	✓	✗	✓	✓	✓	✓	✓	✓	Low
Fernández-De-Las-Peñas, 2012	✓	✓	✓	✓	✓	✓	✓	✗	?	✓	✓	✓	✓	✗	?	✓	Low
Fernandez-Perez, 2012	✓	✓	✓	✓	✓	✓	✓	✗	✓	✓	✓	✓	✓	✗	?	✓	Low
Hilalgo-Lozano et al., 2010	✓	✓	✓	✓	✓	✓	✓	?	?	✓	✓	✓	✓	✗	?	✗	Low
Sari et al., 2012	✓	✓	✓	✗	✓	✓	✓	?	?	✗	✓	✓	✓	?	?	✗	Low
Tali et al., 2014	✓	✓	✓	✓	✓	✗	✓	✗	✓	✓	✓	✓	✓	✓	✓	?	Low

Abbreviations: ✓, yes ✗, no?, unable to determine

Acute whiplash disorder

Fernandez-Perez et al. (2012) compared the prevalence of MTrPs in patients with a high level of disability following acute whiplash injuries with healthy controls [22]. The distribution of MTrPs were statistically significant ($p < 0.05$) in the temporalis, upper trapezius, SCM, levator scapulae, scalenes, and suboccipital muscles between patient and healthy control groups. Active MTrPs in levator scapulae ($p = 0.012$) and upper trapezius ($p < 0.01$) muscles were more prevalent in the patient group when compared to healthy controls. When compared to healthy controls participant's suffering from whiplash associated disorder (WAD) had significantly higher prevalence in the mean total number of MTrPs per person (7.3, SD = 2.8). Patients with WAD had a significantly higher number of active MTrPs per person (3.9, SD = 2.5). No active MTrPs were found in healthy controls ($p < 0.001$). Significant differences in latent MTrPs were also observed between groups ($p = 0.002$). Participants with acute WAD had a mean of 3.4 (SD = 2.7) latent MTrPs per person, whereas healthy subjects had a mean of 1.7 (SD = 2.2) [22]. This study had some reporting, external and internal validity risk of bias.

Unilateral shoulder impingement syndrome

Hidalgo-Lozano et al. (2010) assessed the prevalence of MTrPs in 12 patients with unilateral shoulder impingement syndrome compared to healthy controls [17]. On average each patient had 4.5 (SD = 1) MTrPs and of those, 2.5 (SD = 1) were active MTrPs and 2 (SD = 1) were latent. However, no distinction was made between left and right shoulders. Point prevalence of active MTrPs was most predominant in supraspinatus (67%), infraspinatus (42%) and subscapularis (42%). The distribution of MTrPs in muscles was also significantly higher in individuals with unilateral shoulder impingement syndrome in comparison to healthy controls. Differences in

MTrPs between healthy controls and symptomatic participants were reported for the levator scapulae, supraspinatus, infraspinatus, pectoralis major, and biceps brachii but not subscapularis muscles. Both active and latent MTrPs were present in unilateral shoulder impingement participants with levator scapula (100%), supraspinatus (66%), infraspinatus (83.33%), and subscapularis (66%). This study had some reporting, external and internal validity, and power risk of bias.

Cervical radiculopathy

One study assessed the presence of active and latent MTrPs in patients with cervical radiculopathy [23]. The muscles assessed included trapezius, multifidus, splenius capitis, levator scapulae, rhomboid major, and rhomboid minor. A total of 244 patients where compared to 122 controls. Findings suggest that active MTrPs are more common on patients with cervical radiculopathy than controls. Participants on the control group did not present active MTrPs on assessed muscles. The study also reported no difference between groups (control and cervical radiculopathy) in the distribution of latent MTrPs ($p = 0.249$). This study had some reporting, external and internal validity, and power risk of bias.

Episodic migraine

Tali et al. (2014) studied two groups with the first (18 women and 2 men) suffering from episodic migraines and the second (17 women and 3 men) being healthy controls [24]. Results from this study revealed an increased number of active MTrPs in the migraine group when compared to healthy controls. No significant difference ($p = 0.185$) between groups was found for the prevalence of latent MTrPs. That study identified a higher prevalence of MTrPs (active and latent) in the migraine group in the right trapezius in comparison to the control group [24]. There was no significant difference in MTrPs between left and right side

Table 3 Characteristics of included studies

Study	Study design	Disorder(s)	Healthy Controls Group	Diagnostic Criteria Active MTrPs	Diagnostic Criteria Latent MTrPs	Assessed Muscles	Country, Setting
Alonso-Blanco et al., 2011	Cross-sectional	CTTH	No	1) Presence of a palpable taut band in a skeletal muscle. 2) Presence of a hyperirritable sensitive spot within the taut band. 3) Local twitch response elicited by the snapping palpation of the taut band. 4) Presence of referred pain in response to MTrP compression.	Not assessed	Upper Trapezius Sternocleidomastoid Temporalis Suboccipital	Spain, hospital
Bron et al., 2011	Cross-sectional	SP	No	1) A nodule in a taut band of skeletal muscle. 2) Painful on compression 3) May produce referred pain or sensations 4) Pain recognised by patient as "familiar"	1) A nodule in a taut band of skeletal muscle. 2) Painful on compression 3) May produce referred pain or sensations 4) Pain not recognizable to patient	Upper/middle/lower trapezius Infraspinatus Supraspinatus Subscapularis Teres minor and major Anterior/middle/ posterior deltoids Pectoralis major and minor Biceps brachii Triceps brachii Scalene Subclavius	Spain, primary care practice.
Fernandez-Perez et al., 2012	Cross-sectional cohort	Acute WAD	Yes	1) Palpable taut band within a skeletal muscle 2) Presence of a hypersensitive spot in the taut band 3) Local twitch re-sponse elic-ited by the snapping palpa-tion of the taut band 4) Production of referred pain in response to MTrP manual compression. 5) If referred pain of symptoms reported by the patient is recognized as familiar	1) Palpable taut band within a skeletal muscle 2) Presence of a hypersensitive spot in the taut band 3) Local twitch re-sponse elicited by the snapping pal-pation of the taut band 4) Production of referred pain in response to MTrP manual compression. 5) Symptoms produced are not familiar to the patient	Temporalis Masseter Upper trapezius Levator scapulae Sternocleidomastoid Scalene	Spain, primary care
Fernández-De-Las-Peñas, 2012	Cross-sectional	Non-specific pain	No	1) Presence of a palpable taut band within a skeletal muscle. 2) Presence of a hyperirritable spot in the taut band. 3) Local twitch response elicited by the snapping palpation of the taut band (when possible). 4) Presence of referred pain in response to compression. MTrPs were considered active when the local and referred pains evoked by compression reproduced clinical pain symptoms and also the participant recognized the pain as familiar.	MTrPs were considered latent when the local and the referred pain elicited by digital compression did not reproduce symptoms familiar to the participant.	Temporalis Masseter Upper trapezius Sternocleidomastoid Splenius capitis Oblique capitis inferior Levator scapulae Scalene Pectoralis major Deltoid Infraspinatus Extensor carpi radialis brevis Extensor carpi radialis longus Eetensor digitorum communis Supinator	Spain, Department of PT, OT, rehab and physical medicine.
	Case-control		Yes			Levator scapulae Supraspinatus	Spain, setting unclear

Table 3 Characteristics of included studies *(Continued)*

Study	Study design	Disorder(s)	Healthy Controls Group	Diagnostic Criteria Active MTrPs	Diagnostic Criteria Latent MTrPs	Assessed Muscles	Country, Setting
Hidalgo-Lozano et al., 2010		Unilateral shoulder impingement		1) Presence of a palpable taut band in a skeletal muscle 2) Presence of a hyperirritable tender spot within the taut band 3) Local twitch response elicited by the snapping palpation of the taut band 4) Presence of referred pain in response to MTrP compression. 5) Local and the referred pain evoked by digital compression reproduced the pain symptoms (both in location and pain sensation) and the subject recognized the pain as familiar pain	1) Presence of a palpable taut band in a skeletal muscle 2) Presence of a hyperirritable tender spot within the taut band 3) Local twitch response elicited by the snapping palpation of the taut band 4) Presence of referred pain in response to MTrP compression. 5) Local and referred pain elicited by digital compression did not reproduce symptoms familiar to the subjects	Infraspinatus Subscapularis Pectoralis major Biceps brachii	
Sari et al., 2012	Case-control	Cervical Radiculopathy	Yes	1) Presence of a palpable taut band in a skeletal muscle 2) Presence of hypersensible tender spot in the taut band 3) Local twitch response elicited by the snapping palpation of the taut band 4) Reproduction of the typical referred pain pattern of the MTrP in response to compression; and 5) Spontaneous presence of the typical referred pain pattern and/or patient recognition of the referred pain as familiar. If all of the aforementioned criteria were present the MTrP was considered active	1) Presence of a palpable taut band in a skeletal muscle 2) Presence of hypersensible tender spot in the taut band 3) Local twitch response elicited by the snapping palpation of the taut band 4) Reproduction of the typical referred pain pattern of the MTrP in response to compression	Trapezius, multifidus, splenius capitis, levator scapulae, rhomboid major, and rhomboid minor	Turkey, Outpatient clinic
Tali et al., 2014	Case-control	Episodic migraines	Yes	1) Palpable taut band within a skeletal muscle 2) Presence of a hypersensitive spot in the taut band 3) Local twitch response elicited by the snapping palpation of the taut band 4) Production of referred pain in response to MTrP manual compression. 5) If the MTrP were palpated and produced a headache, familiar or not, it was referred to as an "active MTrP".	1) Palpable taut band within a skeletal muscle 2) Presence of a hypersensitive spot in the taut band 3) Local twitch response elicited by the snapping palpation of the taut band 4) Production of referred pain in response to MTrP manual compression. 5) If the MTrP were palpated and produced local or radiated pain it was referred to as a "latent MTrP".	Sternocleidomastoid Upper trapezius	Israel, Physiotherapy Department

Abbreviations: *CTTH* Chronic tension type headache, *SP* Shoulder pain, *WAD* Whiplash associated disorder, *MTrP* Myofascial trigger point

migraines. This study had some reporting, external validity, and power risk of bias.

Discussion

This systematic review aimed to synthesise evidence on the prevalence of active and latent MTrPs in neck or shoulder disorders. Seven studies were included, each study focused on different populations and conditions. All studies scored 9/16 or higher on the modified Downs and Black checklist, suggesting an overall low risk of bias within included studies. We have identified risk of reporting, external and internal validity and power bias in included studies.

Table 4 Characteristics of the subjects included in the studies

Study	Stage and type of disorder	Patients Sample, n	Sex, % Female	Age (y), Mean ± SD or %	Other Characteristics, Mean ± SD or %	Healthy Controls Sample, n	Sex, % Female	Age (y), Mean ± SD or %	Other Characteristics, Mean ± SD or %
Alonso-Blanco et al, 2011	Chronic TTH	20 Children (6–12 years) 20 Adults (18–47 years)	50% female	Children = 8 ± 2 years Adults = 41 ± 11 years	PH(years)- Children = 1.6 ± 0.8 Adults = 8.6 ± 6.5 HI (NPRS)- Children = 5.0 ± 1.2 Adults = 5.9 ± 1.1 HD (hours/days)- Children = 4.8 ± 2.6 Adults = 7.3 ± 2 HF(days/week)- Children = 4.0 ± 0.9 Adults = 4.3 ± 0.9	0	Not assessed	Not assessed	Not assessed
Bron et al, 2011	Chronic SP	72 patients	69% Female	43.9 ± 12.3 years	Duration- 6–9 months = 23% 9–12 months = 19% 1–2 years = 18% 2–5 years = 19% > 5 years = 19% Recurrence rate- 1st = 36% 2nd = 26% 3rd > = 37%	0	Not assessed	Not assessed	Not assessed
Fernandez-Perez et al, 2012	Acute WAD	20 participants aged over 20 years	50% women	28.7 ± 12.4 (22.9,34.4)	Height, cm: 170.0 ± 10.6 (165.0,175.0) Weight kg: 67.7 ± 16.3 (60.1,75.4) Time from accident, d: 26.6 ± 3.8 (24.8,28.4) Current pain (NPRS): 6.2 ± 2.6 (5.0, 7.5) Worst pain (NPRS): 8.0 ± 2.0 (7.0, 8.9) Lowest pain (NPRS): 3.3 ± 2.9 (1.9, 4.7)	20	50% female	29.1 ± 12.2 (23.3, 34.8)	Height cm: 160.7 ± 39.1 (142.3, 179.0) Weight kg: 64.1 ± 23.3 (53.2, 75.1)
Fernández-De-Las-Peñas, 2012	NSP	16 Blue collar workers 19 White collar worker	Blue = 62% Female White = 75% female	Blue = 44 ± 13 years White = 44 ± 14 years	PH (months)- Blue = 13.2 ± 5.3 White = 9.1 ± 5.5 MP (NPRS)- Blue = 5.0 ± 2.5 White = 3.8 ± 2.6	0	Not Assessed	Not Assessed	Not Assessed
Hidalgo-Lozano et al, 2010	ULSlStage of condition unclear	12 patients	42% female	25 ± 9 years		10	50% female	26 ± 8 years	
Sari 2012	Acute and chronic Cervical radiculopathy	244	52% female	44.6 ± 10.3 years	BMI (kg/m²)- 26.28 ± 5.25 Social status: Married 70%, single 23%, widow 7% Education: University 40%, high school 38%, primary education 18%, uneducated 4% Occupation: Housewife 32%, worker 25%, retired 13%, student 9%, officer 8%, nurse 5%, other 8%	122	N/A	43.8 ± 9.8 years	N/A

Table 4 Characteristics of the subjects included in the studies (Continued)

Study	Stage and type of disorder	Patients Sample, n	Sex, % Female	Age (y), Mean ± SD or %	Other Characteristics, Mean ± SD or %	Healthy Controls Sample, n	Sex, % Female	Age (y), Mean ± SD or %	Other Characteristics, Mean ± SD or %
Tali et al., 2014	EM Stage unclear	20 Physical therapy students	90% female	24.95 ± 1.79 years	Major trauma history 15.6% BMI (kg/m²): 21.68 ± 2.62 HF (days in the past 3 months): 6.60 ± 5.88 AS (NPRS): 6.45 ± 1.50	20 Physical Therapy students	85% female	25.65 ± 1.42 years.	BMI (kg/m2)- 21.69 ± 2.08

Abbreviations: *TTH* tension type headache, *SP* Shoulder pain, *WAD* Whiplash associated disorder, *NSP* Non-specific pain, *EM* Episodic migraines, *ULSI* Unilateral shoulder impingement, *SD* Standard deviation, *PH* Pain history, *HI* Headache intensity, *HD* Headache duration, *HF* Headache frequency, *AS* Average severity, *NPRS* Numeric pain rating scale, *MP* Mean pain, *BMI* Body mass index

Table 5 Point prevalence (Expressed as percentage) of active MTrPs in subjects with shoulder or neck disorders

	Alonso-Blanco et al., 2011		Bron et al., 2011	Fernandez-Perez et al., 2012	Fernández-De-Las-Peñas, 2012		Hidalgo-Lozano et al., 2010	Sari, 2012	Tali et al., 2014	Hidalgo-Lozano et al., 2010
Sample	Adults (N = 20)	Children (N = 20)			White collar (N = 19)	Blue collar (N = 16)				
Information regarding right or left side			Do not specify left and right				Do not specify left and right	Do not specify left and right		Do not specify left and right
Muscles										
Left Temporalis	55	70		20	5.3	6.3				
Right Temporalis	65	75		10	5.3	6.3				
Right SCM	30	25		5	21.1	6.3			5	
Left SCM	40	10		30	21.1	18.8			10	
Left Upper Trapezius	35	20		30	63.2	56.3		13.5	25	
Right Upper Trapezius	80	15		35	63.2	68.8			45	
Suboccipital muscles	100 (bilateral)	80 (bilateral)			OCl- left = 31.6. right = 31.6 SC- left = 15.8. right = 21.1	OCl- left = 12.5. right = 25 SC- left = 31.3. right = 37.5				
Middle Trapezius			43.1							
Lower Trapezius			37.5							
Left Infraspinatus			77.8		31.6	37.5	41.7			41.7
Right Infraspinatus					21.1	43.8				
Supraspinatus			34.7				66.7			66.7
Subscapularis			40.3				41.7			41.7
Teres minor			47.2							
Teres major			36.1							
Left Deltoid			Posterior- 44.4		5.3	18.8				
Right Deltoid			Middle- 50 Anterior- 47.2		10.5	12.5				
Left Pectoralis major			26.4		5.3	18.8	16.7			16.7
Right Pectoralis major					18.8	18.8				
Pectoralis minor			30.6							
Biceps Brachii			20.8				16.7			16.7
Triceps Brachii			19.4							
Left Scalene			16.7	20	21.1	12.5				
Right Scalene				30	15.8	2.3				

The included studies examined the following musculo-skeletal disorders: chronic tension-type headache [5], unilateral shoulder pain [20], upper quadrant pain [21], acute whiplash disorder [22], shoulder impingement syndrome [17], cervical radiculopathy [23], and episodic migraine [24]. Hidalgo-Lozano et al. (2010), Fernandes-de-las-Penas et al. (2012), Fernandes-Perez et al. (2012), and Tali et al. (2014) all compared participants with shoulder or neck disorders to healthy controls and found participants with shoulder and neck disorders had a higher prevalence of MTrPs [17, 21, 22, 24]. Active and latent MTrPs are more common in the upper trapezius muscle, with the exception of Fernández-De-Las-Peñas et al. (2012) who found no significant difference between the distribution on active or latent MTrPs [21].

Alonso-Blanco et al. (2011) and Bron et al. (2011) compared the prevalence of MTrPs between adults and children and the prevalence between right and left shoulders in patients with unilateral shoulder pain respectively [5, 20]. Alonso-Blanco et al. (2011) found that adults had higher prevalence of MTrPs than children, whilst in contrast Bron et al. (2011) found no significant differences between symptomatic and asymptomatic shoulders [20].

All studies, with the exception of two [20, 23] had very small samples sizes. Therefore, the generalisability of results is limited. Bron et al. (2011) and Sari et al. (2012) had the two largest sample sizes (72 and 244 patients respectively) from all 7 studies [20, 23]. However, Bron et al. (2011) study had 69% female participants and did not include a healthy control group which decreases the significance of their findings [20]. Bron et al. (2011) and Hidalgo-Lozano et al. (2010) did not differentiate between the prevalence of left and right MTrPs and they did not acknowledge which side was symptomatic [17, 20]. This made interpreting results more difficult and hindered the synthesis of data from multiple studies.

Studies presented limitations regarding sample size and assessor blinding. All studies were considered to have small sample sizes [25]. A small sample size can lead to biased results. Future studies with larger sample sizes should be designed, and estimated a priori, to ensure more reliable and accurate findings. Only four studies ensured practitioners assessing trigger points were blinded. Blinding the assessor helps reducing the influence of the assessors' perception and believes towards an outcomes measure [26].

Only 4 of the 7 studies included a control group. Findings from control groups inform what outcomes are expected within an asymptomatic population. Additionally, the inclusion of a control group helps to control for other variables (e.g. age, occupation), and also accounts for normal biological variations [27]. Future studies should therefore include a control group, to enhance

our understanding on the role of MTrPs and musculo-skeletal disorders.

There is lack of consensus on how to define myofascial trigger point pain syndrome [28]. The use of different definitions, or the lack of clarity around MTrPs definition, impact on the external validity of reported findings. Included studies used similar (but not always the same) diagnostic criteria for assessing active and latent MTrPs. Currently, the criterion validity of MTrPs diagnostic criteria is poor, as there is no gold standard for diagnosing MTrP. Therefore, it is unknown what the sensitivity and specificity is when using the clinical criteria proposed by Simons et al. [29].

The reliability of physical examination for diagnosing MTrP has been questioned in the literature [30]. One study reported excellent test-retest reliability for physical examination when assessing MTrPs in patients with rotator cuff disorders [31]. On the other hand, two previous systematic reviews [30, 32] questioned the reliability of physical examination for assessing the presence of MTrP due to low methodological quality of included studies. There is definitely a need for an international consensus for standardizing the assessment of MTrP in clinical practice and research [18].

All studies used very similar definitions to define a MTrP (Table 3). Most used the description from "Myofascial Pain and Dysfunction. The trigger point manual. Upper half of body" by Simons et al. [29] The criteria often comprised: *1) presence of a palpable taut band within a skeletal muscle; 2) existence of a hyperirritable spot in the taut band; 3) local twitch response elicited by the snapping palpation of the taut band (when possible); 4) presence of referred pain in response to compression* [29]. The criteria for distinguishing between active and latent MTrPs were also defined by Simons et al. [29]. The difference in active and latent MTrPs was found following compression of the MTrP. If patient's symptoms were reproduced, it is considered to be an active MTrP; whereas no reproduction of symptoms or production of unfamiliar symptoms is considered latent [20].

The results from this review suggest that active and latent MTrPs are highly present in patients with different neck or shoulder disorders. From the 7 included studies, 5 revealed that the upper trapezius was consistently one of the muscles with highest, if not the highest, prevalence of a MTrP. Furthermore, 3 studies examined the prevalence of MTrPs on infraspinatus muscle [17, 20, 21] and, together, these findings suggest that infraspinatus is among one of the most prevalent muscles with active MTrPs across all 3 studies.

All seven studies reported the importance of referred pain mechanism relating to MTrPs, and how it may be an underlying contributing factor to the patient's condition. Alonso-Blanco et al. (2011) found a significantly

Table 5 Point prevalence (Expressed as percentage) of active MTrPs in subjects with shoulder or neck disorders *(Continued)*

	Alonso-Blanco et al., 2011	Bron et al., 2011	Fernandez-Perez et al., 2012	Fernández-De-Las-Peñas, 2012		Hidalgo-Lozano et al., 2010	Sari, 2012	Tali et al., 2014	Hidalgo-Lozano et al., 2010
Subclavius		25							
Left Masseter			10	15.8	0				
Right Masseter			0	5.3	0				
Left Levator scapulae			55	31.6	25	41.7	16.3		41.7
Right Levator scapulae			65	36.8	12.5				
Splenius capitis							14.7		
Rhomboid minor							14.3		
Rhomboid major							10.2		
Multifidus							8.6		

Abbreviations: CTTH – Chronic tension type headache SP – Shoulder pain, WAD – Whiplash associated disorder, NPRS – Numerical pain rating scale, OCI – Oblique capitis inferior, SC – Splenius capitis, SCM -Sternocleidomastoid

higher number of active MTrPs in adults and discussed the similarities observed between the presence of active MTrPs and patterns of their headache symptoms [5]. Hidalgo-Lozano et al. (2011) revealed that the referred pain pattern from the active MTrPs of the levator scapulae, supraspinatus, infraspinatus, subscapularis, pectoralis major, and biceps brachii reproduced patient symptoms [17]. This was also in agreement with Dong et al. (2015) and Koester et al. (2005) who reported shoulder impingement often refers pain down to the mid humerus level, further increasing the validity of MTrPs and their impact on the reported symptoms for this disorder [33, 34]. These studies support the idea that high active MTrPs may contribute to patient's symptoms.

Study limitations and previous systematic reviews

We were unable to perform a meta-analysis due to patients with different disorders being included, and different outcome measures used by the included studies. Due to limited number of articles included in this review, we could not explore differences in the prevalence of MTrPs between acute and chronic conditions. We did not register the protocol of this review, and that increases risk of reporting bias of this review. A previous systematic review assessed the prevalence of MTrPs in spinal disorders [18]. Findings from the review support the theory that MTrPs are more prevalent in patients with musculoskeletal disorders.

Conclusion

Findings from this systematic review suggest that there is limited evidence supporting the high prevalence of active and latent MTrPs in patients with neck or shoulder

disorders. Point prevalence estimates of MTrPs were based on a small number of studies with very low sample sizes and with design limitations that increased risk of bias within included studies. Therefore, future studies assessing patients neck or shoulder disorders, with large samples and stronger study designs are required to provide more reliable pooled estimates of point prevalence of MTrPs in these patients.

Acknowledgements
The authors acknowledge the financial support from Centre for Health, Activity and Rehabilitation Research (CHARR), School of Physiotherapy – University of Otago. Daniel Cury Ribeiro is supported by The Sir Charles Hercus Health Research Fellowship – Health Research Council of New Zealand.

Funding
No funding was obtained for this study.

Authors' contributions
DCR was responsible for the study concept and design of this review. AB, AN, HF, PM, SP were responsible for the study selection and assessment of risk of bias within included studies. All authors participated in acquisition, analysis, and interpretation of data. AB, AN, HF, PM, SP were responsible for drafting the first version of the manuscript. DCR was responsible for drafting the final version of the manuscript. All authors read and approved the final manuscript.

Competing interests
Daniel Cury Ribeiro is a member of the Editorial Board of BMC Musculoskeletal Disorders. The other authors state no conflict of interest to declare.

References
1. Greenberg DL. Evaluation and treatment of shoulder pain. Med Clin N Am. 2014;98(3):487–504.
2. Hoy D, March L, Brooks P, Blyth F, Woolf A, Bain C, Williams G, Smith E, Vos T, Barendregt J, et al. The global burden of low back pain: estimates from the global burden of disease 2010 study. Ann Rheum Dis. 2014;73(6):968–74.

3. Irnich D. Myofascial trigger points: comprehensive diagnosis and treatment: Elsevier Ltd; 2013.

4. Rha DW, Shin JC, Kim YK, Jung JH, Kim YU, Lee SC. Detecting local twitch responses of myofascial trigger points in the lower-back muscles using ultrasonography. Arch Phys Med Rehabil. 2011;92(10):1576–80. e1571

5. Alonso-Blanco C, Fernández-de-las-Peñas C, Fernández-Mayoralas DM, de-la-Llave-Rincón AI, Pareja JA, Svensson P. Prevalence and anatomical localization of muscle referred pain from active trigger points in head and neck musculature in adults and children with chronic tension-type headache. Pain Med. 2011;12(10):1453–63.

6. Shah JP, Thaker N, Heimur J, Aredo JV, Sikdar S, Gerber L. Myofascial trigger points then and now: a historical and scientific perspective. PM R. 2015;7(7): 746–61.

7. Celik D, Mutlu EK. Clinical implication of latent myofascial trigger point. Curr Pain Headache Rep. 2013;17(8):353.

8. Castaldo M, Ge HY, Chiarotto A, Villafane JH, Arendt-Nielsen L. Myofascial trigger points in patients with whiplash-associated disorders and mechanical neck pain. Pain Med. 2014;15(5):842–9.

9. Quintner JL, Bove GM, Cohen ML. A critical evaluation of the trigger point phenomenon. Rheumatology (Oxford). 2015;54(3):392–9.

10. Arias-Buria JL, Valero-Alcaide R, Cleland JA, Salom-Moreno J, Ortega-Santiago R, Atin-Arratibel MA, Fernandez-de-las-Penas C. Inclusion of trigger point dry needling in a multimodal physical therapy program for postoperative shoulder pain: a randomized clinical trial. J Manip Physiol Ther. 2015;38(3):179–87.

11. Hall ML, Mackie AC, Ribeiro DC. Effects of dry needling trigger point therapy in the shoulder region on patients with upper extremity pain and dysfunction: a systematic review and meta-analysis. Physiotherapy. 2017; in press

12. Liu L, Huang QM, Liu QG, Ye G, Bo CZ, Chen MJ, Li P. Effectiveness of dry needling for myofascial trigger points associated with neck and shoulder pain: a systematic review and meta-analysis. Arch Phys Med Rehabil. 2015; 96(5):944–55.

13. Shah JP, Danoff JV, Desai MJ, Parikh S, Nakamura LY, Phillips TM, Gerber LH. Biochemicals associated with pain and inflammation are elevated in sites near to and remote from active myofascial trigger points. Arch Phys Med Rehabil. 2008;89(1):16–23.

14. Ge HY, Monterde S, Graven-Nielsen T, Arendt-Nielsen L. Latent myofascial trigger points are associated with an increased intramuscular electromyographic activity during synergistic muscle activation. J Pain. 2014; 15(2):181–7.

15. Ge HY, Arendt-Nielsen L, Madeleine P. Accelerated muscle fatigability of latent myofascial trigger points in humans. Pain Med. 2012;13(7):957–64.

16. Ibarra JM, Ge HY, Wang C, Martinez Vizcaino V, Graven-Nielsen T, Arendt-Nielsen L. Latent myofascial trigger points are associated with an increased antagonistic muscle activity during agonist muscle contraction. J Pain. 2011; 12(12):1282–8.

17. Hidalgo-Lozano A, Fernández-de-las-Peñas C, Díaz-Rodríguez L, González-Iglesias J, Palacios-Ceña D, Arroyo-Morales M. Changes in pain and pressure pain sensitivity after manual treatment of active trigger points in patients with unilateral shoulder impingement: a case series. J Bodyw Mov Ther. 2011;15(4):399–404.

18. Chiarotto A, Clijsen R, Fernandez-de-Las-Penas C, Barbero M. Prevalence of myofascial trigger points in spinal disorders: a systematic review and meta-analysis. Arch Phys Med Rehabil. 2016;97(2):316–37.

19. Downs SH, Black N. The feasibility of creating a checklist for the assessment of the methodological quality both of randomised and non-randomised studies of health care interventions. J Epidemiol Community Health. 1998; 52(6):377–84.

20. Bron C, Dommerholt J, Stegenga B, Wensing M, Oostendorp RA. High prevalence of shoulder girdle muscles with myofascial trigger points in patients with shoulder pain. BMC Musculoskelet Disord. 2011;12:139.

21. Fernández-De-Las-Peñas C, Gröbli C, Ortega-Santiago R, Fischer CS, Boesch D, Froidevaux P, Stocker L, Weissmann R, González-Iglesias J. Referred pain from myofascial trigger points in head, neck, shoulder, and arm muscles reproduces pain symptoms in blue-collar (manual) and white-collar (office) workers. Clin J Pain. 2012;28(6):511–8.

22. Fernández-Pérez AM, Villaverde-Gutiérrez C, Mora-Sánchez A, Alonso-Blanco C, Sterling M, Fernández-De-Las-Peñas C. Muscle trigger points, pressure pain threshold, and cervical range of motion in patients with high level of disability related to acute whiplash injury. J Orthop Sports Phys Ther. 2012; 42(7):634–41.

23. Sari H, Akarirmak U, Uludag M. Active myofascial trigger points might be more frequent in patients with cervical radiculopathy. Eur J Phys Rehabil Med. 2012;48(2):237–44.

24. Tali D, Menahem I, Vered E, Kalichman L. Upper cervical mobility, posture and myofascial trigger points in subjects with episodic migraine: case-control study. J Bodyw Mov Ther. 2014;18(4):569–75.

25. Higgins J, Green S, editors. Cochrane handbook for systematic reviews of interventions version 5.1.0. [updated march 2011]: The Cochrane Collaboration; 2011.

26. Schulz KF, Grimes DA. Case-control studies: research in reverse. Lancet. 2002; 359(9304):431–4.

27. Portney LG, Watkins MP. Foundations of clinical research: applications to practice. 3rd ed. Pennsylvania: F.A. Davis Company; 2015.

28. Tough EA, White AR, Richards S, Campbell J. Variability of criteria used to diagnose myofascial trigger point pain syndrome - evidence from a review of the literature. Clin J Pain. 2007;23(3):278–86.

29. Simons DG, Travell JG, Simons LS. Travell & Simons' myofascial pain and dysfunction. The trigger point manual. Volume 1. Upper half of body., vol. 1. Upper half of body. 2nd ed. Philadelphia: Lippincott Williams and Wilkins; 1998.

30. Lucas N, MacAskill P, Irwig L, Moran R, Bogduk N. Reliability of physical examination for diagnosis of myofascial trigger points: a systematic review of the literature. Clin J Pain. 2009;25(1):80–9.

31. Al-Shenqiti AM, Oldham JA. Test-retest reliability of myofascial trigger point detection in patients with rotator cuff tendonitis. Clin Rehabil. 2005;19(5):482–7.

32. Myburgh C, Larsen AH, Hartvigsen J. A systematic, critical review of manual palpation for identifying myofascial trigger points: evidence and clinical significance. Arch Phys Med Rehabil. 2008;89(6):1169–76.

33. Dong W, Goost H, Lin XB, Burger C, Paul C, Wang ZL, Zhang TY, Jiang ZC, Welle K, Kabir K. Treatments for shoulder impingement syndrome a prisma systematic review and network meta-analysis. Medicine. 2015;94(10).

34. Koester MC, George MS, Kuhn JE. Shoulder impingement syndrome. Am J Med. 2005;118(5):452–5.

2

Immunological and morphological analysis of heterotopic ossification differs to healthy controls

Klemens Trieb[1*], Andreas Meryk[2], Sascha Senck[3], Erin Naismith[2] and Beatrix Grubeck-Loebenstein[2]

Abstract

Background: Formation of lamellar bone in non-osseus tissue is a pathological process called heterotopic ossification. It is the aim of this study to analyse the morphology and immunological status of patients with heterotopic ossification compared to individual healthy persons.

Methods: Human bone marrow and blood samples were obtained from 6 systemically healthy individuals and 4 patients during resection of heterotopic ossification from bone at hip arthroplasty. Bone was fragmented and treated with purified collagenase. Immunofluorescence surface staining was performed and analyzed with flow cytometry. Microcomputed tomography scanning was done performed at a resolution of 11 and 35 μm isometric voxel size respectively using a two different cone beam X-computer tomography systems and a microfocus X-ray tube. Subsequently the volume data was morphometrically analysed.

Results: The monocytes, stem cells, stroma cells and granulocytes progenitor cells were strongly reduced in the heterotopic ossification patient. Additionally a significant reduction of stromal stem cells cells and CD34 positive stem cells was observed. The frequency of NK-cells, B cells and T cells were not altered in the patients with heterotopic ossification compared to a healthy person. Micromorphometric parameters showed a lower content of mineralized bone tissue compared to normal bone. Mean trabecular thickness showed a high standard deviation, indicating a high variation in trabecular thickness, anisotropy and reducing bone strength.

Conclusions: This work shows altered immunological distribution that is accompanied by a low decrease in bone volume fraction and tissue mineral density in the heterotopic ossification sample compared to normal bone. Compared to healthy subjects, this might reflect an immunological participation in the development of this entity.

Background

Formation of lamellar bone in non-osseus tissue is a pathological process called heterotopic ossification (HO). This can occur in muscle or connective tissue as a result of trauma, surgery, fractures, neurological injury or genetic mutations (fibrodysplasia ossificans progressiva, Albright's hereditary osteodystrophy). It causes major clinical burdens due to limitation of motion, persistent pain and nerve entrapement [1–4]. So far morphometric data on morphometric indices like porosity, tissue mineral density, and trabecular volume is fragmentary for human samples and immunological data are rarely available. Skeletal muscle tissue has a wide capacity for regenaration by myogenic stem cells in combination with mesenchymal stromal cells. It is not clear which factors induce enchondral bone formation during this process. Some studies have proposed endothelial or brown adipogenic cells as a or the source for HO. The reciprocal interactions between bone and the immune system have become more the subject of increased attention in recent years and the so called osteoimmunology describes cytokine induces bone resorption and inflammatory induced ossification [5–14].

Neurogenic HO induced by spinal cord or traumatic brain injury is described but detailed characteristion of immunoligal and morphologic changes are hardly available. It is the aim of this study to analyse the morphology and immunological status of patients with heterotopic ossification compared to individual healthy persons [15].

* Correspondence: klemens.trieb@klinikum-wegr.at
[1]Department of Orthopaedics, Klinikum Wels-Grieskirchen, Grieskirchnerstr 42, 4600 Wels, Austria
Full list of author information is available at the end of the article

Methods

Patients

Human sample collection and preparation

Heterotopic ossification tissue was obtained at resection from four patients and divided for further analysis. The first was obtained from male in the beginning 50s patient who suffered a central ganglion bleeding one year before and developed a central nervous system induced HO in the left musculus vastus. The second was obtained from man in the end 60s suffering from a postdicectomy ischiadical lesion developing peripheral neuroathy induced HO after hip arthroplsaty. The third was obtained from woman in the beginning 20s developing HO after fixation of a femoral neck fracture without neurological impairment. The fourth healthy patient underwent hip replacement (male mid 50s) after an old femur fracture with a removed intramedullary nail. In the gluteus he had a HTO which had to be removed for hip approach, so we gained normal bone (femoral head) and HTO from one patient for analysis. Human bone marrow (BM) samples were obtained from age matched systemically healthy individuals (4 male, 2 female, mean age 52 years) who did not receive immunomodulatory drugs or suffer from diseases known to influence the immune system, including autoimmune diseases and cancer. Informed consent for test and publication was given and documented from each patient after the study received approval of the local institution of the corresponding author and none of the authors has competing interests according to BioMed Central's guidance. Total hip arthroplasty was performed by an antero-lateral minimal invasive approach and bone was harvested from the resected neck and femoral head to isolate bone marrow mononuclear cells (BMMCs) [16]. Bone fragments were washed once with complete RPMI medium (RPMI 1640 supplemented with 10% FCS, 100 U/ml penicillin, and 100 μg/ml streptomycin; Invitrogen) and treated with purified collagenase (CLSPA, Worthington Biochemical; 20 U/ml in complete RPMI medium) for 1 h at 37 °C. After centrifugation purification of BMMCs was done by density gradient centrifugation (Ficoll-Hypaque). This methods are described in detail in previous studies [17].

Flow cytometry

Immunofluorescence surface staining was performed by adding a panel of directly conjugated antibodies to freshly prepared BMMCs. Labelled cells were measured by a FACSCanto II (BD Biosciences) and analyzed with Flowjo.

Microcomputed tomography

During the scanning procedure, fresh samples were stored in air-sealed polymer sample holders to prevent dehydration. The complete samples were scanned at a resolution of 35 μm isometric voxel size using a RayScan 250E cone beam XCT device equipped with a Perkin Elmer flat panel detector (2048 × 2048 pixels with a pixel size 200 μm) and a Viscom 225 kV microfocus X-ray tube. The X-ray scanning parameters were set to 120 kV and 420 μA with an integration time of 1500 ms; a 0.5 mm thick copper filter-plate was applied to prevent beam hardening artefacts. Hydroxyapatite rods (HA; 8 mm diameter, 250 and 750 mg HA/cm^3) were scanned in the same sealed specimen holder to calibrate images for 1) tissue mineral density (TMD) of the trabecular bone to quantifiy trabecula mineralization and 2) bone mineral density (BMD) of trabecular bone in conjunction with the surrounding soft tissue.

A second scan was conducted on cut out samples (ca. 12 mm in diameter) of the respective specimen at resolution of 11 μm isometric voxel size using a GE Phoenix Nanotom 180 cone beam XCT device equipped with a panel detector (2300 × 2300 pixels) and a 180 kV nanofocus X-ray tube. The X-ray scanning parameters were set to 80 kV and 230 μA with an integration time of 600 ms. Image information for each data set was separated into tissue and background using the "advanced threshold" function using Volume Graphics 2.2. Subsequently, volume data was transferred to CTAn (Version 1.16; Bruker) for morphometric analysis. Calculated morphometric indices include bone volume fraction (BV/TV, bone volume/total volume), mean trabecular thickness (TbTh.mean), standard deviation of trabecular thickness (TbTh.SD), mean trabecular separation (TbSp.mean), standard deviation of trabecular separation (TbSp.SD), degree of anisotropy (DA), and connectivity (Con). The computation of these indices is implemented in CTAn and is based on the work of Hildebrand and Ruegsegger [18] and Remy and Thiel [19]. Moreover, TMD and BMD were computed using a calibration curve based on the 16-bit grey values of the two above mentioned Hydroxyapatite rods.

Histology

For histology, formalin-fixed HO tissue was decalcified and embedded in methyl metacrylate. Sections (6 μm) were cut, deplastified and stained with Goldner trichrome for comparative histology.

Statistical analysis

The data obtained in the study are following a non-parametric distribution. Therefore statistical significance was assessed by Spearman correlation analysis, Mann–Whitney test and Wilcoxon matched pairs test, a p-value of less than 0.05 was considered as significant. All data are shown as mean ± standard error of the mean (SEM). Statistical analysis was performed using GraphPad Prism software version 5.0 (GraphPad Software). To determine the significance of differences between two groups, the unpaired two-tailed t test were used, as indicated in the figure legends.

Results

Morphology and histology

The heterotopic ossification is characterized by an inappropriate activation of mesenchymal stem cells in the skeletal muscle tissue, which leads to an extraskeletal bone-containing bone cells, which are derived from several lines. Figure 1 shows the a.p. radiograph of the left hip showing HO formation in the musculus vastus limiting hip flexion and inducing permanent pain. Figure 2 depicts the photograph of the HO after resection and before seperation for different experiments. The histological examination shows the presence of different tissue types, such as mature bones, cartilage and fetal cells. It has been shown that the presence of brown fetal cells reduces the oxygen content and thereby promotes angiogenesis and enchondral ossification, the white fat cells are also present (Fig. 3).

Flow cytometry

Using flow cytometry, the BMMCs of 6 healthy persons can be separated into two populations based on FSC and SSC. The cell population with a low SSC (SSClow) are mainly lymphocytes, monocytes and stem cells, whereas the cells with a higher SSC (SSChigh) are mainly stroma cells and granulocytes progenitor cells. The SSChigh cell population represents 50–70% of all BMMCs but were nearly absent in the patient with heterotopic ossification (Table 1). To further investigate the SSClow population of the BMMCs, we stained with specific markers for monocytes, NK-cells, T cells, B cells and stem cells. The frequency of NK-cells, B cells and T cells were not altered in the patient with HO compared to the healthy controls. However, stromal stem cells and stem cells positive for CD34 were significantly reduced in the HO patients (Figs. 4 and 5). Interestingly we have the same results in the fourth patient comparing normal bone and HTO from the same person. Stromal stem cells (45,4 vs.

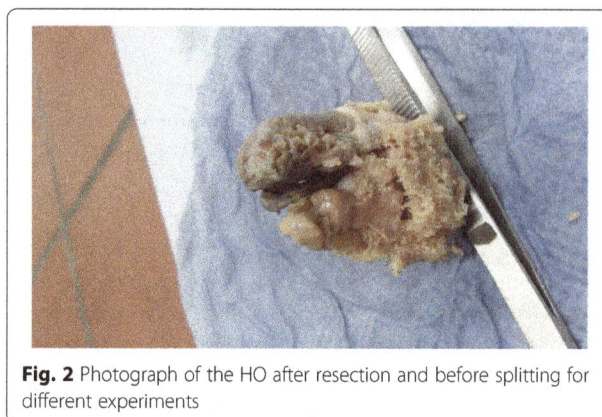

Fig. 2 Photograph of the HO after resection and before splitting for different experiments

25,9) and stem cells positive for CD34 (3,61 vs. 2,09) were reduced in the HO bone, too (Table 1, Fig. 6).

Bone morphometric parameters

Due to the voxel size of 35 µm in the scans of the complete samples, only trabeculae of a thickness larger then 105 µm are considered in the morphometric analysis since at least three voxels are necessary to ascertain that detail detectability is sufficiently high. To investigate the distribution of trabeculae thinner than 105 µm we scanned a cut-out part at a higher resolution at 11 µm voxel size. The values of the extracted microstructural parameters are presented in Table 2.

Despite the rather large volume of sample 1 (ca. 24 cm^3), bone volume fraction (BV/TV) is relative low (14.5%), showing a low content of bone tissue compared to normal 36.46 ± 15.38%), osteoporotic (25.03 ± 6.22%), and metastatic bone (24.29 ± 12.26%) [28]. The high value of mean trabecular separation (TbSp.mean) and its high standard deviation (TbSp.SD) support this finding. Likewise, mean trabecular thickness (TbTh.mean) shows a high standard deviation, indicating a high variation in trabecular thickness from extra skeletal bone to parts of

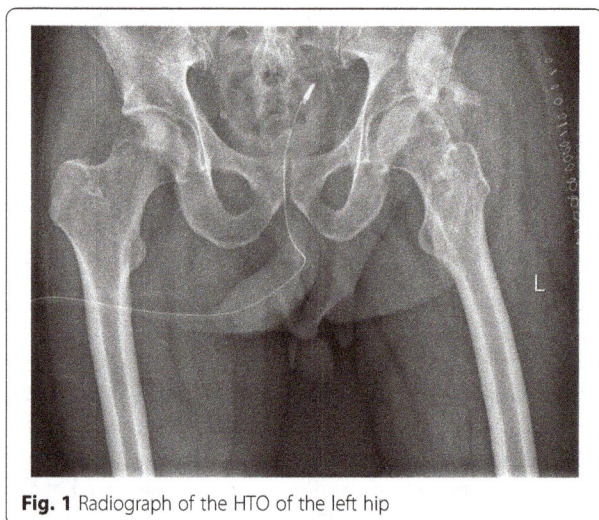

Fig. 1 Radiograph of the HTO of the left hip

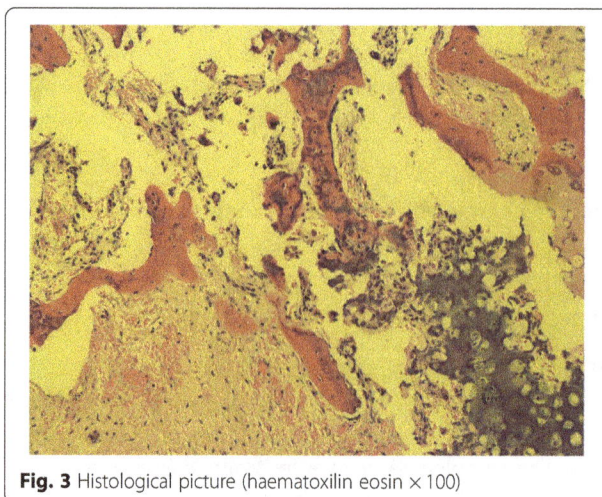

Fig. 3 Histological picture (haematoxilin eosin × 100)

Table 1 Flow cytometry analysis of BMMCs

	Healthy		HTO	
	mean	SEM	mean	SEM
T cells	24,72	2.95	24.75	4.08
CD4	46.35	3.16	42.48	9.15
CD8	44.88	3.28	48.73	7.26
B cells	9.357	1.22	13.20	2.43
SSC high	39.9	3.43	16.77**	5.64
CD34+ Stem cells	12.74	2.70	1.77*	0.46
Monocytes	9.57	2.26	4.16	1.58
NK cells	4.87	0.79	5.92	2.95

$*p < 0,05$; $**p < 0,01$

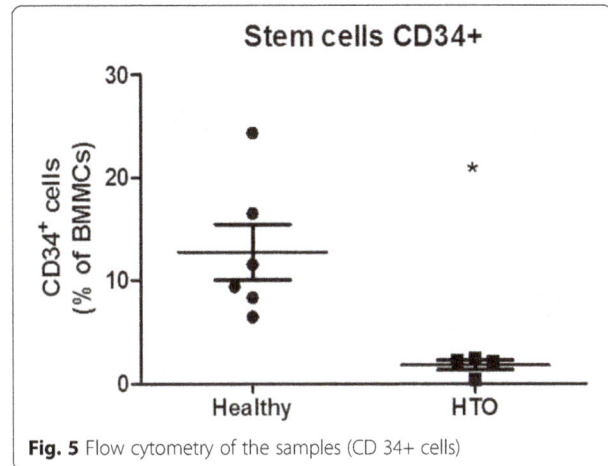

Fig. 5 Flow cytometry of the samples (CD 34+ cells)

the remaining normal bone adjacent to the resection site. While the central region of the sample shows low values of trabecular thickness, regions at the section site and the outer regions encompassing the central part are characterized by bone structures with a higher trabecular thickness (Fig. 7).

Samples 2–4 show higher BV/TV values between 29,69% and 50,91% (see Tab. 1), exceeding reported values for bone volume fraction [28]. TbSp.mean and TbSp.SD are less pronounced compared to the complete sample 1, showing values between 237.85 μm (Sample 2) and 1097.32 μm (Sample 4) for mean trabecular separation. Depending on the microstructure of the investigated subregion, values for TbSp.mean are either increased (Sample 2) or decreased (Sample 1, 3 and 4). This illustrates the high regional variation in the microstructural composition of the respective sample. The same applies to mean trabecular thickness, Sample 2 and 3 showing higher TbTh.mean values

compared to Sample 1. In general, the high standard deviation for TbTh.mean (for overview and detail samples) points to a high variation in the regional distribution of thinner and thicker trabeculae in each sample.

Apart from bone volume fraction, degree of anisotropy (DA) of trabecular bone is another important determinant of biomechanical strength. Using the calculation of DA implemented in CTAn, total isotropy is represented by the value 0 and total anisotropy by 1. In this sample, values between 0.24 and 0.45 point to a rather low low degree of anisotropy, i.e. trabecular alignment along a particular directional axis. However, the low resolution scan of Sample 4 shows a higher DA value. Since, the detail scan of Sample 4 shows a much lower DA value comparable to Samples 1–3, this high value may be explained by very thin trabeculae that are not detected at a lower physical resolution, hence exaggerating the degree of anisotropy. Since thin trabeculae are detected in the detail scan, i.e. those interconnecting larger trabeculae, the total DA is lower. While highly organized bone structures correlate with higher anisotropic values, disordered bone deposition, e.g. of

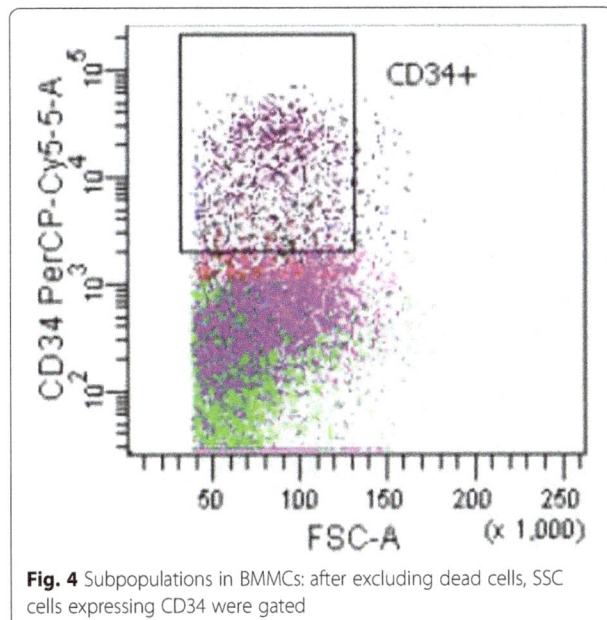

Fig. 4 Subpopulations in BMMCs: after excluding dead cells, SSC cells expressing CD34 were gated

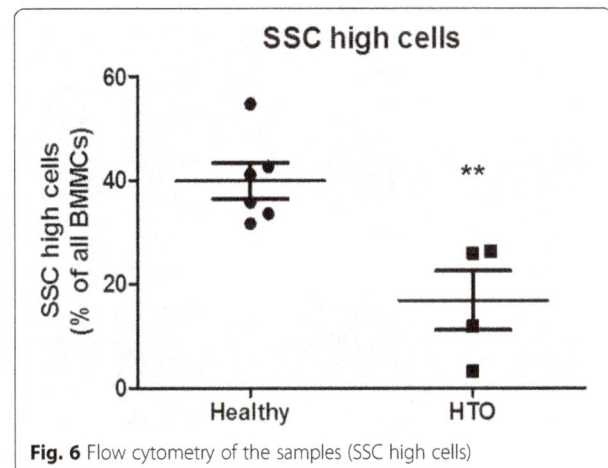

Fig. 6 Flow cytometry of the samples (SSC high cells)

Table 2 Extracted microstructural parameters of the complete sample (35 μm voxel size) and of the cut-out subsample (11 μm voxel size)

	Sample 1	Sample 2	Sample 3	Sample 4
BV/TV (in %)	14,5	39,6	50,9	29,7
TbTh.mean (in μm)	312,1	446,5	352,5	280,5
TbTh.SD (in μm)	192,2	665,5	179,7	135,5
TbSp.mean (in μm)	1634,9	237,9	467,8	1097,3
TbSp.SD (in μm)	1391,5	350,4	312,8	863,8
DA	0,3	0,24	0,34	0,64
TMD (in mg/cm3)	484,3	661,9	635,8	763,5
BMD (in mg/cm3)	109,5	343,6	349,2	283,7

reactive woven bone, is associated with decreased anisotropy [29].

In this study we furthermore quantified the degree of mineralization of bone tissue in the HO sample. Tissue mineral density (TMD) of trabecular bone showed low average values (484.34–763,46 mg HA/cm^3) compared to average TMD of normal trabecular bone of the femoral neck, greater trochanter, and proximal tibia (approximately 900 mg HA/cm^3) [30]. Also bone mineral density (BMD) of trabecular bone in conjunction with the surrounding soft tissue showed a lower average value in sample 1 (109,52 mg HA/cm^3) compared to reported normal bone volumetric BMD for women and men without hip fractures (310 ± 60 mg/cm^3 and 310 ± 60 mg/cm^3, respectively) and with hip fractures (250 ± 40 and 260

± 40 mg/cm^3, respectively) [31]. Nevertheless, BMD values for Sample 2, 3 and Sample 4 show higher values compared to Sample1.

Discussion

A neurogenic heterotopic ossification is a serious complication of traumas or disorders of the central nervous system observed in 20% of patients with this condition [2]. The hip and elbow joints affected predominantly are with severe pain, loss of movement and nerve compression syndromes. In addition, complications of the urinary tract system and pressure ulcers may arise in this disease [1–4]. In addition to conservative therapy with NSAIDs or bisphosphonates, surgical resection is indicated, with local recurrence being described.Neurogenic heterotopic ossification is characterized by ectopic bone formation in the soft tissue and muscle tissue around large joints, especially the hip and elbow joints. The severity of the HO depends on the severity of the brain damage. In the initial stage, NHO is difficult to diagnose and can also be interpreted as phlebitis, arthritis or cellulitis in a differential diagnosis, which often leads to a treatment delay. It is then necessary to take care of the hygiene in the case of concomitant diseases and complications as well as, for example, pressure ulcers, urinary tract infections or pneumonia [1–5].

As a rule, surgical resection occurs within the first year after the occurrence of the disease, whereby the indication for the operation is indicated on the one hand by the size of the ossification, on the other also by pain and possible compression of nerves or blood vessels.

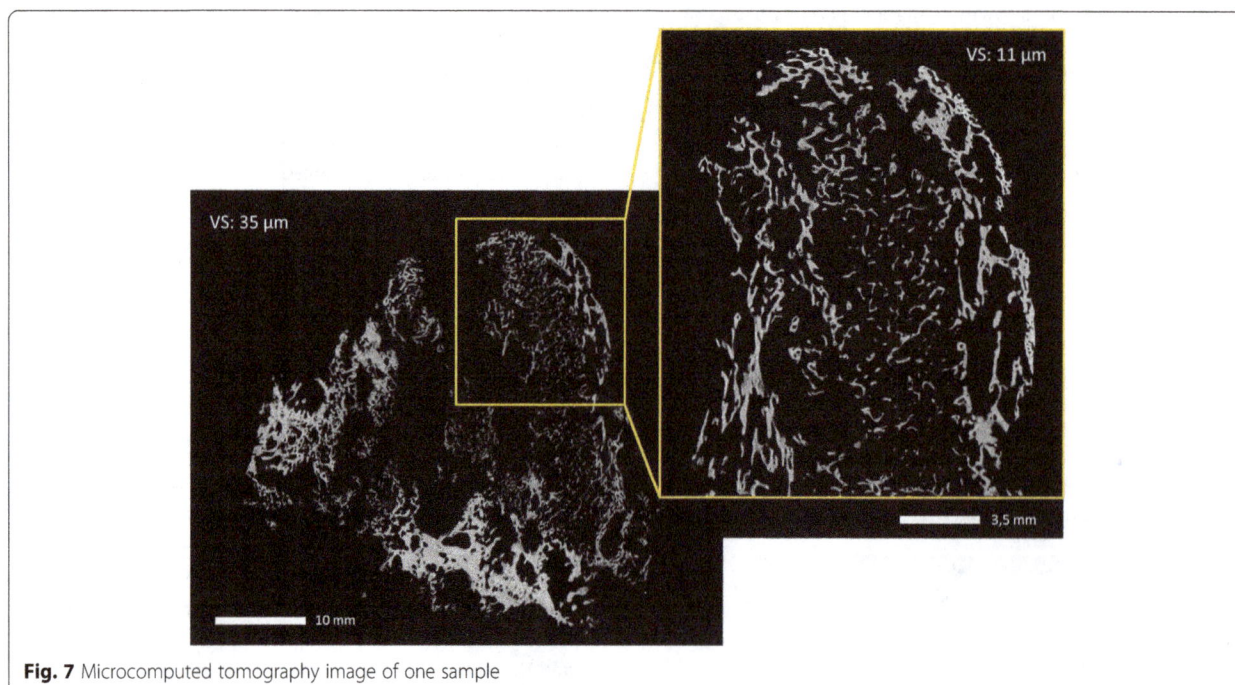

Fig. 7 Microcomputed tomography image of one sample

Good preoperative planning is important to avoid the potential complications such as infection, fracture, recurrent hemorrhage and nerve injury [2, 20, 21].

The time should be chosen so that the ossification is mature, but not yet so great that the complication probability becomes more frequent. Setting the right time for resection is not always easy, especially given the recurrence probability determined by the severity of brain damage. Likewise, too late a resection is bad for the adjacent joint, since this it is then stiffened and subsequent mobilization is made more difficult. There are different reports in the literature such as a series with 20 hips and another with 29 patients, with an improvement in the scope of movement in both studies [21, 22].

The pathophysiology of the NHO is not fully understood. However, there are 3 causes (traumatic, genetic, neurogenic) that can trigger the formation of the HO by activating stem cells for proliferation and differentiation [23]. In these patients, humoral factors can be altered; the exact relationship between the nervous system and the bone is not fully understood. It has been shown that some factors such as vasoactive peptides, neurotransmitters and the vasoactive substance can be altered [24–27]. There are some limitations in this study, one is the limited number of patients and another the descriptive concept. But our findings should induce other groups to initiate studies on this topic to get more information on the involvement of the immune system in HO.

In our study it is shown that immunological distribution in heterotopic ossification is altered compared to healthy subjects, this might reflect an immunological participation in the development of this entity. The result is tissue formation with a low bone volume fraction. Morphometric parameters additionally show that the disordered bone deposition in HO, e.g. of reactive woven bone, produces bone tissue that is characterized by a decrease in bone strength due to a low degree of mineralization and anisotropy. Further studies are needed to understand the mechanisms which induce HO.

Conclusions

This work shows altered immunological distribution that is accompanied by a low decrease in bone volume fraction and tissue mineral density in the heterotopic ossification sample compared to normal bone. Compared to healthy subjects, this might reflect an immunological participation in the development of this entity.

Abbreviations

BM: Bone marrow; BMD: Bone mineral density; BMMC: Bone marrow mononuclear cells; BV/TV: Bone volume/total volume; Con: Connectivity; DA: Degree of anisotropy; HO: Heterotopic ossification; TbSp.mean: Mean trabecular separation; TbSp.SD: Standard deviation of trabecular separation; TbTh.mean: Mean trabecular thickness; TbTh.SD: Standard deviation of trabecular thickness; TMD: Tissue mineral density

Authors' contributions

AM, SS, EN carried out the molecular, morphometric studies, immunoassays and histologic studies, participated in the sequence alignment and drafted the manuscript. KT designed the study and drafted the manuscript and BG participated in its coordination. All authors read and approved the final manuscript.

Competing interests

The authors declare that they have no competing interests.

Author details

[1]Department of Orthopaedics, Klinikum Wels-Grieskirchen, Grieskirchnerstr 42, 4600 Wels, Austria. [2]Institute for Biomedical Aging Research, University of Innsbruck, 5020 Innsbruck, Austria. [3]Computed Tomography Research Group, University of Applied Sciences Upper Austria, 4600 Wels, Austria.

References

1. Potter BK, Burns TC, Lacap AP, Granville RR, Gajewski DA. Heterotopic ossification following traumatic and combat-related amputations. Prevalence, risk factors, and preliminary results of excision J Bone Joint Surg Am. 2007;89:476–86.
2. Sullivan MP, Torres SJ, Mehta S, Ahn J. Heterotopic ossification after central nervous system trauma: a current review. Bone Joint Res. 2013;2:51–7.
3. Alfieri KA, Forsberg JA, Potter BK. Blast injuries and heterotopic ossification. Bone and Joint Research. Aug 2012;1:174–9.
4. Simonsen LL, Sonne-Holm S, Krasheninnikoff M, Engberg AW. Symptomatic heterotopic ossification after very severe traumatic brain injury in 114 patients: incidence and risk factors. Injury. 2007;38:1146–50.
5. Downey J, Lauzier D, Kloen P, Klarskov K, Richter M, Hamdy R, Faucheux N, Scimè A, Balg F, Grenier G. Prospective heterotopic ossification progenitors in adult human skeletal muscle. Bone. 2015;71:164–70.
6. Wittenberg RH, Peschke U, Bötel U. Heterotopic ossification after spinal cord injury: epidemiology and risk factors. J Bone Joint Surg (Br). 1992;74-B:215–8.
7. van Kuijk AA, Geurts AC, van Kuppevelt HJ. Neurogenic heterotopic ossification in spinal cord injury. Spinal Cord. 2002;40:313–26.
8. Ramirez D, Ramirez M, Reginato A, Medici M. Molecular and cellular mechanisms of heterotopic ossification. Histol Histopathol. 2014;29:1281–5.
9. Convente M, Wang H, Pignolo R, Kapaln F, Shore E. The immunological contribution to heterotopic ossification disorders. Curr Osteoporosis Rep. 2015;13:116–24.
10. Brownley RC, Agarwal S, Loder S, Eboda O, Li J, Peterson J, et al. Characterization of heterotopic ossification using radiographic imaging: evidence for a paradigm shift. PLoS One. 2015;10:e0141432. https://doi.org/10.1371/journal.pone.0141432.
11. Ji Y, Christopherson GT, Kluk MW, Amrani O, Jackson WM, Nesti LJ. Heterotopic ossification following musculoskeletal trauma: modeling stem and progenitor cells in their microenvironment. Adv Exp Med Biol. 2011;720:39–50.
12. Leblanc E, Trensz F, Haroun S, Drouin G, Bergeron E, Penton CM. BMP-9-induced muscle heterotopic ossification requires changes to the skeletal muscle microenvironment. Bone Miner Res. 2011;26:1166–77.
13. Kan L, Kessler JA. Evaluation of the cellular origins of heterotopic ossification. Orthopedics. 2014;37:329–40.
14. Medici D, Shore EM, Lounev VY, Kaplan FS, Kalluri R, Olsen BR. Conversion of vascular endothelial cells into multipotent stem-like cells. Nat Med. 2010;16: 1400–6.
15. Kan C, Kann L. The burning questions of heterotopic ossification. Ann Transl Med 215. 3:14–6.
16. Stadler N, Lehner J, Trieb K. Prospective mid-term results of a consecutive series of a short stem. Acta Orthop Belg. 2016;82:372–5.
17. Pangrazzi L, Meryk A, Naismith E, Koziel R, Lair J, Krismer M, Trieb K, Grubeck-Loebenstein B. "Inflamm-aging" influences immune cell survival factors in human bone marrow. Eur J Immunol. 2016; https://doi.org/10.1002/eji.201646570.

18. Hildebrand T, Ruegsegger P. A new method for the model independent assessment of thickness in three dimensional images. J Microsc. 1997;185:67–75.

19. Remy E, Thiel E. Medial axis for chamfer distances: computing look-up tables and neighbourhoods in 2D or 3D. Pattern Recogn Lett. 2002;23:649–61.

20. Meiners T, Abel R, Bohm V, Gerner HJ. Resection of heterotopic ossification of the hip in spinal cord injured patients. Spinal Cord. 1997;35:443–5.

21. Garland DE, Orwin JF. Resection of heterotopic ossification in patients with spinal cord injuries. Clin Orthop Relat Res. 1989;(242):169–76.

22. Moore TJ. Functional outcome following surgical excision of heterotopic ossification in patients with traumatic brain injury. J Orthop Trauma. 1993;7:11–4.

23. Kurer MH, Khoker MA, Dandona P. Human osteoblast stimulation by sera from paraplegic patients with heterotopic ossification. Paraplegisa. 1992;30:165–8.

24. Bidner SM, Rubins IM, Desjardins JV, Zukor DJ, Goltzman D. Evidence for a humoral mechanism for enhanced osteogenesis after head injury. J Bone Joint Surg Am. 1990;72:1144–9.

25. Hohmann E, Elde R, Rysavy J, Einzig S, Gebhard R. Innervation of peristoneum and bone by symphatetic vasoactive intestinal peptide-containing nerve fibers. Science. 1986;232:868–71.

26. Wang L, Tang X, Zhang H, et al. Elevated leptin expressionin rat model of traumatic spinal cord injury and femoral fracture. J Spinal Cord Med. 2011;34:501–9.

27. Forsberg J, Potter B, Safford S, Do E. Inflammatory Markers Portend heterotopic ossification and wound failure in combat wounds? Clin Orthop Relat Res. 2014;472:2845–54.

28. Nazarian A, von Stechow D, Zurakowski D, Müller R, Snyder BD. Bone volume fraction explains the variation in strength and stiffness of cancellous bone affected by metastatic cancer and osteoporosis. Calcif Tissue Int. 2008; 83:368–79.

29. Cole HA, Ohba T, Ichikawa J, Nyman JS, Cates JMM, Haro H, et al. Micro-computed tomography derived anisotropy detects tumor provoked deviations in bone in an orthotopic osteosarcoma murine model. PLoS One. 2014;9:1–7.

30. Wang J, Kazakia GJ, Zhou B, Shi XT, Guo XE. Distinct tissue mineral density in plate and rod-like trabeculae of human trabecular bone. J Bone Min Res. 2015;30:1641–50.

31. Center JR, Nguyen TV, Pocock NA, Eisman JA. Volumetric bone density at the femoral neck as a common measure of hip fracture risk for men and women. JCEM. 2004;89:2776–82.

3

Age and sex related differences in shoulder abduction fatigue

John D. Collins[1] and Leonard O'Sullivan[2]* iD

Abstract

Background: Injury prevalence data commonly indicate trends of higher rates of work-related musculoskeletal disorders in older workers over their younger counterparts, and for females more than males. The purpose of this study was to investigate age and sex-related differences in manifestations of shoulder muscle fatigue in a cohort of young and older working age males and females, in a single experiment design allowing for direct comparison of the fatigue effects between the target groups.

Methods: We report upper trapezius muscle fibre Conduction Velocity (CV) as an indicative measure of muscle fatigability, and isometric endurance time, at three levels of shoulder abduction lifting force set relative to participants' maximal strength.

Results: Upper trapezius conduction velocity was significantly different between the young and old groups ($p = 0.002$) as well as between males and females ($p = 0.016$). Shoulder abduction endurance time was affected by age ($P = 0.024$) but not sex ($p = 0.170$).

Conclusions: The study identified age-related improvement in muscle fatigue resistance and increased resistance for females over males, contrary to injury prevalence trends. The muscle fatigue effects are most likely explained by muscle fibre type composition. Experimental fatigue treatments of the upper trapezius were tested at exposures relative to the participants' strength. Absolute strength is higher when young and is generally higher for males. The findings of this study point towards age and sex-related differences in strength rather than in muscle fatigue resistance as a primary cause for the differences in the injury trends.

Keywords: Musculoskeletal disorders, Age, Sex, Trapezius, Shoulder, Fatigue

Background

Occupational injury and symptom prevalence data often indicate higher rates for older workers and for females [1, 2]. Collins and O'Sullivan [3] previously reported prevalence of neck/shoulder symptoms of Musculo-Skeletal Disorders (MSDs) for young and old age groups in a sedentary occupation, a trend also described by others [4]. In the study by Collins and O'Sullivan symptoms were highest for the oldest cohort and for females compared to their male counterparts. Silvia et al. [5] reported back pain across multiple industrial sectors and again reported higher prevalence for females. Laperriere et al. [6] detailed higher prevalence of self-reported work-related pain for females than males in food service work. Anton and

Weeks [7] described higher rates of MSD symptoms for female grocery workers than their male counterparts. In addition, they reported higher rates for workers aged 35+ years compared to younger age groups. Regarding ageing and MSDs, Slovak et al. [8] analysed data from The Health and Occupational Reporting Network which indicated a fivefold increase in work-related musculoskeletal disorders from ages 15–24 to 45–64. This is of considerable concern in view of the ageing workforce [9]. Many occupational health and ergonomics studies of MSD prevalence focus on heavy manual work, yet MSDs are highly prevalent in low force sedentary work, specifically in relation to the shoulder, for example in computer-based work [2, 4, 10].

The authors propose that there are three primary explanations for age and sex-related differences in muscle-related occupational injuries. The first explanation is due to differences in exposures, where some occupational

* Correspondence: leonard.osullivan@ul.ie
[2]School of Design and Health Research Institute, University of Limerick, Limerick, Ireland
Full list of author information is available at the end of the article

groups with higher risk of developing MSDs are dominated by one sex and/or age group. Controlling for exposure, a second potential explanation of variations are age/sex-related differences in muscle strength. A third possible explanation is due to differences in muscle fibre composition. The current study focuses on evaluating the latter explanation by measuring muscle fibre conduction velocity in a group of old and young participants.

Muscle activity, particularly where forceful exertions exist, has been implicated in many studies as a primary risk factor of muscle fatigue [11, 12]. However, muscle fatigue is not limited to high force contractions as low force static contractions can also cause muscle fatigue [13]. It is therefore important to acknowledge age and sex-based differences in fibre distribution as these characteristics may explain, at least in part, injury prevalence patterns detailed in previous research [3]. If age and sex-related differences in fibre types affect endurance and fatigue, it may be postulated that the magnitude of differences is important from an injury causation perspective.

There is good reason to consider muscle fibre-related differences as a mechanism of increased injury, especially for low force static contractions. The scientific literature on muscle fatigue resistance [14, 15] and muscle fibre type composition indicate age [16] and sex-based differences [17]. Furthermore, studies have investigated muscle fatigue and function specifically for low force muscle activity contractions, which is particularly important considering muscle fibre type differences [12, 13, 17]. According to the Hennmann Principle [18] and the Cinderella hypothesis [19], sustained low-level isometric contractions set up a stereotyped recruitment pattern of Motor Units (MUs) according to the size principle. Low threshold (type I) MUs are constantly active even in situations of continuous low muscle activity which could result in metabolically overloaded 'Cinderella' muscle fibres.

There are numerous studies of age and sex-related differences in muscle performance [14, 15]. However, we have been unable to find any studies specifically assessing age and sex-based differences in muscle fibre conduction velocity of the trapezius. The aim of this study was to investigate manifestations of shoulder muscle fatigue across age and sex. Conduction Velocity (CV) was used as an index of muscle fatigue in this experiment. It is possibly the most accurate physiological parameter of muscle fatigue as it is affected by fibre size and changes in pH, whereby CV values decrease during fatigue contractions and the slope of the CV values is indicative of the rate of fatigue in the muscle [20].

Method
Study design and statistical analysis
This was a laboratory based study of upper trapezius muscle fibre Conduction Velocity (CV) (as a measure of

muscle fatigue and endurance) for three relative levels of shoulder abduction, tested with the shoulder abducted 90^0. The two dependent variables were CV (normalised slope) and Endurance Time (ET). The independent variables were sex, age (young and old) and shoulder abduction exertion load (0, 10 and 20% Maximum Voluntary Contraction (MVC)). The exertion levels were based on previous studies of shoulder fatigue [21]. VO_2 MAX was entered as a covariate to control for differences in aerobic fitness.

Participants
There were 40 participants, 20 males and 20 females, with 10 each in the young and old sex-age groups (young participants mean age 26.0 years ±2.18 SD; older group mean age 59.6 years ±3.17 SD). A power analysis indicated this sample would yield an experimental power of > 0.8.

The experiment was approved by the University of Limerick Research Ethics Committee. Participants were recruited through advertisements on the University campus and through requests for volunteers through fellow researchers' contacts. Participants gave their written informed consent prior to testing. No participant reported any known symptoms of locomotive or musculoskeletal disorders.

Equipment
As muscle CV reduces with time in fatiguing muscles, the slope of the data, normalised to the initial value of the treatment, was selected as the index of fatigue [20]. CV was measured using a disposable 16-array surface electrode at a 5 mm electrode pitch (Model ELSCH016 electrode, OT Bioelettronica). Signals were sampled by a multichannel EMG amplifier (OT Bioelettronica, Torino, Italy). The EMG signals were amplified, band pass filtered (3 dB bandwidth, 10–500 Hz, roll-off of 40 dB/decade), sampled at 2048 Hz, and stored on a PC (12 bit A/D converter). VO_2 MAX was measured using a portable O2 analyser (Model Cosmed k4B^2) and a cycle ergometer to perform the aerobic activity.

Shoulder abduction exertion was measured using a commercial force meter (Mecmesin Advanced Force Gauge AFG-500 N) modified with an adjustable level handle attached to a platform.

Procedure
Part 1 shoulder abduction MVC
The testing posture involved the participant seated, with feet firmly on the ground and their back in an upright posture, the dominant shoulder abducted to 90^0, the elbow fully extended, and the forearm fully pronated. The handle of the force meter was adjusted to the required testing posture. Participants performed an initial warm-up which consisted of a number of repetitive shoulder movements from 0^0 to 90^0 abduction. Instructions to the participants informed them to abduct their

Table 1 Summary of ANOVA/ANCOVA main and interaction effects on endurance time

Dependent variable	Main Effects			Interaction			
	L	S	A	AxS	AxL	SxL	AxSxL
Endurance Time	0.0005**	0.1	0.021*	0.491	0.521	0.15	0.012*
Endurance Time (VO$_2$ MAX as covariate)	0.0001**	0.175	0.024*	0.308	0.548	0.242	0.009**

L = Load (exertion level) S=Sex A = Age
*$p < 0.05$ **$p < 0.01$

pronated arm while grasping the handle of the force meter, to generate their maximum lifting effort and sustaining it for 3 sec, in line with the Caldwell regime [22]. Three trials were conducted with 5 min of rest between each treatment. The maximum result was determined as the participant's MVC.

Part 2 upper trapezius CV and shoulder abduction endurance

The participants' skin was shaven, if required, and prepared with abrasive paste and alcohol wipes to reduce skin impedance [23]. Conductive gel was injected into each space of the array electrode and secured to the skin with tape. The electrode was positioned over the upper trapezius lateral to the innervation zone, between the seventh cervical vertebra and the posterior tip of the acromion. The Innervation Zone (IZ) of the muscle was detected using a bar electrode and the position marked on the skin to position the array.

Each participant completed three static shoulder abduction endurance exertions at 0, 10, and 20% MVC. Contractions were maintained until the participant could no longer sustain the exertion. The target percentage MVC levels were calculated by the experimenter and the participants were instructed to exert the force levels visually via the real-time values on the force meter interface. The 0% MVC exertion involved holding the arm outright without exerting a lifting force on the force meter.

The treatments were randomised for each participant using Latin Square orders, which are unique orders of treatments for each participant. A 10-min resting period followed each endurance test with additional rest given if residual fatigue or discomfort was reported, as per Yassierli and Nussbaum [24].

Part 3 post-test measurements of the covariate VO$_2$ MAX

The starting workload was estimated based on age and level of activity. The cadence was adjusted to achieve a heart rate of 60–85% of maximal capacity (i.e. 220-age) and VO$_2$ MAX was measured in real time using the Cosmed software system.

Statistical analysis

Data were presented as means and Standard Deviation (SD) of the mean. Statistical significance was set at $p < 0.05$. Statistical Analysis was performed using SPSS V 22. The Kolmogorov-Smirnov test applied to the data indicated the shoulder abduction MVC values were normally distributed, but the CV and ET data were not. The log transformation was successful in normalising these data. Independent samples t-tests were used to compare the MVC data between the young versus old age groups, and separately for males versus females. ANOVA was used to test the main and interaction effects on both CV and ET, and repeated with ANCOVA to include VO$_2$ max as the covariate.

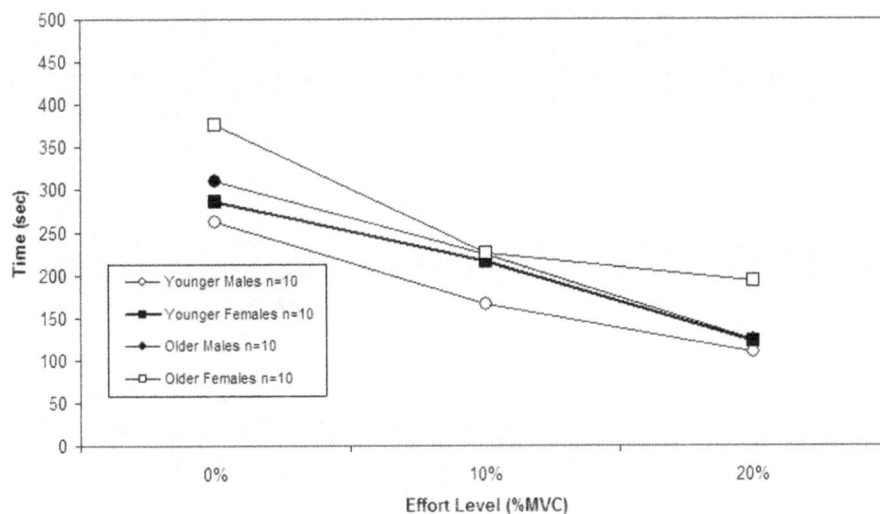

Fig. 1 Mean endurance times illustrating the statistically significant effects for Load, Age, and the Age x Sex x Load interaction ($p < 0.05$)

Table 2 Summary of ANOVA/ANCOVA main and interaction effects on normalised rate of change of CV

Dependent variable	Main Effects			Interaction			
	L	S	A	AxS	AxL	SxL	AxSxL
Conduction Velocity	0.049*	0.035*	0.003*	0.621	0.044*	0.187	0.845
Conduction Velocity (VO$_2$ MAX as a covariate)	0.13	0.016*	0.002**	0.292	0.035*	0.154	0.827

L = Load S=Sex A = Age
*p < 0.05 **p < 0.01

Results

Mean shoulder abduction MVC of the young group was 73.1 N ± (27.30 SD) and mean MVC of the older individuals was 64.01 N ± (24.15 SD). This difference was not statistically significant. Mean shoulder abduction MVC for males was 87.8 N (± 21 SD) and for females 49.3 N (± 12.3 SD), which were significantly different (t-test $p = 0.0001$).

Regarding endurance times, Table 1 details the results of the statistical analysis while Fig. 1 depicts the plots of the mean values by age, sex and load. Age had a highly significant effect on Endurance Time ($p = 0.02$), with higher times for the older age group. T there was no significant effect ($p = 0.1$) for sex. The three-way interaction was also significant ($p = 0.01$).

Regarding the upper trapezius conduction velocity data, Table 2 details the results of the statistical analysis while Table 3 and Fig. 2 detail the mean and standard deviation of the data for the experimental conditions. Age had a significant effect ($p = 0.002$) with greater slopes (higher fatigue) for the younger groups. Sex also had a significant effect ($p = 0.016$) with males showing greater slopes (higher fatigue). There was a significant Age x Load interaction ($p = 0.035$).

Discussion

The principal findings of this study are an apparent age-related improvement in muscle endurance and increased fatigue resistance for females over males. These trends have been previously observed in individual studies of age or sex for muscles groups. There are two key strengths to this study over previous fatigue studies of this nature. Firstly, it is a single experimental study of the same fatigue conditions involving both males and females of both age groups. This enables a direct comparison of the fatigue

differences between these groups, which, to our knowledge, is not present in the literature for working age adults. The second key strength of this study is the measurement of muscle fatigue via muscle fibre conduction velocity for the experimental fatigue conditions tested, and for a shoulder muscle commonly associated with MSDs.

The age-related improvement in fatigue identified in this study may be due to differences in muscle fibre type compositions [25]. Aged muscles have been characterised as muscles with a type I fibre dominance [26] resulting in increased fatigue resistance [27]. Type I fibre fatigue resistance is indicated to be due to their myosin heavy chain cross bridges [28, 29]. Merletti et al. [30] detail that reduction in the motor unit firing rate also plays a role in improvement of age-related muscle fatigue resistance. Muscle fibre type differences also most likely explain the increased fatigue resistance for females. Although there is a similar distribution of fast and slow fibre types for males and females, there is, however, a significant sex-related difference in the total area occupied by type I fibres [28, 31], which increases oxidative capacity of these fibres, increasing fatigue resistance for female muscle. Fulco et al. [32] propose that female muscle has increased muscle oxidative phosphorylation, while Crowther and Gronka [33] have identified that the muscle fibres recruited first in voluntary contractions have a higher oxidative capacity than those recruited last. Sex-based differences have also been observed in muscle function [28], but explanations for these differences remain underdeveloped. In accordance with the Henneman Theory and the Cinderella Hypothesis, female muscle would contain a greater oxidative capacity prolonging fatigue. Each of these suggestions may explain the sex-related difference in the current study, however, additional tests incorporating greater loads would be advantageous in supplementing these attributes.

This study reinforces the need for clinicians and policymakers to emphasise workplace and policy-level occupational health strategies to correct the clear trends of elevated work-related injuries/symptoms for certain groups of workers. This can be achieved through group level exposure monitoring, and/or through improved workplace risk assessments/monitoring sensitivity of more vulnerable workers.

A weakness of the study is the sample size. Each group contained only ten participants, but it should be noted that this is greater than the full sample size of many other EMG-based lab studies. The sample sizes were

Table 3 Mean endurance times and SD by load age and sex

Load (Exertion level)	Group	Male		Female	
		Mean	SD	Mean	SD
0% MVC	Young	262	99	285	145
	Older	310	149	377	168
10% MVC	Young	166	66	215	109
	Older	224	80	225	34
20% MVC	Young	109	31	122	48
	Older	124	39	193	25

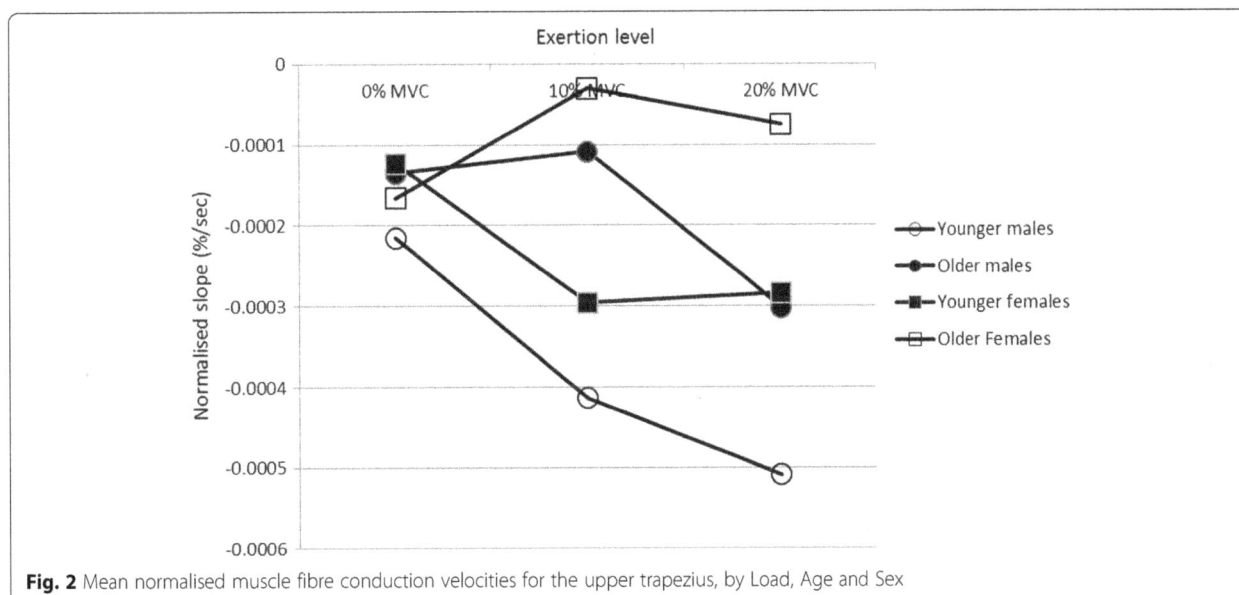

Fig. 2 Mean normalised muscle fibre conduction velocities for the upper trapezius, by Load, Age and Sex

considered adequate for statistical analysis in this experiment. However, a larger sample would clarify borderline near significant results, which may be indicative of type II errors. The testing posture, while typical of static arm positions in many construction and industrial tasks, may not represent many typical arm postures involving low levels of shoulder flexion/abduction, for example in computer work, also representing a limitation of the study. The mean age of the older participants was 59 years, which is not representative of the older general population, however it is representative of the older working age population where many people retire by the age of 65 years. Further studies should be performed with older participants than studied in this experiment to assess the wider generalisability of these findings.

Conclusions

The overall conclusion from this research was that the older cohort exhibited decreased shoulder strength, longer endurance times, and signs of slower progression of muscular fatigue, suggesting type I fibre dominance in aged muscles. Females exhibited higher endurance times and slower progression of muscular fatigue than the males. The importance of this work is that it identified that the groups with increased fatigue resistance (older age & females) are indicated to be those typically with lower muscle strength in the working population. A key inference from the study is that when controlling for exposure, the trends in age and sex-related differences in shoulder MSD prevalence might not primarily be due to muscle fibre type related differences, but rather differences in muscle strength.

Authors' contributions
JC was a Ph.D. researcher on this study. He planned, performed and analysed the study, and drafted the paper. LOS was the supervisor of the research. He assisted in the planning and oversight of the research, and provided feedback on the manuscript. Both authors read and approved the final manuscript.

Competing interests
The authors declare that they have no competing interests.

Author details
[1]School of Design, University of Limerick, Limerick, Ireland. [2]School of Design and Health Research Institute, University of Limerick, Limerick, Ireland.

References
1. Davis K, Dunning K, Jewell G, Lockey J. Cost and disability trends of work-related musculoskeletal disorders in Ohio. Occup Med (Lond). 2014;64:608–15.
2. Ekman A, Andersson A, Hagberg M, Hjelm EW. Gender differences in musculoskeletal health of computer and mouse users in the Swedish workforce. Occup Med (Lond). 2000;50:608–13.
3. Collins JD, O'Sullivan L. Musculoskeletal disorder prevalence and psychosocial risk exposures by age and gender in a cohort of office based employees in two academic institutions. Int J Ind Ergon. 2015;46:85–97.
4. Janwantanakul P, Pensri P, Jiamjarasrangsri V, Sinsongsook T. Prevalence of self-reported musculoskeletal symptoms among office workers. Occup Med (Lond). 2008;58:436–8.
5. Silvia C, Barros C, Cunha L, Carnide F, Santos M. Prevalence of back pain problems in relation to occupational group. Int J Ind Ergon. 2016;52:52–8.
6. Laperriere E, Messing K, Bourbonnais R. Work activity in food service: the significance of customer relations, tipping practices and gender for preventing musculoskeletal disorders. Appl Ergon. 2017;58:89–101.
7. Anton D, Weeks DL. Prevalence of work related musculoskeletal symptoms among grocery workers. Int J Ind Ergon. 2016;54:139–45.
8. Slovak A, Carder M, Money A, Turner S, Agius R. Work-related musculoskeletal conditions: evidence from the THOR reporting system 2002–2005. Occup Med (Lond). 2009;59:447–53.
9. Algarni FS, Gross DP, Senthilselvan A, Battie MC. Ageing workers with work-related musculoskeletal Injuries. Occup Med (Lond). 2015;65:229–37.
10. Moen BE, Wieslander G, Bakke JV, Norbäck D. Subjective health complaints and psychosocial work environment among university personnel. Occup Med (Lond). 2013;63:38–44.
11. Li ZZ, Zhang WK, Ma W, L. Chen Z. Muscular fatigue and maximum endurance time assessment for male and female industrial workers. Int J Ind Ergon. 2014;44:292–7.

12. Troiano A, Naddeo F, Sosso E, Camarota G, Merletti R, Mesin L. Assessment of force and fatigue in isometric contractions of the upper trapezius muscle by surface EMG signal and perceived exertion scale. Gait Posture. 2008;28: 179–86.

13. Farina D, Falla D. Estimation of muscle fibre conduction velocity from two-dimensional surface EMG recordings in dynamic tasks. Biomedical Signal Processing and Control. 2008;3:138–44.

14. Sundberg C, Kuplic A, Hassanlouei H, Hunter S. Mechanisms for the age-related increase in fatigability of the knee extensors in old and very old adults. J Appl Physiol. 2018;91:2686–94.

15. Deering R, Senefeld J, Pashibin T, Hunter S. Muscle function and fatigability of trunk flexors in males and females. Biol Sex Differ. 2017;8:1–12.

16. Avin KG, Frey Law LA. Age-related differences in muscle fatigue vary by contraction type: a meta-analysis. J Am Phys Ther Assoc. 2011;91:1153–65.

17. Zhanga Z, Li Way K, Zhang W, Ma L, Chen Z. Muscular fatigue and maximum endurance time assessment for male and female industrial workers. Int J Ind Ergon. 2014;44:292–7.

18. Henneman E, Somjen G, Carpenter DO. Functional significance of cell size in spinal motoneurons. J Neurophysiol. 1965;28:560.

19. Hägg G. Static work loads and occupational myalgia—a new explanation model. In: Anderson P, Hobart D, Danoff, Electromographical kinesiology. Amsterdam: Elsevier; 1999.

20. Merletti R, Parker P. Electromyography: physiology, engineering and non-invasive applications. New York: Wiley-IEEE Press; 2004.

21. Wahlstrom J. Ergonomics, musculoskeletal disorders and computer work. Occup Med (Lond). 2005;55:168–76.

22. Caldwell L, Chaffin D, Dukes Dobos F, Kroemer K, Labach L, Snook S, Wasserman D. A proposed standard procedure for static muscle strength testing. Am Ind Hyg Assoc J. 1974;35:201–6.

23. Hermens HJ, Freriks B, Disselhorst-Klug C, Raru G. Development of recommendations for SEMG sensors and sensor placement procedures. J Electromyogr Kinesiol. 2000;10:361–74.

24. Yassierli. Nussbaum. MA., Muscle fatigue during intermittent isokinetic shoulder abduction: Age effects and utility of electromyographic measures. Ergonomics. 2007; 50; 1110–1126.

25. Trappe S, Gallagher P, Harber M, Carrithers J, Fluckey J, Trappe T. Single muscle fibre contractile properties in young and old men and women. J Physiol. 2003;552:47–58.

26. Nilwirk R, Snijders T, Leenders M, Groen BB, van Kranenburg J, Verdijk LB, van Loon LJ. The decline in skeletal muscle mass with aging is mainly attributed to a reduction in type II muscle fibre size. Exp Gerontol. 2013;48:492–8.

27. Merletti R, Benvenuti F, Doncarli C, Disselhorst-Klug C, Ferrabone R, Hermens H, Kadefors R, Lâubli T, Orizio C, Sjâ-gaard G, Zazula D. The European project -neuromuscular assessment in the elderly worker: achievements in electromyogram signal acquisition, modelling and processing. Med Biol Eng Comput. 2004;42:429–31.

28. Yu F, Hedström M, Cristea A, Dalén N, Larsson L. Effects of ageing and gender on contractile properties in human skeletal muscle and single fibres. Acta Physiol. 2007;190:229–41.

29. Callahan DM, Miller MS, Sweeny AP, Tourville TW, Slauterbeck JR, Savage PD, Maugan DW, Ades PA, Beynnon BD, Toth MJ. Muscle disuse alters skeletal muscle contractile function at the molecular and cellular levels in older adult humans in a sex-specific manner. J Physiol. 2014;592:4555–73.

30. Merletti R, Farina D, Gazzoni M, Schieroni MP. Effect of age on muscle functions investigated with surface electromyography. Muscle Nerve. 2002;25:65–76.

31. Staron RS, Hagerman FC, Hikida RS, Murray TF, Hoster DP, Crill MT, Ragg KE, Toma K. Fiber type composition of the vastus Lateralis muscle of young men and women. Journal of Histochemistry Cytochemistry. 2000;48:623–30.

32. Fulco CS, Rock PB, Muza SR, Lammi E, Braun B, Cymerman A, Moore LG, Lewis SF. Gender alters impact of hypobaric hypoxia on adductor pollicis muscle performance. J Appl Physiol. 2001;91:100–8.

33. Crowther CG, Crowther GJ, Gronka RK. Fiber recruitment affects oxidative recovery measurements of human muscle in vivo. Med Sci Sports Exerc. 2002;34:1733–7.

4

Effects of erythropoietin for precaution of steroid-induced femoral head necrosis in rats

Yong-Qing Yan[1], Qing-Jiang Pang[1] and Ren-Jie Xu[2,3*]

Abstract

Background: Steroids such as glucocorticoid have been widely used for their excellent anti-inflammatory, anti-immune, and anti-shock properties. However, the long-term use in high doses has been found to cause necrosis of femoral head and other serious adverse reactions. Thus, it is of great importance to safely use these medications on patients without inducing bone necrosis.

Methods: In this preclinical study, we examined the effects of erythropoietin (EPO) to attenuate the induction of steroid-induced femoral bone necrosis using rats to build up the in-vivo models. Rats were randomly divided into three groups: negative control group (group A), disease group (group B), and EPO group (group C). 20 mg/kg methylprednisolone was administrated into group B and group C for 6 weeks with two intramuscular injections per week per rat. Group C was further given daily intraperitoneal injections of rHuEPO during this period. Group A received only injection of saline at the same schedule. 12 weeks after the initial drug administration, the rats' femoral tissues were harvested for HE staining, immunohistochemistry studies for PECAM-1(also CD31) expression and Western Blotting for VEGF expression.

Results: Histology studies showed that compared with the disease group, EPO group had significant improvement and bone morphology being much closer to the negative control group. Immunohistochemical studies revealed that EPO group had statistically much more expression of PECAM-1 than the other groups did. Western Blot demonstrated that the EPO group had significantly higher VEGF expression than the disease group.

Conclusion: Results suggested that simultaneous injection of EPO could partially prevent steroid-induced ANFH.

Keywords: Erythropoietin, Steroid, Necrosis, Rat, Femoral head

Background

Osteonecrosis is often observed in hips, knees, shoulders, and ankles, in which avascular necrosis of the femoral head (ANFH) is the most common one. Approximately 80% of patients suffering from ANFH progress to a collapse of the femoral head, resulting in impaired hip joint function and permanent disability if did not receive appropriate treatments [1].

Glucocorticoid (GC) administration is the most common non-traumatic cause of ANFH [2]. About 25% of patients receiving hormone therapy would eventually develop osteonecrosis [3], therefore early prevention is of most importance. However, the exact pathogenesis remains to be fully elucidated. There are several hypotheses including fat embolization, intramedullary pressure changes, coagulation disorders, circulatory impairment and cell dysfunction and apoptosis [4–6]. Amongst these mechanisms, the vascular hypothesis, in which local microvascular impairment leads to a decrease in blood flow in the femoral head, has become more widely accepted [7–11].

Erythropoietin (EPO) is a glycoprotein excreted by the kidneys. Its main function is to stimulate the proliferation and differentiation of reticulocytes. Further studies proved that erythropoietin could also promote angiogenesis [12].

* Correspondence: fredxurj@sina.com
[2]Department of Orthopaedics, Suzhou Municipal Hospital/The Affiliated Hospital of Nanjing Medical University, No 26, Daoqian Street, Suzhou 215000, Jiangsu, People's Republic of China
[3]Department of Orthopaedics, the First Affiliated Hospital, Orthopaedic Institute, Soochow University, Suzhou 215000, Jiangsu, People's Republic of China
Full list of author information is available at the end of the article

Studies have shown that erythropoietin is a multifunctional factor that exerts extensive protective effects in a variety of non-hematopoietic organs [13–16], which can promote cell regeneration and vessel formation; resist inflammation, oxidation, and apoptosis; and accelerate vessel formation, cell proliferation, and cell protection [17–19]. Recently, erythropoietin has been reported to be capable of promoting bone healing [20]. To summarize, apoptosis of bone cells, microcirculation impairment and cell dysfunction could be possible mechanisms in ANFH. And EPO can inhibit cell apoptosis promoting angiogenesis and proliferation which might counteract side effect of GCs. Therefore, we hypothesize that EPO might have some positive effects on preventing steroid-induced ANFH.

Methods

Materials

Human erythropoietin (10,000 U, Shenyang Sunshine Pharmaceutical Co., Ltd. Shenyang, China); Goat polyclonal to PECAM-1 Antibody (1:50, Santa Cruz, CA, USA); Rabbit anti-sheep SP immunohistochemical staining kit and citrate antigen retrieval solution (pH 6.0) (Fuzhou Maixin Biotech. Co., Ltd., Fuzhou, China); Hematoxylin (Sigma, St. Louis, USA); PVDF membranes (Millipore Company, MA, USA); Polylysine solution (0.1%) and DAB Horseradish Peroxidase Color Development Kit (Beijing Golden Bridge Biotechnology Co., Ltd., Beijing, China); Prestained Color Protein Molecular Weight Marker (Fermentas, Waltham, MA, USA); Tris-Hcl/SDS solutions (1.5 mM, pH 8.8; and 0.5 mM, pH 6.8, Sangon Biotechnology, Shanghai, China); Acrylamide/Bis solution (30%, Bio-Rad, California, USA); BeyoECL Plus kit, SDS-PAGE Sample Loading Buffer (5×), Western blot, IP cell lysates, PMSF together with BCA protein assay kit (Beyotime Biotechnology, Shanghai, China); Skim milk powder (Yili Group, Inner Mongolia, China); VEGF Antibody (Abcam, Cambridge Science Park, UK); β-actin Antibody, goat anti-Rabbit IgG-HRP, and goat anti-Mouse IgG-HRP (Bioworld, Minnesota, USA).

Eighteen SD male rats and eighteen SD female rats were supplied by Hangzhou hi-biotechnology Co., Ltd. (Hangzhou, China).

Animal models

The adoption of 36 rats in this study was approved by Institutional Animal Care and Use Committee and complied with NIH animal usage guidance. These eighteen male rats and eighteen female rats were randomly assigned into three groups (6 male rats and 6 female rats for each group) using a random number table: the negative control group, disease group, and EPO group. Methylprednisolone (20 mg/kg bodyweight) was muscularly intramuscularly injected into one of the hind legs of each rat from both group B and Group C twice a week for 6 weeks. Every rat from the Group C was further given a daily intraperitoneal injection of rHuEPO (500 u/d/kg-bodyweight) during these 6 weeks. The group A only received injection of saline at the same schedule. Rats were housed in cages together for 12 weeks (including 6 weeks after completing treatment) and had freely available food as well as water for the whole period.

The animals were sacrificed after 12 weeks. Under general anesthesia a lethal dose of pentobarbital (80 mg/kg BW) was injected. Femurs of both hind legs were dissected under sterile conditions and further investigations were conducted (72 femurs in total). Some harvested femoral tissues from each group were dehydrated accordingly and embedded in wax before being sliced into thin slices for HE stain (6 femurs for each group) and immunohistochemistry studies (12 femurs for each group). The rest samples (3 femurs for each group) were used for Western blot experiments.

Histological examination

Some tissue slices embedded in wax from each rat were de-waxed using xylene and then gradually re-hydrated using ethanol. The rehydrated tissue slices were stained for 8–10 min with 2% Hematoxylin solution and then for 1–2 min with 2% eosin solution. The stained tissue slices were dehydrated by ethanol. The dehydrated tissue slices were washed with xylene for three times before being blocked for observation under the microscope.

Immunohistochemistry

Some tissue slices embedded in wax from each rat were de-waxed using xylene and then gradually re-hydrated using ethanol. The re-hydrated tissue slices were washed with 0.3% H_2O_2 methanol solution and then with phosphate buffer. The resulting tissue slices were incubated in 1% bovine serum albumin (BSA) at 20 °C for 15 min. The slices were further incubated with rabbit anti-rat CD31 polyclonal antibodies according to the manufacturer's instruction. Briefly, the incubation with the primary antibody was conducted at 4 °C for 16 h, and the following incubation with the secondary antibody was conducted at room temperature for 20 min. DAB Horseradish Peroxidase Color Development Kit was used to develop the coloring and Hematoxylin was used to stain the cell Nuclei. The negative control slices were treated with the same procedure mentioned above except that these samples were incubated with PBS instead of the primary antibody before being incubated with the secondary antibody. The stained tissue slices were dehydrated using ethanol. The dehydrated tissue slices were washed with xylene for three times before being blocked for observation under the microscope. Three different visual fields were randomly selected for each immunohistochemical slice under the magnification of 400× to count positive expression of blood vessels.

Western blot

Some harvested femoral heads were ground in a grinding mortar in the presence of liquid N_2. After the liquid N_2 evaporated from the mortar, 300 μL single detergent lysate (containing 3 μL PMSF) was added for further grinding at 4 °C for 30 min. The supernatant was sampled and stored at − 80 °C after the lysate was centrifuged at 12,000 rpm for 10 min at 4 °C. Electrophoresis was performed for the collected supernatant samples using acrylamide gel electrophoresis (PAGE) gels in 15% PAGE gel electrophoresis. After the electrophoresis, the resulting PAGE gels were harvested and trimmed to strips according to the Marker. After the gel strips were washed with distilled water, wet transfer method was used for transferring separated proteins to PVDF transfer membranes. The resulting PVDF membranes were blocked through incubation in TBST containing 5% skim milk powder at room temperature for 2 h, followed by incubation with the primary antibodies at

4 °C for overnight and then the secondary antibodies at room temperature for 1 h. TBST was used to wash the PVDF membranes three times (10 min each) before the PVDF membranes were incubated with BeyoECL Plus kit for 5 min. After the fluorescent bands became obvious, the excess substrate solution was blotted using filter paper. The PVDF membranes were covered with plastic wrap and then pressed with X-ray film before detection and visualization.

Statistical analysis

All numerical data are presented as mean ± standard deviation. Statistical analyses were performed with PASW Statistics for Windows18.0 (SPSS Inc., Chicago, IL), and differences between groups were tested with one-way ANOVA followed by Post hoc LSD method. A P value of < 0.05 indicates a statistically significant difference.

Results

Observation of HE staining results

Figure 1 showed the representative optical images of HE stained femoral head bone slices in the negative control

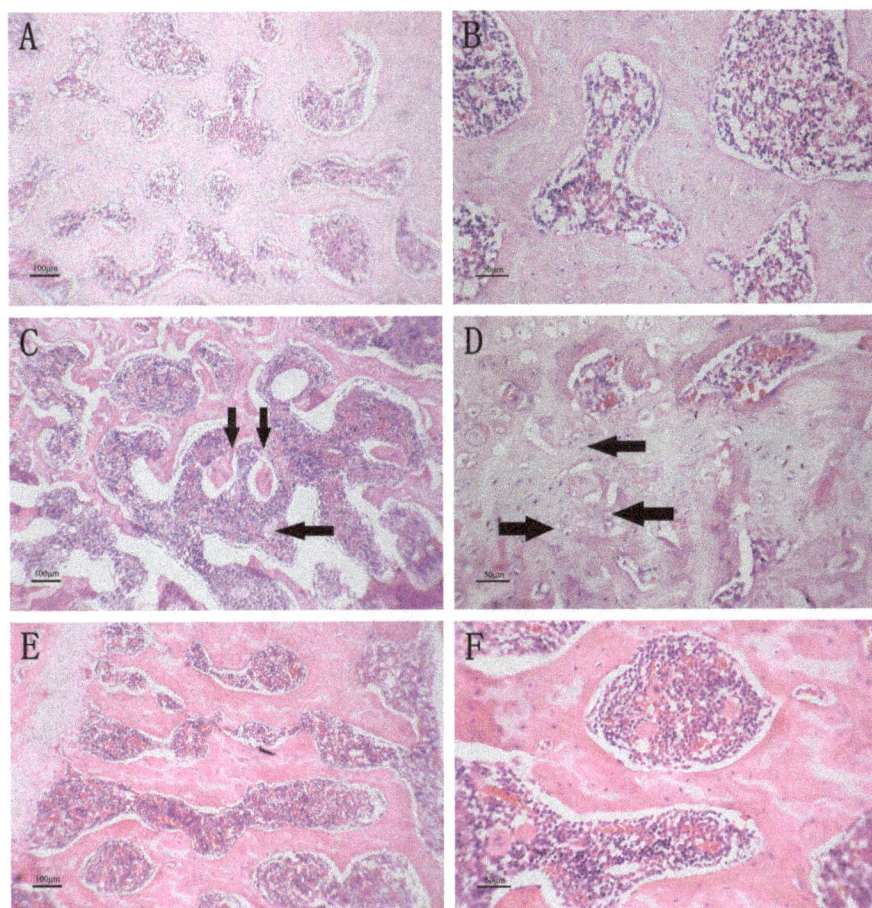

Fig. 1 Representative optical images of HE stained femoral head bone slices from rats in negative control group (**a** and **b**), disease group (**c** and **d**), and EPO group (**e** and **f**). Magnification 100× for (**a**, **c** and **e**) (scale bars 100 μm), and 250× for (**b**, **d**, and **f**) (scale bars 50 μm)

group (group A), disease group (group B), and EPO group (group C). Group A: an integral circular or oval arched structure and high connectivity without osteoclasts, narrowed bone trabeculae, or fractures was observed in bony trabeculae of Fig. 1a and b. Group B: on contrast, bony trabeculae were obviously sparse, narrowed and fractured with decreased connectivity (Fig. 1c and d). The arch structure partially disappeared and became irregular in shape (marked with an arrow in Fig. 1c). Some cell nuclei had shrunken, dissolved or disappeared (marked with an arrow in Fig. 1d), while more osteoclasts were present. Group C: Fig. 1e and f clearly showed that there were significant improvements observed on the rats from the group C as compared with the group B (Fig. 1e and f). The bony trabeculae were relatively regular in shape. The connectivity was markedly superior to that in group B. Some bony trabeculae had become coarse. The fracture rate was obviously decreased, while connection and repair had occurred in the defects.

Immunohistochemical expression of PECAM-1

Figure 2a-c showed the representative images of immunohistochemical slices for rats in group A, B and C. Immunohistochemical staining for PECAM-1 was clearly and selectively present in the blood vessel endothelial cells. Positivity was indicated by the presence of yellow particles. In group A, PECAM-1expression was strong, and the blood supply of the femoral head was sufficient (Fig. 2a). The rats in group B (Fig. 2b) had statistically significantly lower blood vessel density in the femoral

heads than those in the group A ($p < 0.01$, Fig. 2d, Table 1). However, the blood vessel density in the femoral heads of the rats receiving EPO injection was statistically significant higher than those of the group B ($p < 0.05$, Fig. 2c, Table 1).

Expression of VEGF in western blot

Figure 3a revealed the expression of VEGF in the femoral heads for all three groups of rats determined by Western blot. The data was quantified and normalized according to the control protein of β-actin (Fig. 3b). The rats in group B had apparently less expression of VEGF in their femoral heads. The injection of methylprednisolone at 20 mg/kg bodyweight caused a statistically significant decrease on the secretion of VEGF in the Group B as compared with the group A ($p < 0.05$, Table 2). This observed decrease was rescued by the co-administration of rHuEPO at 500 u/d/kg-bodyweight ($p < 0.05$, Table 2). Indeed, the ratio of VEGF/β-actin for group C was slightly larger than that for the control group, although the difference was not statistically significant ($p > 0.05$, Table 2).

Discussion

In this study, we successfully induced ANFH in the rats of disease group by intramuscularly injecting methylprednisolone. Obvious cell apoptosis and avascular necrosis were observed in the HE stained slices of disease group [21, 22], while results of EPO group resembled that of the negative control group.

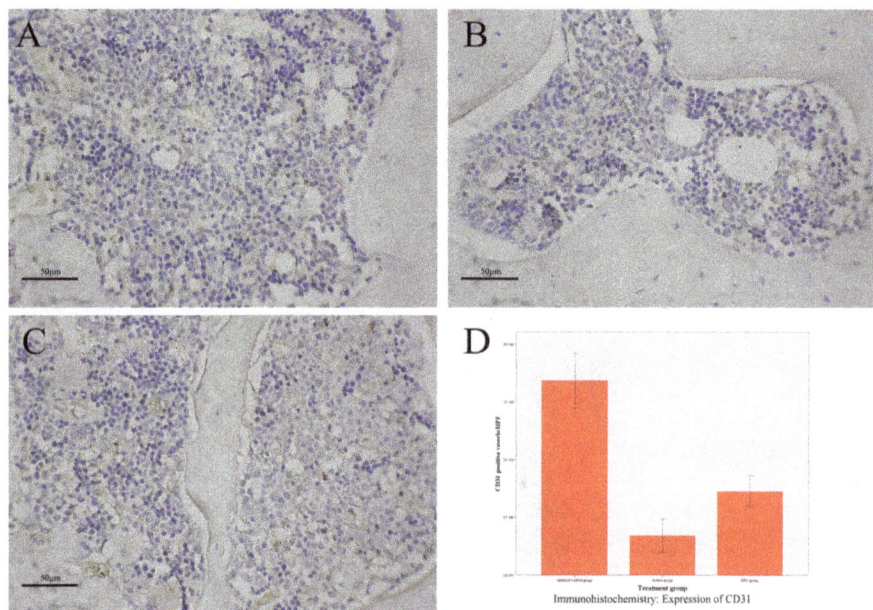

Fig. 2 Representative optical images of immunohistochemical femoral head bone slice from rats (**a**, **b** and **c**) in negative control group (**a**), disease group (**b**), and EPO group (**c**); and the expression of CD31 in the femoral head bone determined from immunohistochemistry (**d**). Scale bar: 50 μm. * for $p < 0.05$, and ** for $p < 0.01$

Table 1 Immunohistochemistry results

	Group A	Group B	Group C
counts/HPF ($\bar{x} \pm s$)	26.83 ± 7.02	13.41 ± 4.27	17.28 ± 4.03
F		61.397	
p		< 0.01	
Multiple Comparison	Group A-B	Group B-C	Group A-C
p (LSD)	< 0.01**	0.03*	< 0.01

Sufficient blood supply is reported critical for bone regeneration and skeletal tissue engineering [23]. Some scholars have revealed two main mechanisms, angiogenesis and vasculogenesis responsible for the formation of new blood vessels, also known as neovascularization [23]. Regarding EPO, both of these mechanisms might play roles in the present studies, which could promote bone regeneration via an improved microenvironment and nutrient supply [24]. In this study, the simultaneous injection of EPO clearly slowed down the progress of ANFH. There was evidenced with the observation on HE stained slices of femoral heads in the EPO group of rats. PECAM-1 is highly expressed in vascular

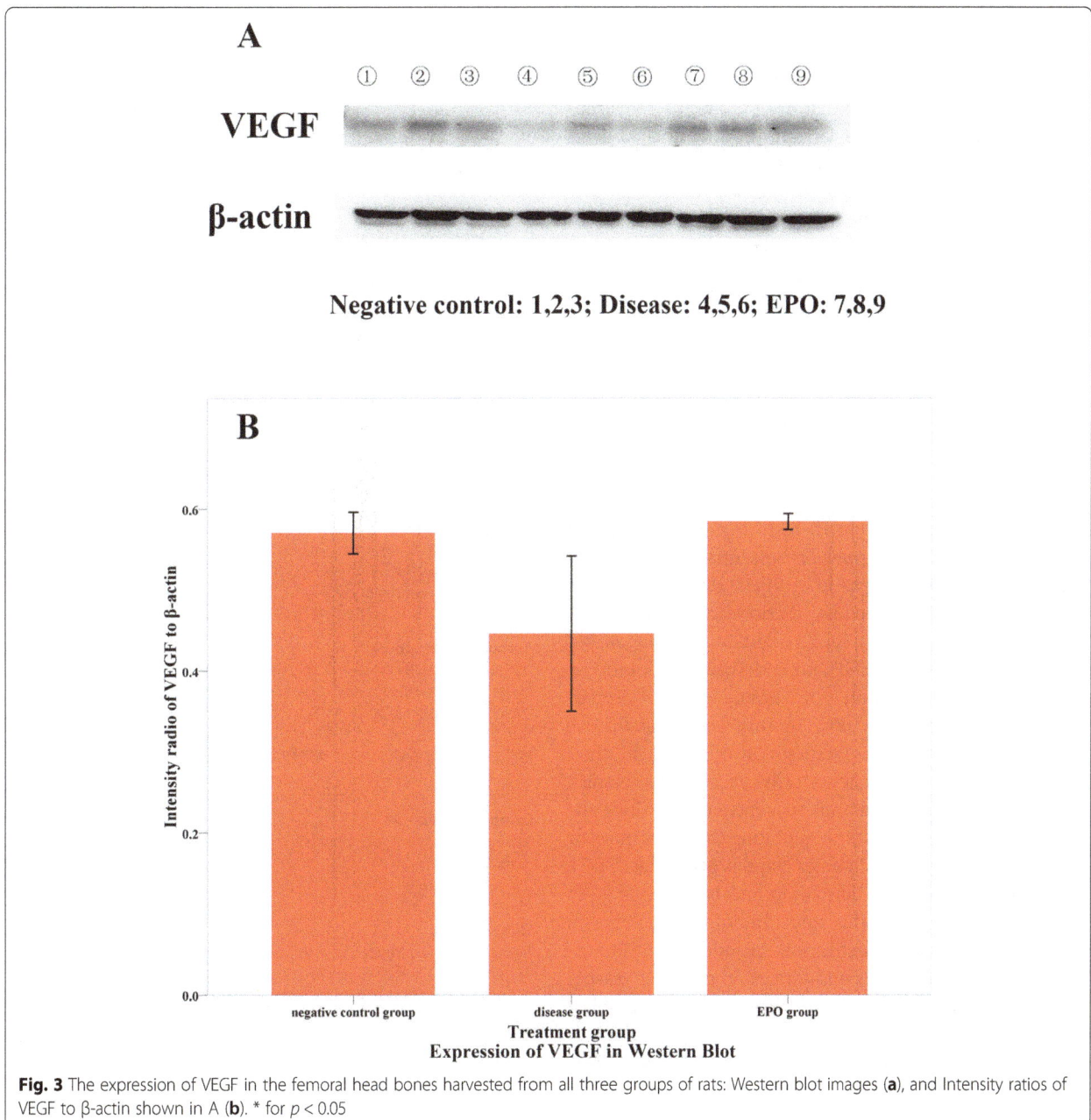

A

Negative control: 1,2,3; Disease: 4,5,6; EPO: 7,8,9

B

Fig. 3 The expression of VEGF in the femoral head bones harvested from all three groups of rats: Western blot images (**a**), and Intensity ratios of VEGF to β-actin shown in A (**b**). * for $p < 0.05$

Table 2 Western blotting results

	Group A	Group B	Group C
VEGF/β-actin ($\bar{x} \pm s$)	0.570 ± 0.022	0.446 ± 0.048	0.584 ± 0.005
F		7.025	
p		0.027	
Multiple Comparison	A-B	B-C	A-C
p (LSD)	0.022	0.014	0.742

endothelial cells, which was used in the immunohisto-chemical study to define the blood vessel density. The results revealed that the blood vessel density in the femoral heads of the disease group was significantly lower than those in the EPO group, while the results were similar in the control group and the EPO group. For disruption of bone blood supply and essential nutrient supply are the direct cause of femoral head necrosis [11], the effect could be inferred that EPO promotes neovascularization. Besides neovascularization, other mechanisms and signaling pathways may be involved in the protective function of EPO. Shiozawa et al. [25] reported EPO promoting the production of BMPs in hematopoietic stem cells by activating the Jak-Stat signaling pathways as well as enhancing bone formation by activating mesenchymal cells to osteoblasts. Kim [26] found that EPO increased the osteoclast numbers and decreased the bone resorption activity in model by increasing the expression of NFATc1 while decreasing cathepsin K expression in mTOR signaling pathway. Hu et al. [27] discovered EPO could inhibit p38MAPK, reduce the TNF-α level, alleviate the inflammatory injury, and alleviate inhibit apoptosis.

Reducing the cell apoptosis, restoring the bone blood supply and nutrient supply are essential in successful treatment or management of ANFH [28, 29]. VEGF is an angiogenic factor which has a critical role in bone formation and bone healing [30]. In addition to angiogenesis, studies indicated that VEGF and endothelial cells induces osteogenic differentiation of bone marrow-derived mesenchymal stem cells [31]. In this work, the disease group had apparently less expression of VEGF in their femoral heads, which matches other researchers' results. Li et al.[10] found that dexamethasone, could reduce the synthesis of VEGF protein by inhibiting the bone marrow multipotent cell. Recent studies have proved that VEGF may play a role in bone formation and bone repair [32]. Based on the reports of this study and other scholars, we speculate the possible mechanisms including: (1) EPO increases VEGF expressions and formation of blood vessels, which leads to promoting bone formation and osteoblast differentiation; (2) Besides, EPO might perform osteogenic action and inhibit apoptosis mediated via multiple signaling pathway, which is based on reports of other scholars and remains to be further researched.

Reports questioning the promoting functional effects of EPO in bone have also been published [33]. Despite the controversy of how EPO affects bone tissue, most scholars hold the view that the effect of EPO on bone tissue is site specific and dose-dependent [34]. So in this research, 20 IU/mL EPO was applied, which was demonstrated effective both in vivo and vitro [35].

Conclusions

In summary, this study suggested the use of rHuEPO at the same time with steroid has achieved a certain precaution effect for steroid-induced ANFH. However, its long-term effect and preventive mechanism require further research and observation.

Abbreviations
ANFH: Avascular Necrosis of the Femoral Head; BMP: Bone Morphogenetic Protein; DAB: Diaminobenzidine; EPO: Erythropoietin; GC: Glucocorticoid; HE staining: Hematoxylin-Eosin Staining; HPF: High power Field; JAK-STAT: The Janus Kinase-Signal Transducer And Activator of Transcription; LSD: Least—Significant Difference; mTOR: The Mammalian Target of Rapamycin; NFATC1: Nuclear Factor of Activated T Cells C1; one-way ANOVA: One-way Analysis of Variance; PAGE: Polyacrylamide Gel Electrophoresis; PBS: Phosphate Buffered Saline; PECAM-1(also CD31): Platelet Endothelial Cell Adhesion Molecule; PVDF: Polyvinylidene Fluoride; rHuEPO: Recombinant Human Erythropoietin; TNF-α: Tumor Necrosis Factor α; VEGF: Vascular Endothelial Growth Factor; MAPK: Mitogen Activated Protein Kinases

Acknowledgements
Medjaden Bioscience and Dr. Lloyd Luo from Siena University Hospital, Italy offered help in translating and improving.

Funding
This study was financially supported by Natural Science Foundation of Zhejiang Province (LY12H06002); Ningbo Clinical Key Specialty (Project No: 2013–88) and Ningbo Natural Science Foundation (2013A610255), Suzhou Science and Technology Development Plan (SYSD2010146), and Young medical key talent of Jiangsu Province (QNRC2016242).

Authors' contributions
YQY, QJP and RJX conceived and designed the research. YQY and RJX performed the experiments, collected data and conducted research. YQY, QJP and RJX analyzed and interpreted data. YQY wrote the initial manuscript. YQY, QJP and RJX revised the manuscript. RJX was primarily responsible for the final content. All authors have reviewed and approved the final manuscript.

Competing interests
None of the authors associated with this study have any conflicts of interest to report.

Author details
[1]Department of Orthopaedics, Ningbo No.2 Hospital, Xibei Street No.41 Ningbo, 315010 Zhejiang, People's Republic of China. [2]Department of Orthopaedics, Suzhou Municipal Hospital/The Affiliated Hospital of Nanjing Medical University, No 26, Daoqian Street, Suzhou 215000, Jiangsu, People's Republic of China. [3]Department of Orthopaedics, the First Affiliated Hospital, Orthopaedic Institute, Soochow University, Suzhou 215000, Jiangsu, People's Republic of China.

References

1. Kuroda Y, Matsuda S, Akiyama H. Joint-preserving regenerative therapy for patients with early-stage osteonecrosis of the femoral head. Inflammation & Regeneration. 2016;36(1):1–8.
2. Huang G, Wei Y, Zhao G, Xia J, Wang S, Wu J, Chen F, Chen J, Shi J. Microarray-based screening of differentially expressed genes in glucocorticoid-induced avascular necrosis. Mol Med Rep. 2017;15(6):3583–90.
3. Mont MA, Hungerford DS. Non-traumatic avascular necrosis of the femoral head. J Bone Joint Surg Am. 1995;77(3):459–74.
4. Calder JD, Buttery L, Revell PA, Pearse M, Polak JM. Apoptosis--a significant cause of bone cell death in osteonecrosis of the femoral head. J Bone Joint Surg Br. 2004;86(8):1209–13.
5. Bekler H, Uygur AM, Gökçe A, Beyzadeoğlu T. The effect of steroid use on the pathogenesis of avascular necrosis of the femoral head: an animal model. Acta Orthop Traumato. 2007;41(1):58–63.
6. Moriishi T, Maruyama Z, Fukuyama R, Ito M, Miyazaki T, Kitaura H, Ohnishi H, Furuichi T, Kawai Y, Masuyama R, et al. Overexpression of Bcl2 in osteoblasts inhibits osteoblast differentiation and induces osteocyte apoptosis. PLoS One. 2011;6(11):e27487.
7. Lafforgue P. Pathophysiology and natural history of avascular necrosis of bone. Joint Bone Spine. 2006;73(5):500–7.
8. Samara S, Dailiana Z, Chassanidis C, Koromila T, Papatheodorou L, Malizos KN, Kollia P. Expression profile of osteoprotegerin, RANK and RANKL genes in the femoral head of patients with avascular necrosis. Exp Mol Pathol. 2014;96(1):9–14.
9. Feng Y, Yang S, Xiao B, Xu W, Ye S, Xia T, Zheng D, Liu X, Liao Y. Decreased in the number and function of circulation endothelial progenitor cells in patients with avascular necrosis of the femoral head. BONE. 2010;46(1):32–40.
10. Li J, Fan L, Yu Z, Dang X, Wang K. The effect of deferoxamine on angiogenesis and bone repair in steroid-induced osteonecrosis of rabbit femoral heads. Exp Biol Med (Maywood). 2015;240(2):273–80.
11. Powell C, Chang C, Naguwa SM, Cheema G, Gershwin ME. Steroid induced osteonecrosis: an analysis of steroid dosing risk. Autoimmun Rev. 2010;9(11):721–43.
12. Ribatti D, Presta M, Vacca A, Ria R, Giuliani R, Dell'Era P, Nico B, Roncali L, Dammacco F. Human erythropoietin induces a pro-angiogenic phenotype in cultured endothelial cells and stimulates neovascularization in vivo. BLOOD. 1999;93(8):2627–36.
13. D'Andrea AD, Lodish HF, Wong GG. Expression cloning of the murine erythropoietin receptor. CELL. 1989;57(2):277–85.
14. Erbayraktar S, Yilmaz O, Gokmen N, Brines M. Erythropoietin is a multifunctional tissue-protective cytokine. Curr Hematol Rep. 2003;2(6):465–70.
15. Brines ML, Ghezzi P, Keenan S, Agnello D, de Lanerolle NC, Cerami C, Itri LM, Cerami A. Erythropoietin crosses the blood-brain barrier to protect against experimental brain injury. Proc Natl Acad Sci U S A. 2000;97(19):10526–31.
16. Celik M, Gökmen N, Erbayraktar S, Akhisaroglu M, Konakc S, Ulukus C, Genc S, Genc K, Sagiroglu E, Cerami A. Erythropoietin prevents motor neuron apoptosis and neurologic disability in experimental spinal cord ischemic injury. Proc Natl Acad Sci U S A. 2002;99(4):2258–63.
17. Westenfelder C, Biddle DL, Baranowski RL. Human, rat, and mouse kidney cells express functional erythropoietin receptors. Kidney Int. 1999;55(3):808–20.
18. Ogilvie M, Yu X, Nicolas-Metral V, Pulido SM, Liu C, Ruegg UT, Noguchi CT. Erythropoietin stimulates proliferation and interferes with differentiation of myoblasts. J Biol Chem. 2000;275(50):39754–61.
19. Juul SE, Ledbetter DJ, Joyce AE, Dame C, Christensen RD, Zhao Y, DeMarco V. Erythropoietin acts as a trophic factor in neonatal rat intestine. GUT. 2001;49(2):182–9.
20. Holstein JH, Menger MD, Scheuer C, Meier C, Culemann U, Wirbel RJ, Garcia P, Pohlemann T. Erythropoietin (EPO): EPO-receptor signaling improves early endochondral ossification and mechanical strength in fracture healing. Life Sci. 2007;80(10):893–900.
21. Xi H, Tao W, Jian Z, Sun X, Gong X, Huang L, Dong T. Levodopa attenuates cellular apoptosis in steroid-associated necrosis of the femoral head. Exp Ther Med. 2017;13(1):69–74.
22. Mutijima E, De MV, Deprez M, Malaise M, Hauzeur JP. The apoptosis of osteoblasts and osteocytes in femoral head osteonecrosis: its specificity and its distribution. Clin Rheumatol. 2014;33(12):1791–5.
23. Hankenson KD, Dishowitz M, Gray C, Schenker M. Angiogenesis in Bone Regeneration. Injury. 2011;42(6):556–61.
24. Joshi D, Tsui J, Ho TK, Selvakumar S, Abraham DJ, Baker DM. Review of the role of erythropoietin in critical leg ischemia. Angiology. 2010;61(6):541–50.
25. Shiozawa Y, Jung Y, Ziegler AM, Pedersen EA, Wang J, Wang Z, Song J, Wang J, Lee CH, Sud S, et al. Erythropoietin couples hematopoiesis with bone formation. PLoS One. 2010;5(5):e10853.
26. Kim J, Jung Y, Sun H, Joseph J, Mishra A, Shiozawa Y, Wang J, Krebsbach PH, Taichman RS. Erythropoietin mediated bone formation is regulated by mTOR signaling. J Cell Biochem. 2012;113(1):220–8.
27. Hu L, Yang C, Zhao T, Xu M, Tang Q, Yang B, Rong R, Zhu T. Erythropoietin ameliorates renal ischemia and reperfusion injury via inhibiting tubulointerstitial inflammation. J Surg Res. 2012;176(1):260–6.
28. Weinstein RS. Glucocorticoid-induced osteonecrosis. Endocrine. 2012;91(4):225–43.
29. Assouline-Dayan Y, Chang C, Greenspan A, Shoenfeld Y, Gershwin ME. Pathogenesis and natural history of osteonecrosis. Semin Arthritis Rheum. 2002;32(2):94–124.
30. Carlevaro MF, Cermelli S, Cancedda R, Cancedda FD. Vascular endothelial growth factor (VEGF) in cartilage neovascularization and chondrocyte differentiation: auto-paracrine role during endochondral bone formation. J Cell Sci. 2000;113(1):59–69.
31. Zheng LZ, Cao HJ, Chen SH, Tang T, Fu WM, Huang L, Chow DHK, Wang YX, Griffith JF, He W. Blockage of Src by specific siRNA as a novel therapeutic strategy to prevent destructive repair in steroid-associated osteonecrosis in rabbits. J Bone Miner Res. 2015;30(11):2044–57.
32. Hu K, Olsen BR. Osteoblast-derived VEGF regulates osteoblast differentiation and bone formation during bone repair. J Clin Invest. 2016;126(2):509.
33. Singbrant S, Russell MR, Jovic T, Liddicoat B, Izon DJ, Purton LE, Sims NA, Martin TJ, Sankaran VG, Walkley CR. Erythropoietin couples erythropoiesis, B-lymphopoiesis, and bone homeostasis within the bone marrow microenvironment. Blood. 2011;117(21):5631–42.
34. Shiozawa Y, Taichman RS. Bone: elucidating which cell erythropoietin targets in bone. Nat Rev Endocrinol. 2015;11(5):263–4.
35. JH R. The effect of erythropoietin on bone. Acta Orthop Suppl. 2014;85(353):1–27.

5

Total hip arthroplasty following failure of tantalum rod implantation for osteonecrosis of the femoral head with 5-to 10-year follow-up

Qi Cheng[1], Jin-long Tang[1], Jiang-jiang Gu[1], Kai-jin Guo[1], Wang-shou Guo[2], Bai-liang Wang[2] and Feng-chao Zhao[1]*

Abstract

Background: Total hip arthroplasty (THA) with failure of tantalum rod implant for osteonecrosis of the femoral head (ONFH) will be the only choice for patients. However,it remains unknown whether tantalum rod implantation has an adverse effect on the survival time of implants following conversion to THA. The aim of this study was to retrospectively evaluate the clinical and radiographic outcomes of conversion to THA in patients who were previously treated with implantation of a tantalum rod.

Methods: This study included 31 patients (39 hips), who underwent conversion to THA due to failure of core decompression with an implanted tantalum rod. Among these 31 patients, 26 patients were male and five patients were female. The mean age of these patients was 49.3 years old (range: 36–64 years old). The control group included 33 patients (40 hips), who underwent total hip replacement without tantalum rod implantation. The hip Harris score, implant wear, osteolysis, radiolucencies and surgical complications were recorded during the follow-up. The distribution of tantalum debris in the proximal, middle and distal periprosthetic femoral regions, radiolucent lines and osteolysis were analyzed on post-operative radiographs.

Results: There were no significant differences in Harris score, liner wear and complications between the two groups ($P > 0.05$). Osteolysis and radiolucent lines more likely occurred in patients with tantalum debris distributed in three regions than in one or two regions ($P < 0.05$).

Conclusions: The mid-term clinical outcome of patients who underwent THA with tantalum rod implantation was not different from those without a tantalum rod, suggesting that tantalum debris did not increase the liner wear rate. However, the distribution of periprosthetic tantalum debris in the proximal, middle and distal femoral regions may increase the risk of femoral osteolysis and radiolucent lines.

Keywords: Core decompression, Trabecular metal implant, Conversion total hip arthroplasty, Hardware removal

Background

Osteonecrosis of the femoral head (ONFH) is a progressive disease due to decreased vascular supply to the subchondral bone of the femoral head, resulting in osteocyte death and collapse of the articular surface. This disease typically affects adults in the third to fifth decades of life,

and incapacitates patients due to pain and decreased hip range of motion [1]. If the disease remains untreated at the early stage, approximately 70–80% of the patients will develop to secondary hip osteoarthritis, and total hip arthroplasty (THA) will be the only choice for patients with ONFH [2].

The primary goal during the early stages of ONFH is to preserve the hip joint, and several techniques have been implemented [3–5]. In recent years, core decompression combined with insertion of a porous tantalum rod has been developed for preventing and curing

* Correspondence: 18361386805@163.com
[1]Department of Orthopedic Surgery, The Affiliated Hospital of Xuzhou Medical University, No. 99 Huaihai West Road, Xuzhou, Jiangsu 221002, People's Republic of China
Full list of author information is available at the end of the article

ONFH. Tantalum rods have a similar elastic modulus to the bone and the compressive strength of the cancellous bone, thereby providing good tissue compatibility. However, the clinical outcomes, postoperative weight-bearing time and role of porous tantalum implants remain controversial [2, 6, 7]. The failure of tantalum rods for ONFH has been reported in the last few years. The failure rates range from 2 to 56% [8–10]. Once the subchondral bone collapses, disease progression is difficult to reverse. Cracks to the femoral head, the narrowing of the joint space and the deterioration of joint function occur sequentially, and hip arthroplasty becomes the only remaining therapeutic option for these patients.

Approximately 5–18% of all hip arthroplasties are performed on patients with a primary diagnosis of osteonecrosis [11]. THA with failure of tantalum rod implants has recently been indicated in relatively young patients with a long lifespan, who may have a higher rate of revision surgeries than elderly patients. However, the mid-term follow up results of the implants have not been reported. In addition, it remains unknown whether tantalum rod implantation has an adverse effect on the survival time of implants following conversion to THA. Thus, we retrospectively evaluated the clinical and radiographic outcomes of the conversion to THA with a mid-term follow-up period of 5–10 years in patients previously treated with tantalum rod implantation. In addition, the clinical outcomes of these patients were compared with patients who underwent a similar THA without the insertion of a tantalum rod.

Methods
Patients
The Ethical Committee of our institution approved the present study. This retrospective study included 44 osteonecrotic hips in 35 consecutive patients, who were treated with THA following failure of core decompression with an implanted tantalum rod (Zimmer, USA) in the Affiliated Hospital of Xuzhou Medical University and China-Japan Friendship Hospital between June 10, 2007 and July 15, 2012. Patient data were collected retrospectively for more than 5 years. One patient (2 hips) died of diseases unrelated to the surgery and 3 patients (3 hips) were lost to follow-up. The 31 patients (39 hips; 5 women and 26 men) were available for review. The average age of these patients was 49.3 years old (range: 36–64 years old). The etiology of the osteonecrosis was idiopathic or unknown in 13 hips, and was due to the use of corticosteroids in six hips, alcohol abuse in 16 hips, and a traumatic event in four hips. The mean time between tantalum rod implantation and conversion to THA was 33.1 months (range: 16–63 months). Twenty-three hips in 20 patients were treated with ceramic-on-ceramic (CoC) implants, and 16

hips in 11 patients were treated with ceramic-on-polymer (CoP) implants. Anatomy stems (Ribbed, Link, Germany) were used in 14 hips and tapered stems (CLS, Zimmer, USA) were used in 25 hips. This study also included 40 hips in 33 patients with ONFH, and assigned this as the control group. Patients in the control group underwent primary THA for ONFH with the same type of implants during the same period.

Surgical procedure
All patients were placed in the lateral decubitus position. For the standard posterolateral approach, a skin incision was made through the fascia over the greater trochanter, and the lateral cortical portion of the rods was exposed. The gluteus maximus was split, the external rotators were detached, and an incision was made on the hip capsule. The tantalum rod was removed through two methods. In the antegrade method, after exposing the femoral head and dislocating the hip, an oscillating saw blade was used to split the femoral neck. Based on the diameter of the implants, a medical metal-cutting trephine was chosen and placed over the proximal end of the tantalum rod. The rod was trephined from the level of the head to the lateral cortex of the femur in an antegrade direction. Then, the tantalum rods were removed without major bone loss. In the retrograde method, the rod was trephined from the lateral cortex of the femur to the level of the head in a retrograde direction, and the tantalum rods were removed without splitting the femoral neck. After the rod was removed, the tantalum particles imbedded in the bone were washed with normal saline. The lateral cortical hole was packed with a bone graft from the femoral head (Fig. 1).

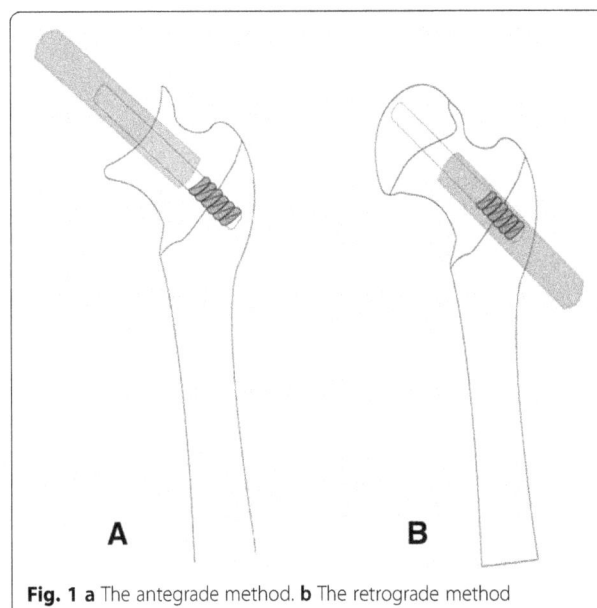

Fig. 1 a The antegrade method. **b** The retrograde method

For all patients, THA was performed using cementless femoral stems and an acetabular cup according to the standard surgical procedure. For patients with bilateral surgeries, the same implants were used. In the tantalum rod group, a 28-mm head with CoC implants was used in 11 hips, and a 32-mm head with CoC implants was used in 12 hips. In the control group, a 28-mm head with CoC implants was used in 10 hips and a 32-mm head with CoC implants was used in 15 hips. For CoP implants, a 28-mm head was used in seven hips and a 32-mm head was used in nine hips in the tantalum rod group. A 28-mm head was used in 10 hips and a 32-mm head was used in five hips in the control group.

Clinical evaluation

All patients underwent clinical and radiographic examinations at one and three months, postoperatively, and at 6-month intervals thereafter. The clinical results were assessed using the Harris Hip Score (HHS) [12]. Thigh pain, complications and squeaking phenomenon, particularly those arising from CoC bearings, were also recorded. Anteroposterior (AP) pelvic and unilateral hip radiographs were routinely performed during the follow-up period. At 1-month follow-up, radiographs were evaluated to determine the inclination and anteversion of the acetabular component based on the AP film. A point M was marked at the 1/5th of the distance along the maximum diameter (D) of the projected ellipse of the wire marker. The AB line was a perpendicular line that passed through the M point and intersected the circle at A and B. The perpendicular distance (p) was measured from point A to point B. The formula of planar anteversion was calculated as follows: anteversion = arc of sin (p/0.8D). CD was a line that connected the ischial tuberosity at C and D. The nclination was the angle (θ) between the diametrical axis D and the line CD (Figs. 2, 3 and 4). For hips in the tantalum rod group, the distribution of tantalum debris was assessed at one week after surgery based on the AP unilateral hip radiographs. The femoral stem was divided into the proximal, middle and distal regions. The proximal region was defined by the region above the horizontal line of the lower point in the lesser trochanter. The middle and distal regions were separated equally between the lower point in the lesser trochanter and the tip of the stem. Femoral stem osteolysis and radiolucencies were classified, as previously described by Gruen et al [13] Furthermore, the acetabular components were evaluated according to the DeLee and Charnley classification of acetabular osteolysis and radiolucencies [14]. Periprosthetic osteolysis is defined as a circular or oval area of distinct bone loss with a diameter of > 2 mm [15]. A radiolucent line between the implant and the surrounding bone, usually parallel to the implant surface. Radiolucencies mostly remain constant and reflect a connective tissue layer. Bony demarcation of radiolucencies on the bone side, also known as sclerotic zones without irregularities or bone resorption. They are therefore considered to be a sign of absence of osseointegration. Subsequent osteolysis and radiolucencies has been recognized as the major cause of long term failure in total hip replacement. Acetabular liner wear was calculated using an Avenger Digital Caliper (Avenger Products, Boulder City, Nev) [16]. AP unilateral hip radiographs performed at one week postoperatively were used as a baseline, and wear measurements were performed on the most recent radiographs. The shortest distance between the acetabular cup interface and the center of the head of the prosthesis was measured, which was considered to be the point of maximum wear. Then, the initial thickness of the polyethylene cup was measured along the line of greatest wear. Measurements were corrected for magnification. The difference between two corrected values was calculated to determine the distance of the liner wear. The accurate value of this method is 0.075 mm. All X-Ray examinations were interpreted by one fellowship-trained academic musculoskeletal radiologist, who had 15 years of experience in interpreting hip XR examinations.

Statistical analysis

All statistical analyses were performed using SPSS version 19.0 software (SPSS, Inc., Chicago, Illinois, USA). Demographic and clinical data were analyzed using Student t-test or Pearson's chi-squared test between different groups. A P-value < 0.05 was considered statistically significant.

Results
Clinical results

Table 1 summarizes the clinical characteristics of patients in the tantalum rod group and control group. There were no significant differences in gender, age at time of surgery,

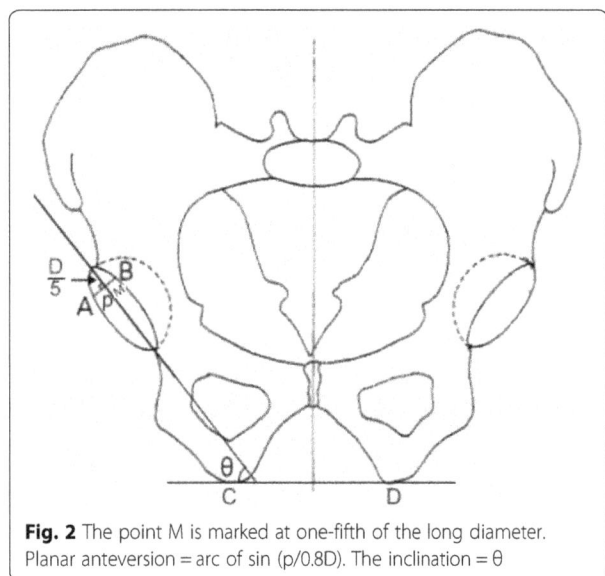

Fig. 2 The point M is marked at one-fifth of the long diameter. Planar anteversion = arc of sin (p/0.8D). The inclination = θ

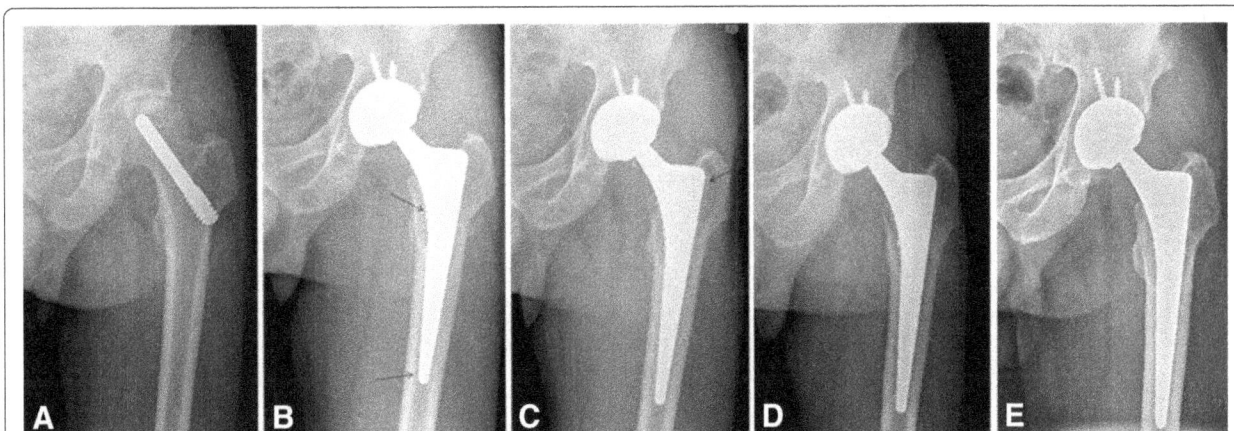

Fig. 3 Radiographs of the left hip of a 46-year-old man with osteonecrosis of the femoral head (ONFH) after failure of the tantalum implant with conversion to total hip arthroplasty with ceramic-on-ceramic bearing. **a** Pre-operative radiograph. **b** Radiograph at 1-year, postoperatively, shows no osteolysis. Tantalum debris can be observed in the proximal, middle and distal regions (black arrows). **c** An anteroposterior view of the left hip at two years after total hip arthroplasty reveals a well-defined sclerotic edge near the medulla of the greater trochanter (black arrow). **d** Radiograph at four years, postoperatively, shows that the acetabular and femoral components are solidly fixed in a satisfactory position, with the radiolucencies in zones 1 and 7. **e** Radiograph at six years, postoperatively, shows no evidence of prosthesis loosening. The Harris score was 93 points at the last follow up

BMI, primary diseases and the type of femoral stems between the two groups ($P > 0.05$, for five comparisons; Table 1).

All patients were followed up for 7.4 years (range: 5–10 years). There were no differences in pre- or post-operative HHS values with CoC or CoP between the tantalum rod group and the control group ($P > 0.05$). Squeaking phenomenon was observed in five hips in the tantalum group and four hips in the control group. There were no significant differences in squeaking phenomenon between the groups ($P > 0.05$). No thigh pain, infections, dislocations, periprosthetic fractures and revision occurred during the follow-up period.

Radiographic analysis
Ceramic-on-ceramic implants
There were no differences in acetabular inclination angle and acetabular anteversion angle between the tantalum rod group and the control group ($P > 0.05$). Acetabular periprosthetic osteolysis was not observed during the follow-up period. Femoral periprosthetic osteolysis or radiolucencies was observed in four hips in the tantalum rod group, but was not found in the control group (Fig. 1). The occurrence of femoral periprosthetic osteolysis or radiolucencies was significantly higher in the tantalum rod group than in the control group ($P < 0.05$). Osteolysis or radiolucencies was only involved in zones 1 and 7 in four hips (Fig. 1).

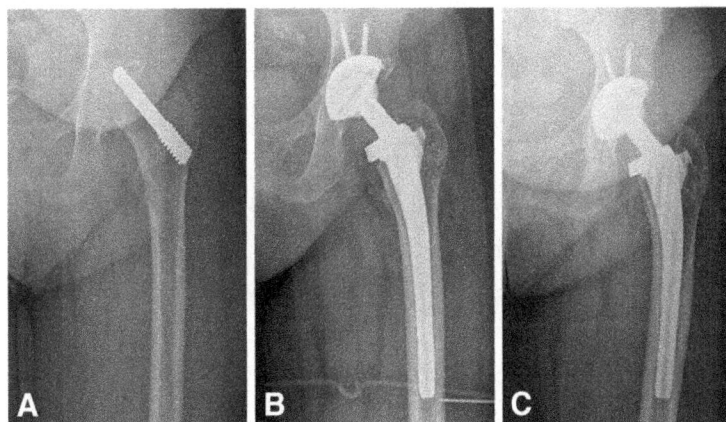

Fig. 4 Radiographs of the left hip of a 51-year-old woman with ONFH after insertion of the tantalum implant with later conversion to total hip replacement with a ceramic-on-polyethylene bearing. **a** Pre-operative radiograph. **b** Anteroposterior postoperative radiograph at 1-year follow-up shows no osteolysis or radiolucencies. Tantalum debris can be observed in the femoral proximal region. **c** Radiograph at the 7-year follow-up shows no changes

Table 1 Clinical demographics of patients

Variable	Tantalum rod group		Control group	
	CoC	CoP	CoC	CoP
Patient (hip)	20 (23)	11 (16)	19 (25)	14 (15)
Gender				
Male	18	8	15	11
Female	2	3	4	3
Age (yr), mean (range)	41.4 (36–52)	46.2 (42–64)	43.2 (37–64)	45.6 (40–68)
Body mass index (kg/m^2), mean (range)	25.2 (22.3–26.4)	24.7 (20.3–29.1)	24.6 (21.5–25.6)	23.2 (20.8–25.9)
Etiology				
Idiopathic	9	4	10	5
Corticosteroid	4	2	3	3
Alcohol	10	6	8	4
Trauma	0	4	4	3
Femoral Stem				
Anatomy stem	8	6	6	4
Tapered stem	15	10	19	11

CoC ceramic-on-ceramic, *CoP* ceramic-on-polymer

The mean liner wear rate in the tantalum rod group was 20.3 um/yr. (range: 15.1–27.8 um/yr), which was not significantly different from that in the control group (mean: 18.9 um/yr.; range: 14.2–26.7 um/yr.; $P > 0.05$, Table 2).

Ceramic-on-polymer implants

There were no differences in acetabular inclination angle and acetabular anteversion angle between the tantalum rod group and the control group ($P > 0.05$). Acetabular periprosthetic osteolysis or radiolucencies was not observed during the follow-up period. Femoral periprosthetic osteolysis or radiolucencies was observed in two hips in the tantalum rod group and one hip in the control group (Fig. 2). The osteolytic rate in the tantalum

rod group was not significantly different from that in the control group ($P > 0.05$). Osteolysis or radiolucencies was involved in zones 1 and 7 in all three hips, and extended to zone 2 in one hip. The mean liner wear rate in the tantalum rod group was 68.9 μm/yr. (range: 34.5–89.6), which was not significantly different form that in the control group (mean: 56.5 μm/yr.; range: 23.5–102.7; $P > 0.05$, Table 3).

The analysis of osteolysis or radiolucencies in the different tantalum debris groups

Tantalum debris was mainly located in the femoral region. For all hips in the tantalum rod group, tantalum debris in the proximal region was found. Moreover,

Table 2 Outcomes and complications in the two groups with ceramic-on-ceramic

Variable	Tantalum rod group ($n = 23$)	Control group ($n = 25$)	P-value
Preoperative HHS	55.7 (49–63)	55.9 (34–68)	0.773
Postoperative HHS	95.1 (91–100)	94.2 (88–100)	0.202
Acetabular component			
Inclination	38.6 (32–44)	37.8 (33–45)	0.430
Anteversion	18.1 (13–25)	17.4 (10–27)	0.386
Femoral head (mm)			0.585
28	11	10	
32	12	15	
Squeaking phenomenon	5	4	0.719
Osteolysis or radiolucencies	4	0	0.022
liner wear rate (um/yr)	20.3 (15.1–27.8)	18.9 (14.2–26.7)	0.295

HHS Harris Hip Score

Table 3 Outcomes and complications in the two groups with ceramic-on-polymer

Variable	Tantalum rod group (n = 16)	Control group (n = 15)	P-value
Preoperative HHS	54.4 (38–63)	55.8 (47–65)	0.949
Postoperative HHS	95.3 (88–100)	94.3 (83–98)	0.328
Acetabular component (°)			
Inclination	37.2 (31–43)	38.4 (32–48)	0.347
Anteversion	19.2 (14–28)	17.6 (11–26)	0.163
Femoral head (mm)			0.200
28	7	10	
32	9	5	
Osteolysis or radiolucencies	2	1	1.000
liner wear rate (µm/yr)	68.9 (34.5–89.6)	56.5 (23.5–102.7)	0.155

HHS Harris Hip Score

tantalum debris was also present in the middle region in 11 hips and in the whole regions in 14 hips. For methods used to remove the tantalum rod, the debris distribution rates were significantly lower in the antegrade method (44.4%, 8/18) than in the retrograde method (81.0%, 17/21) ($P < 0.05$). The incidence rate of osteolysis or radiolucencies at the last follow-up time was 7.1% (1/14) in the proximal region, 0% (0/11) in the proximal and middle region, and 35.7% (5/14) in the whole region. Osteolysis or radiolucencies more likely occurred in the whole region ($P < 0.05$). However, there were no differences in the occurrence of osteolysis or radiolucencies between the other two groups without the distal region ($P > 0.05$, Table 4).

Discussion

ONFH typically affects young patients in their one third to fifth decades of life, and a considerable proportion of patients suffer from bilateral hip involvement. Core decompression and tantalum rod implantation is a commonly used prophylactic surgery for the treatment of ONFH in pre-collapse osteonecrosis (prior to Ficat and ARCO stage II, and Steinberg stage III). However, the clinical outcomes and role of porous tantalum implants in preventing necrosis progression remains controversial [17, 18]. Although core decompression for Steinberg stage I and

Steinberg stage II disease was successful as a definitive procedure in > 80% and 60% of patients, respectively, approximately 30–71% of treatments fails and converts to THA [11, 18]. The conversion to THA is technically demanding in terms of removing the metallic rod, increased blood loss, prolonged operative time, bone loss and the potential risk of femoral fracture [19, 20]. Olsen et al. [6] compared the clinical outcome of 21 patients (21 hips), who received THA following a failed index procedure for tantalum rod implantation, with a cohort of 21 patients (21 hips), who received primary THA for the same diagnosis. They found that there were no significant differences in the survival, clinical, or radiographic outcomes between two groups during a mean follow-up period of 24 months. However, the mid-term clinical outcome of THA following failure of tantalum rod implantation for the treatment of ONFH remains unclear. In the present study, the mid-term outcomes of conversion to THA in patients previously treated with tantalum rod implantation were investigated. It was found that the mid-term clinical outcomes of THA with tantalum rod implantation were accepted, and the tantalum debris did not increase the liner wear rate. However, the distribution of periprosthetic tantalum debris in the whole region of the femoral stem may increase the risk of femoral osteolysis and radiolucencies.

Table 4 Characteristics of six patients with osteolysis in the tantalum rod group

Case	Gender	Age (years)	prosthesis	Femoral head (mm)	Tantalum debris	Follow-up (years)	Osteolytic or radiolucency zones	HHS (points)
1	Male	46	CoC	28	Proximal, middle and distal	6	1,7	93
2	Female	51	CoP	28	Proximal, middle and distal	8	1,7	92
3	Male	57	CoP	32	Proximal, middle and distal	9	1, 2 and 7	93
4	Male	52	CoC	32	Proximal, middle and distal	6	1,7	90
5	Male	48	CoC	28	Proximal	8	1,7	95
6	Female	50	CoC	28	Proximal, middle and distal	6	1,7	91

CoC ceramic-on-ceramic, *CoP* ceramic-on-polymer, *HHS* Harris Hip Score

It was also found that there was no difference in the liner wear rate of CoC bearings between the tantalum rod group and control group at the > 5 year follow-up. The wear rate (20.3 um/yr. in the tantalum rod group and 18.9 μm/yr. in the control group) of implants with ceramic bearings is similar to that reported in literature. For example, Lewis et al. [21] reported a wear rate of 20 μm/year for ceramic bearing and 100% survivorship at a mean follow-up period of 10.9 years (56 hips/55 patients). Amanatullah et al. [22] reported that the mean liner rate was 30.5 μm/year in ceramic-ceramic implants (125 hips) and 94.4% survivorship (196 hips) at a mean follow-up of five years. For high cross-linked polyethylene, the liner wear rates range from 37 μm/year to 60 μm/year during a follow-up period of at least 10 years [23–25]. The porous tantalum debris, which is produced by reaming, is mainly visible in the femoral canal. Therefore, tantalum debris may not potentially cause third-body wear, and no correlation between the existence of tantalum debris and liner wear rate was found.

The osteolytic rate was 17.4% in the present ceramic cohort in the tantalum rod group, which was obviously higher than that in literature. For example, D'Antonio et al. [26] reported that osteolysis or radiolucencies occurred in 26% of metal-on- polyethylene patients (72 hips), but this did not occur in patients with alumina bearings (144 hips). Lau et al. [27] reported that there were no cases with acetabular or femoral osteolysis in 126 hips with third generation ceramic bearings during a > 10-year follow-up. Furthermore, it was found that the osteolytic rate was 12.5% in the present CoP group with tantalum rod implantation, which was similar to that (6.7%) in the control group. Furthermore, it has been reported that acetabular polyethylene cups with annual wear rates of under 80 mm^3, between 80 and 140 mm^3, and more than 140 mm^3 were associated with very little, low-to-moderate, and high levels of osteolysis [28]. Dowd et al. [29] found that polyethylene wear rates of < 0.1 mm/y were not associated with osteolysis or radiolucencies, but wear rates higher than 0.3 mm/y were associated with 100% incidence of osteolysis in a 10-year follow up study. In the present study, the wear rate in the tantalum rod group with a CoP implant was very low (68.94 um/y). Thus, its adverse effect was limited. The porous tantalum debris retained in the cavity could be tolerated by the liner, but this did not cause third-body wear. However, radiographic findings revealed that there was a significant correlation between the distribution range of tantalum debris and femoral osteolysis or radiolucencies, and in CoC or CoP implants, especially for tantalum debris that extend to all regions around prosthesis. Olsen et al. [6] reported that a high rate of retained tantalum debris on post-operative radiographs may be a risk of accelerated time of THA revision. Tantalum particles at high concentrations may cause an inflammatory reaction and disrupt the balance between bone tissue formation and break down [30, 31]. Furthermore, the retained debris at the interface of the cementless prosthesis and femur can cause mechanical instability, which is a risk factor of periprosthetic osteolysis and aseptic loosening [32].

Despite the substantial improvements in cementless THA implants, periprosthetic osteolysis and subsequent aseptic loosening can not be avoided as time goes by. Osteolysis usually leads to implant loosening and the need for revision arthroplasty, which is associated with poorer clinical outcome and shorter survival, compared with primary THA [33]. Following the failure of tantalum rod implantation, many younger people with ONFH have to choose THA to complete pain-free activities of daily living. Thus, it is important to improve the survival time of primary THA and postpone the time of revision in patients with ONFH. A suitable trephine should be used to remove a trabecular metal screw [19], and a high-speed burr should be used to clear the joint space, in order to decrease the amount of tantalum debris retained in the periprosthetic cavity. Furthermore, in order to decrease the debris, the rod should be trephined from the level of the head to the lateral cortex of the femur in an antegrade direction.

The present study has some limitations. First, the study included patients with ONFH from many etiologies such as alcoholism, steroid use and hip trauma. It remains unclear whether different etiologies affect osteolysis or radiolucencies. Second, it remains difficult for plain radiology to detect pelvic and femur osteolysis. Therefore, the incidence of osteolysis and radiolucencies in the present study may be less than that evaluated by computed tomography (CT) [34]. Third, this study only measured femoral head penetration, but volumetric wear was not measured.

Conclusion

In conclusion, it was found that the mid-term clinical outcomes of THA following failure in the tantalum rod group were good in patients with ONFH, when compared with THA without tantalum rods. The tantalum debris did not increase the liner wear rate. However, it should be noted that the distribution of periprosthetic tantalum debris in whole femoral stem regions may be associated with osteolysis at mid-term follow-ups.

Abbreviations
AP: Anteroposterior; CoC: Ceramic-on-ceramic; CoP: Ceramic-on-polymer; CT: Computed tomography; HHS: The Harris Hip Score; ONFH: Osteonecrosis of the femoral head; THA: Total hip arthroplasty

Acknowledgements
We would like to acknowledge the helpful comments on this paper received from our reviewers.

Funding
This work was supported by the National Nature Foundation of China (No.81672184), Peak Talents Foundation in Jiangsu Province(2015-WSN-065),

the Key Program of Science and Technique Development Foundation in Jiangsu Province (BE2016642).

Authors' contributions
QC drafted the manuscript. JT, JG, KG, WG and BW performed data collection and data analysis. QC and FZ conceived of the study, participated in the design of the study, performed data interpretation, and participated in coordination. All authors read and approved the final manuscript.

Competing interests
The authors declare that they have no competing interests.

Author details
[1]Department of Orthopedic Surgery, The Affiliated Hospital of Xuzhou Medical University, No. 99 Huaihai West Road, Xuzhou, Jiangsu 221002, People's Republic of China. [2]Department of Joint Surgery, China-Japan Friendship Hospital, Beijing 100029, People's Republic of China.

References

1. Fernández-Fairen M, Murcia A, Iglesias R, et al. Analysis of tantalum implants used for avascular necrosis of the femoral head: a review of five retrieved specimens. J Appl Biomater Funct Mater. 2012;10:29–36.
2. Liu Y, Liang Y, Zhou S, et al. Tantalum rod implantation for femoral head osteonecrosis: survivorship analysis and determination of prognostic factors for total hip arthroplasty. Int Orthop. 2016;40:1397–407.
3. Zhang Q, Liu L, Wei S, et al. Extracorporeal shockwave therapy in osteonecrosis of femoral head: a systematic review of now available clinical evidences. Medicine. 2017;96:5897.
4. Arai R, Takahashi D, Inoue M, et al. Efficacy of teriparatide in the treatment of nontraumatic osteonecrosis of the femoral head: a retrospective comparative study with alendronate. BMC Musculoskelet Disord. 2017;18:24.
5. Morita D, Hasegawa Y, Okura T, et al. Long-term outcomes of transtrochanteric rotational osteotomy for non-traumatic osteonecrosis of the femoral head. Bone Joint J. 2017;99:175.
6. Olsen M, Lewis PM, Morrison Z, et al. Total hip arthroplasty following failure of core decompression and tantalum rod implantation. Bone Joint J. 2016; 98:1175–9.
7. Zhang X, Wang J, Xiao J, et al. Early failures of porous tantalum osteonecrosis implants: a case series with retrieval analysis. Int Orthop. 2016; 40:1827–34.
8. Veillette CJ, Mehdian H, Schemitsch EH, et al. Survivorship analysis and radiographic outcome following tantalum rod insertion for osteonecrosis of the femoral head. J Bone Joint Surg Am. 2006;88:48.
9. Floerkemeier T, Thorey F, Daentzer D, et al. Clinical and radiological outcome of the treatment of osteonecrosis of the femoral head using the osteonecrosis intervention implant. Int Orthop. 2011;35:489–95.
10. Shuler MS, Rooks MD, Roberson JR. Porous tantalum implant in early osteonecrosis of the hip: preliminary report on operative, survival, and outcomes results. J Arthroplast. 2007;22:26.
11. Kaushik AP, Das A, Cui Q. Osteonecrosis of the femoral head: an update in year 2012. World J Orthop. 2012;3:49–57.
12. Banaszkiewicz PA. Traumatic arthritis of the hip after dislocation and acetabular fractures: treatment by Mold arthroplasty: an end-result study using a new method of result evaluation. J Bone Joint Surg Am. 1969;51:737.
13. Gruen TA, Mcneice GM, Amstutz HC. "modes of failure" of cemented stem-type femoral components: a radiographic analysis of loosening. Clin Orthop Relat Res. 1979;141:17.
14. Banaszkiewicz PA. Radiological demarcation of cemented sockets in Total hip replacement. Clin Orthop Relat Res. 1962;121:20–32.
15. Kim YL, Nam KW, Yoo JJ, et al. Cotyloplasty in cementless total hip arthroplasty for an insufficient acetabulum. Clin Orthop Surg. 2010;2:148–53.
16. Livermore J, Ilstrup D, Morrey B. Effect of femoral head size on wear of the polyethylene acetabular component. J Bone Joint Surg Am. 1990;72:518–28.
17. Liu Y, Liu S, Su X. Core decompression and implantation of bone marrow mononuclear cells with porous hydroxylapatite composite filler for the treatment of osteonecrosis of the femoral head. Arch Orthop Trauma Surg 2013; 133: 125–133.
18. Liu Y, Su X, Zhou S, et al. A modified porous tantalum implant technique for osteonecrosis of the femoral head: survivorship analysis and prognostic factors for radiographic progression and conversion to total hip arthroplasty. Int J Clin Exp Med. 2015;8:1918.
19. Owens JB, Ely EE, Guilliani NM, et al. Removal of trabecular metal osteonecrosis intervention implant and conversion to primary total hip arthroplasty. J Arthroplast. 2012;27:1251–3.
20. Lee GW, Park KS, Kim DY, et al. Results of Total hip arthroplasty after Core decompression with tantalum rod for osteonecrosis of the femoral head. Clin Orthop Relat Res. 2016;8:38–44.
21. Lewis PM, Albelooshi A, Olsen M, et al. Prospective randomized trial comparing alumina ceramic-on-ceramic with ceramic-on-conventional polyethylene bearings in total hip arthroplasty. J Arthroplast. 2010;25:392–7.
22. Amanatullah DF, Landa J, Strauss EJ, et al. Comparison of surgical outcomes and implant wear between ceramic-ceramic and ceramic-polyethylene articulations in total hip arthroplasty. J Arthroplast. 2011;26:72–7.
23. Jr CAE, Jr RHH, Huynh C, et al. A prospective, randomized study of cross-linked and non–cross-linked polyethylene for total hip arthroplasty at 10-year follow-up. J Arthroplast. 2012;27:2–7.
24. Battenberg AK, Hopkins JS, Kupiec AD, et al. The 2012 frank Stinchfield award: decreasing patient activity with aging: implications for crosslinked polyethylene wear. Clin Orthop Relat Res. 2013;471:386–92.
25. Greiner JJ, Callaghan JJ, Bedard NA, et al. Fixation and wear with contemporary acetabular components and cross-linked polyethylene at 10-years in patients aged 50 and under. J Arthroplast. 2015;30:1577.
26. D'Antonio JA, Capello WN, Naughton M. Ceramic bearings for Total hip arthroplasty have high survivorship at 10 years. Clin Orthop Relat Res. 2012; 470:373–81.
27. Lau YJ, Sarmah S. 3rd generation ceramic-on-ceramic cementless total hip arthroplasty: a minimum 10-year follow-up study. Hip Int. 2017;21:5–9.
28. Oparaugo PC, Clarke IC, Malchau H, et al. Correlation of wear debris-induced osteolysis and revision with volumetric wear-rates of polyethylene: a survey of 8 reports in the literature. Acta Orthop Scand. 2001;72:22.
29. Dowd JE, Sychterz CJ, Young AM, et al. Characterization of long-term femoral-head- penetration rates. Association with and prediction of osteolysis. J Bone Joint Surg Am. 2000;82:1102.
30. Bitar D, Parvizi J. Biological response to prosthetic debris. World J Orthop. 2015;6:172–89.
31. Goodman SB, Gibon E, Yao Z. The basic science of Periprosthetic Osteolysis. Instr Course Lect. 2013;62:201.
32. Amirhosseini M, Andersson G, Aspenberg P, et al. Mechanical instability and titanium particles induce similar transcriptomic changes in a rat model for periprosthetic osteolysis and aseptic loosening. Bone Rep. 2017;7:17–25.
33. Schwarz EM, Campbell D, Totterman S, et al. Use of volumetric computerized tomography as a primary outcome measure to evaluate drug efficacy in the prevention of peri-prosthetic osteolysis: a 1-year clinical pilot of etanercept vs. placebo. J Orthop Res. 2003;21:1049–55.
34. Kim YH, Park JW, Patel C, et al. Polyethylene wear and osteolysis after cementless total hip arthroplasty with alumina-on-highly cross-linked polyethylene bearings in patients younger than thirty years of age. J Bone Joint Surg Am. 2013;95:1088.

6

Implantation of a bone-anchored annular closure device in conjunction with tubular minimally invasive discectomy for lumbar disc herniation: a retrospective study

Frederic Martens[1], Geoffrey Lesage[1], Jeffrey M. Muir[2] and Jonathan R. Stieber[3]*

Abstract

Background: Minimally invasive techniques for lumbar discectomy have been recommended as superior to open techniques due to lower blood loss, lower rates of infection and shorter recovery. There are, however, concerns that this approach does not sufficiently remove the herniated nuclear material, thus leaving the patient susceptible to reherniation requiring reoperation. The purpose of this study was to examine the safety and viability of an annular closure device in limiting reherniation and reoperation in a cohort of patients undergoing minimally invasive lumbar discectomy with the assistance of an annular closure device.

Methods: We retrospectively analysed the results from patients treated by a single surgeon between March 2011 and December 2017. All patients had been diagnosed with a large (≥ 5 mm) defect and were treated via minimally invasive surgical techniques. Outcomes included demographic data, the procedural duration and the rates of symptomatic reherniation and reoperation.

Results: 60 patients were included in the study. The mean age was 42 years (range: 19–66); mean BMI was 24.1 (range: 16.7–36.3). Mean surgical duration was 29 min (range: 16–50). Reoperation was required in 5% (3/60) of patients, although only 3% (2/60) experienced symptomatic reherniation at the index level. No other complications were reported.

Conclusions: In our study, the use of an annular closure device during minimally invasive lumbar discectomy in a population of patients with large herniations was associated with low rates of reherniation and reoperation at the index level. While more research is required, the results of this study demonstrate the safety and viability of the annular closure device as an adjunct to minimally invasive discectomy.

Keywords: Annular closure device, Limited discectomy, Lumbar disc herniation, Microscopic discectomy, Minimally invasive, Tubular retractor

Background

Surgical discectomy has been proven as an effective treatment for lumbar intervertebral herniation; however, despite refinements of surgical approach and technique, there remains a persistent risk of recurrent reherniation at the index level [1–3]. Indeed, complications necessitating reoperation following discectomy occur in between 15 and 25% of cases [4–8].

Traditional discectomy techniques, first pioneered over 80 years ago, have been associated with generally good results but have also raised concerns regarding increased rates of surgical site infection [9, 10] and increased blood loss [11]. Such concerns have spurred the development of minimally invasive surgical (MIS) techniques that offer similar patient outcomes but without the added risks associated with traditional methods [11, 12]. Larger diameter tubes, bladed retractors, and advancements in technique

* Correspondence: jonathan.stieber@nyumc.org
[3]Clinical Assistant Professor of Orthopaedic Surgery, New York University School of Medicine, 485 Madison Avenue, 8th Floor, New York, NY 10022, USA
Full list of author information is available at the end of the article

have expanded the indications and complexity of minimally invasive spine surgery and have permitted the placement of biomechanical intervertebral devices for fusion purposes [13]. In limited discectomy, MIS techniques first centered around endoscopic access via a muscle-dilating, tubular approach. While more technically demanding than traditional open discectomy, the use of tubular discectomy spread more widely after the adaptation of the instrumentation and technique to direct visualization utilizing an operative microscope. While clinical outcomes have been shown to be equivalent between open and tubular techniques, there are concerns regarding reherniation rates, as minimal removal of nuclear material is thought by some authors to contribute to post-discectomy reherniation and, ultimately, reoperation [13, 14].

Maximizing clinical outcomes thus requires a balance between aggressive versus limited removal of nuclear material. On one hand, comparisons of limited versus traditional lumbar discectomy have demonstrated that while traditional discectomy, with its more extensive removal of disc material, substantially decreases the rate of recurrent disc herniation, aggressive nucleus removal leads to inferior clinical outcomes and patient satisfaction when compared with limited techniques, primarily due to disc collapse and subsequent back pain [15]. Conversely, other studies have demonstrated higher rates of reherniation in cases where limited techniques with minimal removal of disc material resulted in reherniation rates up to 27.3% of cases [15]. These observations were confirmed in a comprehensive review of the literature that found that limited techniques were associated with a higher rate of recurrent disc herniation but a lower rate of long-term recurrent back pain [16].

Ideally, the ability to combine the benefits of both traditional and limited techniques should be sought, to enable surgeons to routinely perform limited disc removal while also minimizing the risk of reherniation, a need that is underscored when considering patients with large annular defects (≥ 5 mm). As such, a novel annular closure device (ACD) has been developed to allow surgeons to retain maximal nuclear volume without increasing the risk of reherniation. The Barricaid® annular closure device has been in use for over a decade and has demonstrated an ability to decrease the rates of reherniation while allowing maximal preservation of nuclear volume at the time of surgery. While the early evidence from studies indicates that the use of this ACD results in a substantial reduction in reherniation rates [2], the use of this device with minimally invasive discectomy techniques remains uncharacterized. Proper placement of the ACD presents challenges unique to MIS techniques, as the facet joints must be preserved without predisposing injurious traction of the neural elements or incidental durotomy. To address these questions, we examined the feasibility, safety and risk of peri-operative complications of tubular minimally invasive insertion of the ACD as an adjunct to microdiscectomy with limited nucleus removal in a cohort of patients with large annular defects.

Methods

Study design

This study was a retrospective review of patients who underwent a lumbar discectomy procedure utilizing a limited surgical approach and an annular closure device. Ethics approval for this study was received from the participating institution. All participants provided informed consent prior to data collection.

Patient eligibility

Patients were eligible for inclusion if they underwent a limited lumbar discectomy procedure between March 2011 and December 2017. Implantation of the ACD as an adjunct to limited tubular minimally-invasive lumbar discectomy was indicated in patients who met the following indications: 1) unilateral, single level lumbar disc herniation demonstrated on computed tomography and/or magnetic resonance imaging; 2) persistent radiculopathy and positive tension signs in both straight and crossed leg raising tests; 3) concordant radicular neurological deficits; and 4) intra-operative measurement of a large annular defect measuring 5–12 mm in width. Contraindications included posterior disc height ≤ 5 mm, spondylolisthesis greater than 25% (Grade II or higher) and osteoporosis.

Annular closure device

The Barricaid® (Intrinsic Therapeutics, Inc., Woburn, MA, USA) is an annular closure device that has been CE-marked since 2009. The use of this ACD has been described in detail elsewhere [1, 2, 17]. In brief, the device is implanted following lumbar discectomy and is designed to retain nucleus pulposis within the disc space. The device consists of a flexible polymer (polyethylene terephthalate) occlusion component intended to block the opening in the annulus and prevent migration of the nucleus from within the disc, affixed to a titanium (Ti6Al4V ELI) bone-anchor that secures the occlusion component to one of the adjacent vertebral bodies (Fig. 1). A platinum iridium (radiopaque) marker on the occlusion component permits radiographic visualization and confirmation of its position. The device is available in 8-, 10-, and 12-mm widths and comes pre-loaded onto a disposable insertion tool (Fig. 2). The ACD is designed for herniations caused by extrusion of the nuclear material; however, as the device is anchored to the bony endplate, avulsion of the cartilaginous endplate material as part of the herniation [18] does not represent a

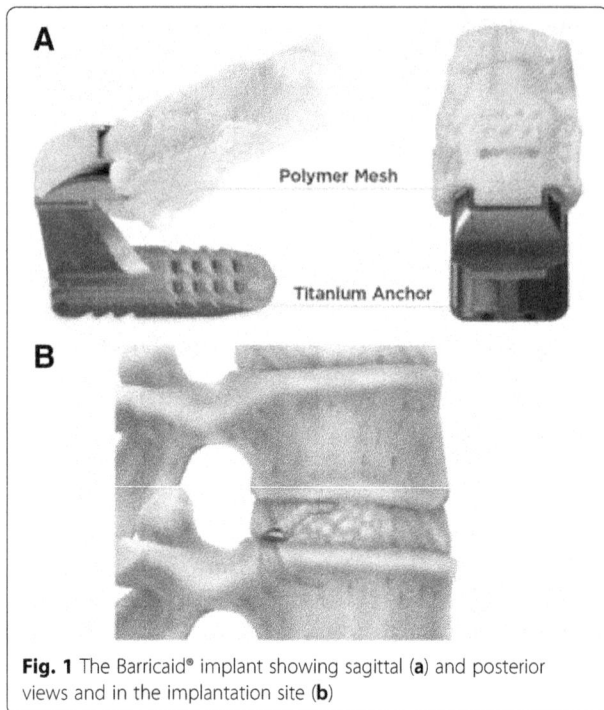

Fig. 1 The Barricaid® implant showing sagittal (**a**) and posterior views and in the implantation site (**b**)

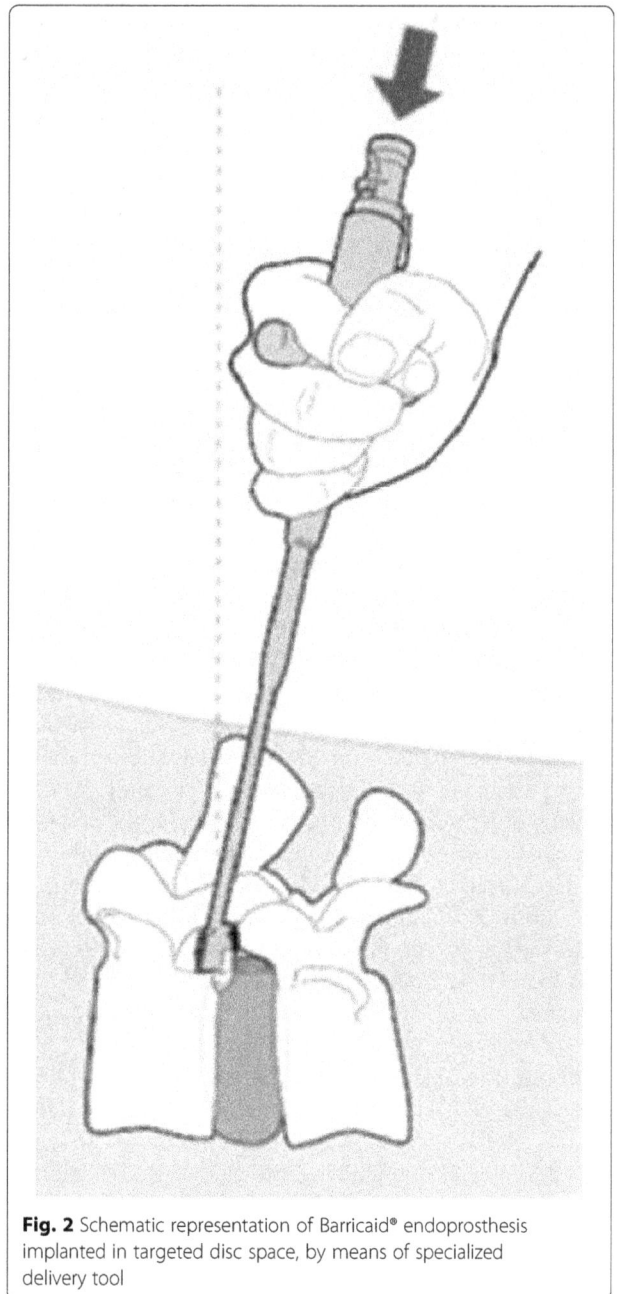

Fig. 2 Schematic representation of Barricaid® endoprosthesis implanted in targeted disc space, by means of specialized delivery tool

contraindication. In such cases, the anchoring to the bony endplate is sufficient to secure the device in place and prevent further reherniation of the disc material.

Surgical procedure

Microdiscectomy was performed utilizing a 22 mm diameter fixed tube per standard technique using a tubular microdiscectomy system (METRx™ MicroDiscectomy System, Medtronic Memphis, TN, USA) in either a knee-on-chest position or utilizing a Wilson frame according to surgeon preference. Intraoperative fluoroscopy was utilized in order to obtain lateral images necessary for precise ACD sizing and implantation in addition to normal localization (Fig. 3). In order to facilitate proper ACD placement, the tube was aligned in the plane of the disc space. Visualization was achieved via an operative microscope. A limited discectomy was then performed, removing only extruded fragments and loose pieces of disc material within the disc space utilizing a pituitary rongeur.

Following discectomy, the annular defect was assessed and measured with specifically-designed measuring tools. The height and width of the defect were measured by inserting dedicated defect measurement tools of varying sizes into the annular defect. Defect size was thus determined based on the best fit of the measurement tools (Figs. 4 and 5). In order to properly accommodate the ACD, the posterior disc height must measure at least 5 mm, per the Barricaid patient inclusion criteria and evidence in the literature that demonstrates the high incidence of symptomatic recurrent lumbar disc herniation

in patients with large annular defects [15]. While there is no absolute limit on the height of the disc that can be implanted, the height of the annular defect should not exceed 6 mm. The width of the defect should not exceed the width of the mesh selected for insertion (8 mm, 10 mm or 12 mm).

Intraoperative data recorded during surgery included procedural duration and the volume of disc material retrieved. Patients were discharged with standard post-operative precautions. No additional bracing or non-standard activity restrictions were prescribed for any patient.

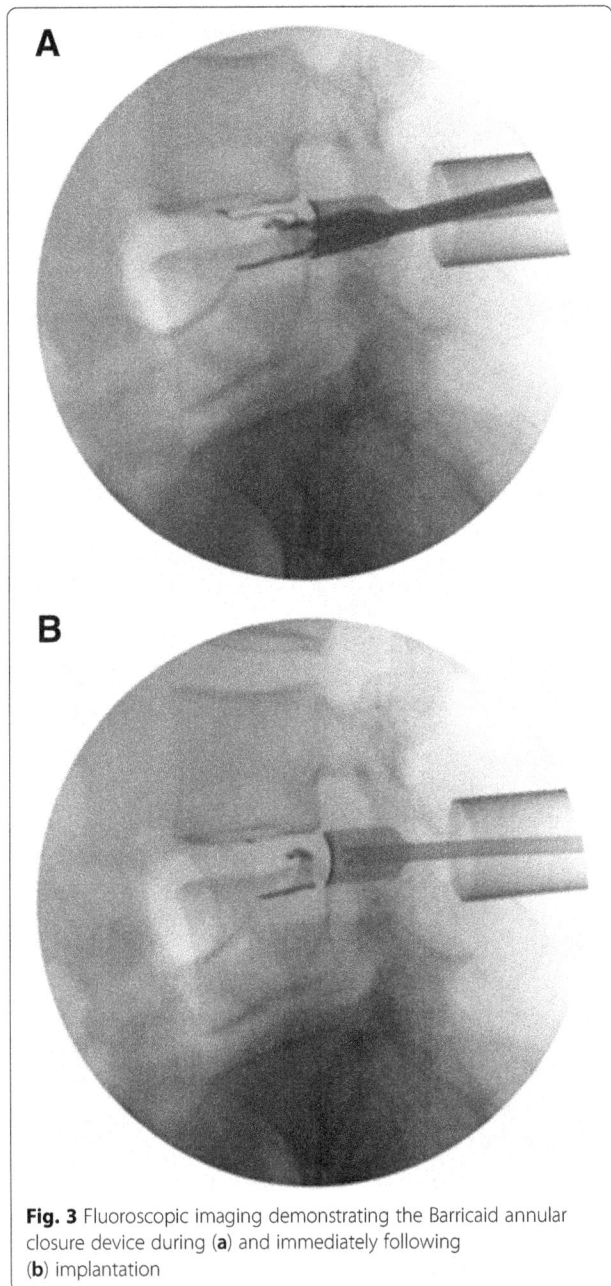

Fig. 3 Fluoroscopic imaging demonstrating the Barricaid annular closure device during (**a**) and immediately following (**b**) implantation

Outcome measures

The primary outcomes for this study were the rate of symptomatic reherniation and reoperation at 6-month, 1-year and 2-year follow-up appointments. Symptomatic reherniation was defined as symptomatic sciatica with or without neurological deficit, with corroborating magnetic resonance (MR) imaging evidence. Secondary outcomes included operative time. Additionally, demographic data (gender, age, body mass index (BMI), surgical level) was also collected for each patient. Patients were followed up at serial timepoints up to 2-years and annually thereafter. Follow-up appointments included radiographic, MRI and

CT imaging to confirm the integrity and positioning of the ACD.

Statistical analysis

Alpha was set *a priori* at 0.05 for all statistical comparisons. Mean values were compared using independent samples t-tests, single-factor ANOVA or chi-squared tests, as appropriate. Mean values are expressed as mean (standard deviation).

Results

Study cohort demographics

A total of 60 patients were included in this study. The mean age of the participants was 42 years (range: 19–66); 58% (35/60) were female. The mean BMI was 24.1 (range: 16.7–36.3). All patients were diagnosed intraoperatively with large annular defects (≥5 mm) and met the indication for implantation of the ACD. Vertebral levels L4/L5 (38%, 23/60) and L5/S1 (52%, 37/60 were addressed surgically.

Outcome measures

The mean operative time was 29 min (range: 16–50) from incision to wound closure. At 6-months post-procedure, no reoperations had occurred. At 1-year follow-up, symptomatic reherniation at the index level was reported in 3% (2/60) of patients, with reoperation at the index level likewise required in 2 patients (3%). In both cases, the reherniation occurred on the contralateral side of the implant. Reoperation at a level other than the index level was required in one additional patient, where herniation occurred on the contralateral side at a different level approximately 16 months following their initial discectomy.

At 2-years post-procedure, only 1 additional patient (2-year total: 3/60, 5%) required reoperation, although not at the index level or side. Three-year follow-up data was available for 29 patients and indicated that no additional reherniations or reoperations at any level were reported.

Discussion

Despite advancements in the surgical technique, patients undergoing discectomy continue to be at risk for both recurrent disc herniation and subsequent disc degeneration with resulting back pain, both of which can compromise surgical outcomes and lead to revision surgical treatment. One method of minimizing the likelihood of reherniation is annular closure. One available device, the Barricaid ACD, is designed to maintain the favorable functional outcomes and patient satisfaction observed with limited discectomy, while also minimizing the risk of recurrent disc herniation in patients with large annular defects. We examined the rate of symptomatic

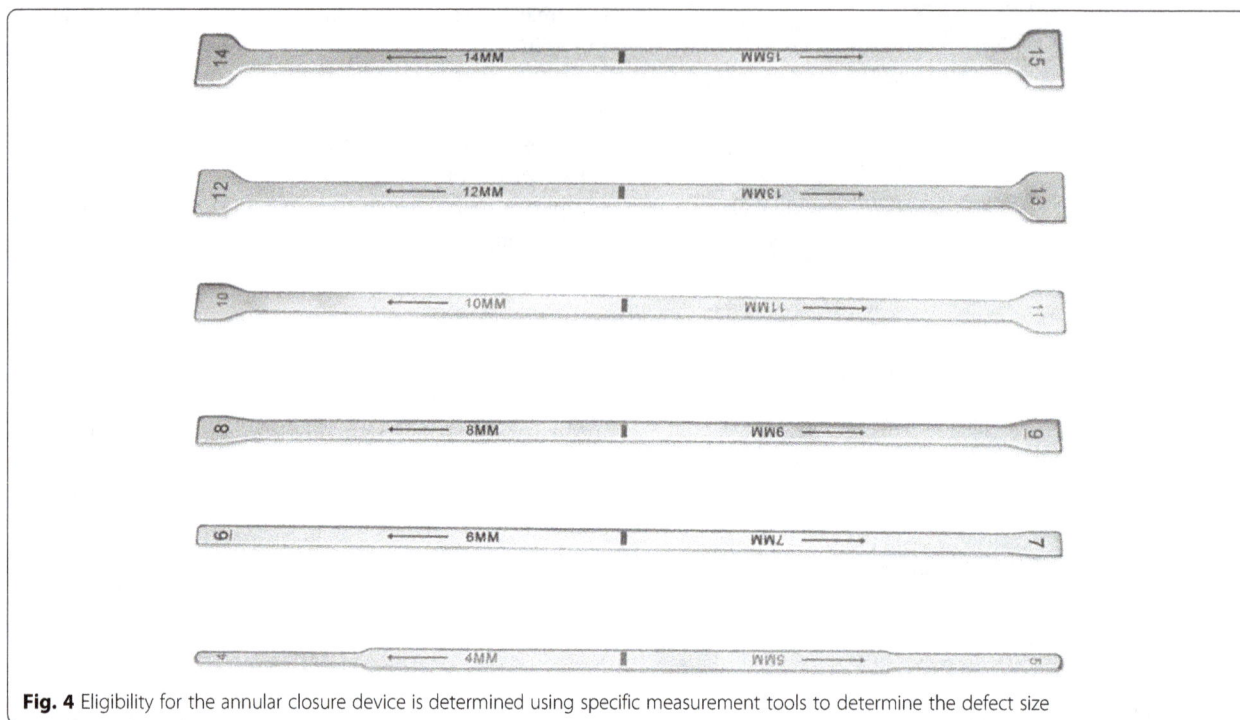

Fig. 4 Eligibility for the annular closure device is determined using specific measurement tools to determine the defect size

reherniation and reoperation in a cohort of patients who underwent lumbar discectomy via a minimally-invasive approach and found that the use of the ACD was associated with lower rates of reherniation and reoperation when compared with rates observed elsewhere [15, 19].

The clinical advantages of tubular minimally invasive discectomy versus conventional discectomy have been examined in different clinical studies with the tubular approach found to be safe and effective [10, 20]. For both patients and surgeons, there continues to be widespread appeal for this approach. For MIS techniques combined with closure of the annulus, safe insertion of

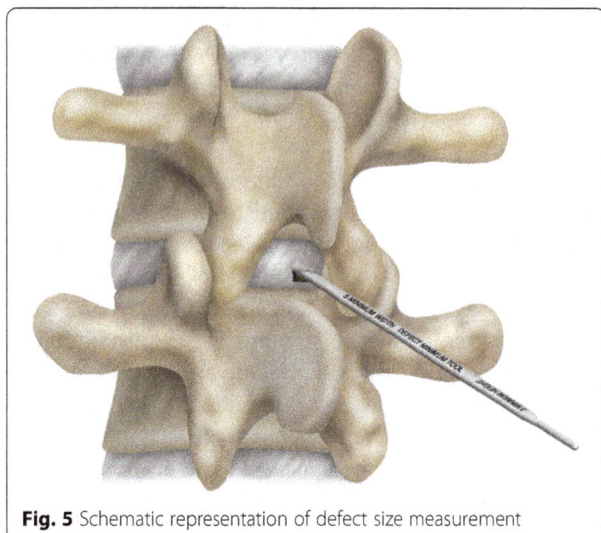

Fig. 5 Schematic representation of defect size measurement

the device may be accomplished through the use of a 22 mm tube. Although implantation through smaller tubes is possible, the increased visibility obtained with the use of the customized combined suction-retractor facilitates safe passage of the ACD adjacent to the neural elements. The ACD can be appropriately placed without damage to the facet joint or sacrificing the stability of the posterior elements. While implantation of the ACD requires greater attention be paid to the location of the incision and the angle of approach than for traditional microdiscectomy, there is no increase in procedural time associated with the ACD and no increased risk of injury. Several studies have demonstrated the time-neutral nature of minimally-invasive discectomy [21, 22]. Indeed, the procedural time for this study (30 mins) was less than that measured in previous studies of minimally-invasive discectomy [22].

Symptomatic reherniation at the index level was observed in our study to have occurred in 2 of 60 patients (3%) by the 1-year mark, a rate that mirrors that of other studies of minimally-invasive discectomy but is significantly lower than that of other studies of large annular defects. In studies of limited discectomy for large annular defects, reherniation rates of up to 18% have been reported [15], suggesting that limited techniques may be lacking when used to treat large defects. Studies of MIS techniques, in contrast, have reported reherniation at rates similar to our study. A recent systematic review of MIS techniques for lumbar discectomy [23] found a pooled rate of reherniation of 2%, although the included studies did not focus on patients with large annular defects. That our study was able to demonstrate similar rates of reherniation in a smaller population of large annular defects is noteworthy, as is the long-term data available from our cohort. In our study, reherniation occurred within 1 year of the index procedure, with only one additional reoperation reported beyond 1-year. This finding is consistent with other studies of this ACD, which found significantly lower rates of reherniation and reoperation up to 2 years in ACD patients versus traditional discectomy [24]. In fact, our cohort was followed-up annually and in the 29 patients with a minimum of 3 years of follow-up, no subsequent instances of reherniation or reoperation were reported. That these patients reported no complications over that long period of time speaks to the value of the ACD in stabilizing the disc and preventing the herniation of the remaining disc material. The ability of the ACD to decrease reherniation rates has been demonstrated in other studies of this device [1, 2, 17, 19, 25] but the current study represents the first reported use of the Barricaid ACD with minimally-invasive techniques. As such, the potential for long-term stability following the use of this device warrants further and more rigorous study.

Our study demonstrated the excellent safety record associated with this device in this minimally-invasive setting, with no adverse events in 60 procedures, reflecting the overall safety of the procedure in general [20]. Previous studies using this ACD [17, 19, 26] have demonstrated similar results. MIS itself has been the subject of a comprehensive systematic review, evaluating the rate of complications in MIS lumbar discectomy versus open surgical methods [27]. These authors pooled results from 42 studies and found that MIS techniques were associated with lower rates of nerve root injury, wound complications and reoperation when compared with open techniques. MIS was also associated with decreases in length of stay, blood loss and the peri-operative risk of infection when compared with open techniques [12, 22]. The combined safety profiles of the ACD and MIS techniques – plus the current evidence of no adverse events when these techniques are combined – suggests that the use of the ACD with MIS techniques is a safe and effective method for addressing large lumbar annular defects.

Our study has limitations. Primarily, the observational nature of our study and the lack of a matched control group limit the veracity with which the results can be extrapolated. This study; however, successfully demonstrates the potential of the ACD during minimally-invasive lumbar discectomy, in a cohort of age-appropriate patients. Although more rigorous data collection in the form of a randomized, controlled trial in this cohort is required, these early results suggest a potential role for the ACD in

minimally-invasive lumbar discectomy. There is also the potential for selection bias in this study, as the patients were all treated by the same surgeon and may represent a group of patients with an inherently greater likelihood of positive outcomes. However, the demographics of this cohort are reflective of the population of patients that would undergo such a procedure. As such, the likelihood of patients being selected for success is minimal, as the cohort represents one that would be operated on using these techniques under normal clinical circumstances.

Conclusion

Our study demonstrated the viability of an annular closure device as an adjunct to minimally-invasive tubular lumbar discectomy in patients with large (≥ 5 mm) annular defects. We demonstrated decreased rates of symptomatic reherniation and reoperation in a representative cohort, when compared with known rates. While more rigorous study in higher level studies is required, the early results demonstrate the potential of the ACD in this operative setting.

Abbreviations
ACD: Annular closure device; BMI: Body mass index; MIS: Minimally-invasive surgery; MR: Magnetic resonance

Acknowledgements
The authors would like to thank Hilde Keymeulen for her assistance with data collection and analysis.

Funding
Financial support for the referenced clinical study and writing of this manuscript was provided by Intrinsic Therapeutics, Inc., Woburn, MA. None of the authors have a financial interest in any of the products or companies discussed.

Authors' contributions
JS completed the initial data analysis and wrote the first draft of the manuscript. GL assisted in study design, data analysis and contributed significantly in writing of the first draft. FM performed all surgical procedures and was a major contributor in writing the manuscript. JMM completed secondary data analysis and wrote the current draft of the manuscript. All authors read, edited and approved the final manuscript.

Competing interests
The authors declare that they have no competing interests.

Author details
[1]Department of Neurosurgery, OLV Ziekenhuis, Moorselbaan 164, 9300 Aalst, Belgium. [2]Motion Research, 3-35 Stone Church Rd., Suite 215, Hamilton, ON L9K 1S4, Canada. [3]Clinical Assistant Professor of Orthopaedic Surgery, New York University School of Medicine, 485 Madison Avenue, 8th Floor, New York, NY 10022, USA.

References
1.　Bouma GJ, Barth M, Ledic D, Vilendecic M. The high-risk discectomy patient: prevention of reherniation in patients with large anular defects using an anular closure device. Eur Spine J. 2013;22:1030–6.

2. Ledic D, Vukas D, Grahovac G, Barth M, Bouma GJ, Vilendecic M. Effect of anular closure on disk height maintenance and reoperated recurrent herniation following lumbar discectomy: two-year data. J Neurol Surg A. 2015;76(3):211–8.
3. McGirt MJ, Eustacchio S, Varga P, Vilendecic M, Trummer M, Gorensec M, et al. A prospective cohort study of close interval computer tomography and magnetic resonance imaging after primary lumbar discectomy. Spine (Phila Pa 1976). 2009;34(19):2044–51.
4. Atlas SJ, Deyo RA, Keller RB, Chapin AM, Patrick DL, Long JM, et al. The Maine Lumbar Spine Study, Part II. 1-year outcomes of surgical and nonsurgical management of sciatica. Spine (Phila Pa 1976). 1996;21(15): 1777–86.
5. Cherkin DC, Deyo RA, Loeser JD, Bush T, Waddell G. An international comparison of back surgery rates. Spine (Phila Pa 1976). 1994;19(11):1201–6.
6. Kim CH, Chung CK, Park CS, Choi B, Kim MJ, Park BJ. Reoperation rate after surgery for lumbar herniated intervertebral disc disease: nationwide cohort study. Spine (Phila Pa 1976). 2013;38(7):581–90.
7. Lehmann TR, Titus MK. Refinements in technique for open lumbar discectomy. In: Proceedings of the International Societ for the Study of the Lumbar Spine (ISSLS). Singapore, June 1997.
8. Weber H. Lumbar disc herniation. A controlled, prospective study with ten years of observation. Spine (Phila Pa 1976). 1983;8(2):131–40.
9. Evaniew N, Khan M, Drew B, Kwok D, Bhandari M, Ghert M. Minimally invasive versus open surgery for cervical and lumbar discectomy: a systematic review and meta-analysis. CMAJ Open. 2014;2(4):E295–305.
10. Dasenbrock HH, Juraschek SP, Schultz LR, Witham TF, Sciubba DM, Wolinsky JP, et al. The efficacy of minimally invasive discectomy compared with open discectomy: a meta-analysis of prospective randomized controlled trials. J Neurosurg Spine. 2012;16(5):452–62.
11. Majeed SA, Vikraman CS, Mathew V. S AT. Comparison of outcomes between conventional lumbar fenestration discectomy and minimally invasive lumbar discectomy: an observational study with a minimum 2-year follow-up. J Orthop Surg Res. 2013;8:34.
12. Clark AJ, Safaee MM, Khan NR, Brown MT, Foley KT. Tubular microdiscectomy: techniques, complication avoidance, and review of the literature. Neurosurg Focus. 2017;43(2):E7.
13. Palmer S. Use of a tubular retractor system in microscopic lumbar discectomy: 1 year prospective results in 135 patients. Neurosurg Focus. 2002;13(2):E5.
14. Hubbe U, Franco-Jimenez P, Klingler JH, Vasilikos I, Scholz C, Kogias E. Minimally invasive tubular microdiscectomy for recurrent lumbar disc herniation. J Neurosurg Spine. 2016;24(1):48–53.
15. Carragee EJ, Spinnickie AO, Alamin TF, Paragioudakis S. A prospective controlled study of limited versus subtotal posterior discectomy: short-term outcomes in patients with herniated lumbar intervertebral discs and large posterior anular defect. Spine J. 2006;31(6):653–7.
16. McGirt MJ, Ambrossi GL, Datoo G, Sciubba DM, Witham TF, Wolinsky JP, et al. Recurrent disc herniation and long-term back pain after primary lumbar discectomy: review of outcomes reported for limited versus aggressive disc removal. Neurosurgery. 2009;64(2):338–44. discussion 44-5
17. Parker SL, Grahovac G, Vukas D, Vilendecic M, Ledic D, McGirt MJ, et al. Effect of an annular closure device (Barricaid) on same level recurrent disc herniation and disc height loss after primary lumbar discectomy: Two-year results of a multi-center prospective cohort study. J Spinal Disord Tech. 2016;In press.
18. Rajasekaran S, Bajaj N, Tubaki V, Kanna RM, Shetty AP. ISSLS prize winner: the anatomy of failure in lumbar disc herniation: an in vivo, multimodal, prospective study of 181 subjects. Spine (Phila Pa 1976). 2013;38(17):1491–500.
19. Kursumovic A, Rath S. Performance of an annular closure device in a 'Real-World', heterogeneous, at-risk. Lumbar Discectomy Population Cureus. 2017;9(11):e1824.
20. Arts MP, Brand R, van den Akker ME, Koes BW, Bartels RH, Peul WC. Tubular diskectomy vs conventional microdiskectomy for sciatica: a randomized controlled trial. JAMA. 2009;302(2):149–58.
21. Lau D, Han SJ, Lee JG, Lu DC, Chou D. Minimally invasive compared to open microdiscectomy for lumbar disc herniation. J Clin Neurosci. 2011; 18(1):81–4.
22. Harrington JF, French P. Open versus minimally invasive lumbar microdiscectomy: comparison of operative times, length of hospital stay, narcotic use and complications. Minim Invasive Neurosurg. 2008;51(1):30–5.
23. Drazin D, Ugiliweneza B, Al-Khouja L, Yang D, Johnson P, Kim T, et al. Treatment of recurrent disc herniation: a systematic review. Cureus. 2016;8(5):e622.
24. Thome C, Klassen PD, Bouma GJ, Kursumovic A, Fandino J, Barth M, et al. Annular closure in lumbar microdiskectomy for prevention of reherniation: a randomized clinical trial. The Spine Journal. 2018;in press.
25. Lequin MB, Barth M, Thome C, Bouma GJ. Primary limited lumbar discectomy with an annulus closure deice: one-year clinical and radiographic results from a prospective, multi-center study. Korean J Spine. 2012;9(4):340–7.
26. Lequin MB, Barth M, Thome C, Bouma GJ. Primary limited lumbar discectomy with an annulus closure device: one-year clinical and radiographic results from a prospective, multi-center study. Korean J Spine. 2012;9(4):340–7.
27. Shriver MF, Xie JJ, Tye EY, Rosenbaum BP, Kshettry VR, Benzel EC, et al. Lumbar microdiscectomy complication rates: a systematic review and meta-analysis. Neurosurg Focus. 2015;39(4):E6.

7

Optimal viewing angles of intraoperative fluoroscopy for detecting screw penetration in proximal humeral fractures: a cadaveric study

Qiuke Wang[†], Yifei Liu[†], Ming Zhang, Yu Zhu, Lei Wang[*] and Yunfeng Chen[*]

Abstract

Background: To identify the optimal viewing angles for every proximal screw in PHILOS plate-fixed proximal humeral fractures.

Methods: Three fresh-frozen human cadaveric bodies with six intact shoulders were studied. All three bodies were put in the beach chair position and PHILOS plates were placed on the proximal humerus. Head screws penetrating 1 mm into the joint were fitted one by one. Fluoroscopy was conducted in the 180° horizontal plane and the 120° coronal plane to analyze each screw's penetration in every shoulder. Images were taken every 5°, then all images were analyzed to identify the sensitive angles.

Results: The range of optimal viewing angles to visualize penetration of every head screw was identified. In the coronal plane, the angles in the range between 0° and 10° were sensitive to all screws except No. 8 and No. 9. Furthermore, penetration of screws No. 8 and 9 could not be identified on any axillary view, but could be identified in the horizontal plane from − 30° to − 10° and from 10° to 35° respectively.

Conclusions: We recommend a 0°–10° axillary view with 30° arm abduction combined with two horizontal angles in the range of − 30° to − 10° and 10° to 35° for routine fluoroscopy during surgery. Our results will be helpful in avoiding primary screw penetration.

Keywords: Proximal humeral fracture, Screw penetration, Complication, Fluoroscopy, Surgery, Trauma

Background

Proximal humeral fracture accounts for approximately 5% of all bone fractures, and the rate is rising with the increasing age of the population [1–3]. Although roughly 80% of these fractures can be treated conservatively, the rest, which are considered as displaced fractures, are recommended to be fixed by surgery [4]. Since locking plates, especially the PHILOS plate (Proximal Humerus Internal Locking System, Depuy Synthes, Warsaw, IN, USA), are becoming more and more popular to achieve satisfactory outcomes in fixing proximal humeral

fractures [5–8], a high rate of complications has been reported related to the use of plates, of which screw penetration is the most frequent [4, 6, 9–11]. Patients with screw penetration may experience severe pain and require subsequent revision surgery to remove the internal plate, which has a significant effect on rehabilitation. Screw penetration includes both primary and secondary screw penetration. The incidence of primary screw penetration is proximately 14% [5] it occurs during surgery and is considered to be an avoidable complication, preventable by careful operation and appropriate fluoroscopic detection during surgery. However, knowledge of the appropriate fluoroscopic detection is inadequate. Spross et al. [12] found that only the combination of four projections of fluoroscopic detection (neutral, 30° external rotation, 30° internal rotation and axial in 30°)

* Correspondence: wanglei2264@126.com; drchenyunfeng@sina.com
[†]Qiuke Wang and Yifei Liu contributed equally to this work.
Department of Orthopedic Surgery, Shanghai Jiao Tong University Affiliated Sixth People's Hospital, 600 Yishan Road, Shanghai 200233, People's Republic of China

could achieve 100% sensitivity and that standard radiographs (anteroposterior and outlet) missed almost half the instances of primary screw penetration in fractures fixed with the PHILOS plate. The process required to complete four angles of fluoroscopic detection during surgery is tedious and time-consuming, which means that primary screw penetration can easily be missed during routine surgeries. Two studies of Theopold et al. reported that intraoperative 3D fluoroscopy enabled 100% detection of the screw perforations [13, 14]. However, 3D fluoroscopy equipment was not available in most operating rooms while regular X-ray projector (c-arm) was always equipped.

The aim of our study therefore was to explore the optimal viewing angles of intraoperative fluoroscopy for every proximal screw in PHILOS plate-fixed proximal humeral fractures, and then suggesting some intra-operative fluoroscopy angles for avoiding screw penetration.

Methods

This study was approved by ethics of committee of Shanghai sixth people's hospital, the approval number is 2016-ky-005, and all donors had signed agreement about further cadaveric research and education before body donation. Three fresh-frozen human cadaveric bodies with six intact shoulders were obtained, which comprised 2 females and 1 male, with a mean age of 72.2 years (range 64–82). All the specimens included the entire scapula, clavicle, humerus and intact associated soft tissues. Gross examination was performed and clinical histories were reviewed to exclude any history of bone diseases.

Preparation of specimens

All three bodies were put in a beach chair position to simulate the intraoperative situation. The PHILOS plates were placed on the proximal humerus, 5 mm lateral to the bicipital groove and 8 mm distal to the tip of the greater tuberosity, in all shoulders through the standard deltopectoral approach. Two non-locking screws were initially placed in the shaft holes to fix the plates in position. Second, we simulated the methods used in the study by Spross et al. [12]; the subscapularis muscle was tenotomized close to the lesser tuberosity and the anterior capsule was vertically incised to gain full sight into the joint and of the humeral head, so that drilling of head screws could be visually controlled to avoid perforating the head. Lastly, the lengths of the head screws were chosen according to the measurement of the lengths of the drill holes, and nine head screws were placed in the humeral head in each shoulder.

Imaging investigation

Head screws were numbered to facilitate identification and recording (Fig. 1). The No. 1 screw was removed (prepared above) and a longer screw was inserted to penetrate the head, the length was controlled to penetrate 1 mm beyond the surface of the head under direct vision (Fig. 2). After exchanging the screws, the joint was sutured and the arm was placed in a neutral position. To simulate the anteroposterior projections, the c-arm was positioned in the anteroposterior direction (perpendicular to coronal plane of the body and c-arm on the horizontal plane) and it was set as 0°. Then the c-arm was rotated clockwise (overlooked), and an image was obtained every 5° up to 90°, resulting in 18 images being obtained. After that, the c-arm was reset at 0° and rotated anti-clockwise up to 90°, and again an image was obtained every 5°. In total, 37 images were obtained in the 180° horizontal plane. In order to facilitate data recording, for the left shoulder we set the angle on the right as "+" and on the left as "-"; we then used the opposite convention for the right shoulder (Fig. 3). During this process, the body and the arm were kept still.

In order to simulate the axillary view, the c-arm was placed on the coronal plane of the body and the arm

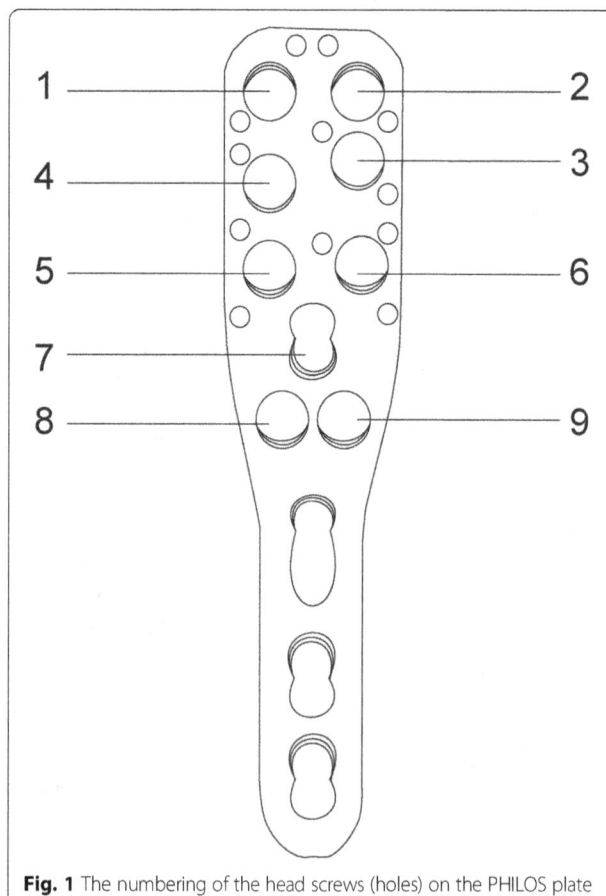

Fig. 1 The numbering of the head screws (holes) on the PHILOS plate

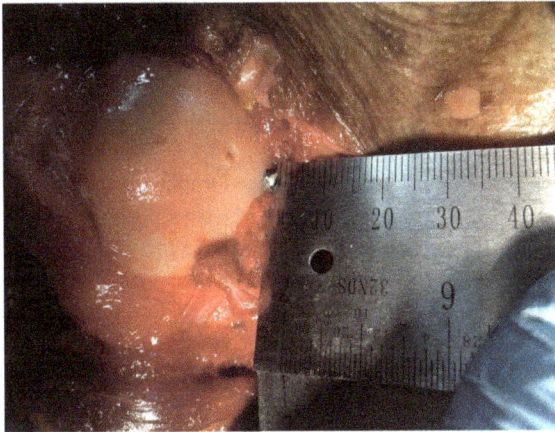

Fig. 2 Each head screw penetrates the humeral head to 1 mm under visual control

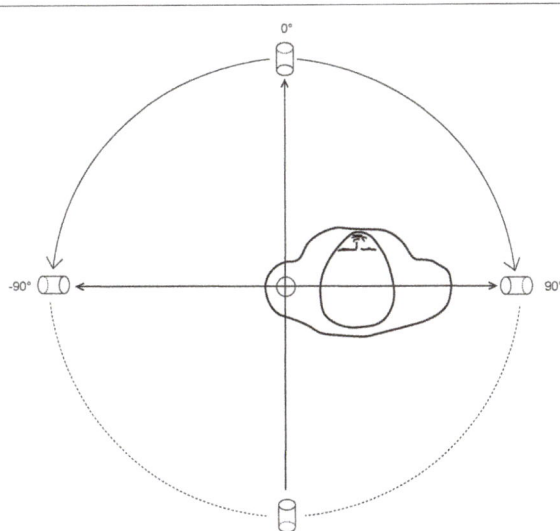

Fig. 4 Taking the left shoulder as an example, the arm was positioned at 30° of abduction, and radiographic projection was conducted in a 120° coronal plane. Radiographic images were taken every 5°

was placed at 30° of abduction (Fig. 4). Taking the left shoulder as an example, the standard axillary view was set as 0°, then the c-arm was rotated clockwise (sighted from the anterior to the posterior of the body), and an image was obtained every 5° up to 90° (equivalent to the axillary view with the arm at 120° of abduction). After that, the c-arm was reset at 0° and rotated anti-clockwise up to 30° (equivalent to the axillary view with the arm at 0° abduction) and an image was obtained every 5°. A total of 25 images were obtained on the 120° coronal plane, and as above, in the left shoulder we set the angle on the right as "+" and on the left as "-", while for the right shoulder, the opposite convention was used. During this process, the body was kept still with the arm in 30° of abduction.

Overall, a total of 62 images were obtained for the penetration of No. 1 screw. The same method was then applied for the imaging investigation of penetration of the next 8 screws, to give a total of 558 images from one shoulder. All 6 shoulders underwent the same process and 558 × 6 images were collected.

Imaging analysis

All images were numbered and were independently and randomly reviewed for screw penetration (yes/no) by two experienced attending doctors. The two doctors were blinded to the experimental design and process. All discordant cases were reevaluated by a third examiner, and the results were assigned by consensus of the three examiners. Based on these results, for each shoulder, we were able to draw a viewing angle range to detect penetration of every head screw.

Statistical analysis

Statistical analysis was performed using the statistical program SPSS version 20.0 (IBM Corp., Armonk, NY, USA). The optimal viewing angle range of every screw was set between the average minimum and maximum of the six shoulders. In this study each screw has an angle range in each shoulder, so the average of the six angle ranges was calculated for each screw, with the lower boundary set as the average of the lower boundary of the six angle ranges and the higher boundary as the average of the higher boundary of the six angle ranges. In order to simplify clinical application, all the angles were measured to the nearest multiple of five greater

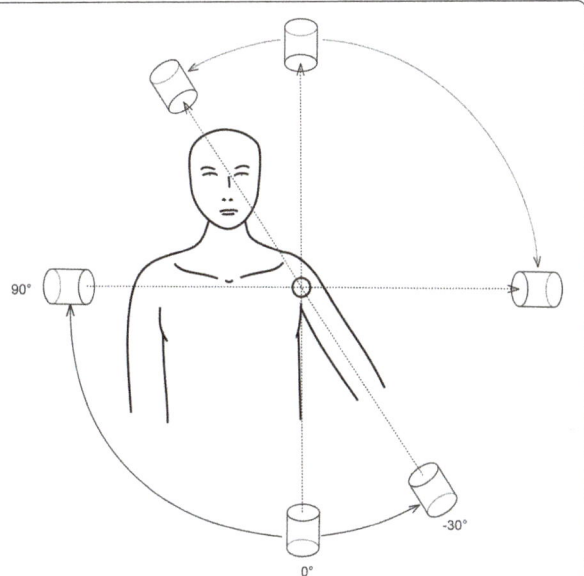

Fig. 3 Taking the left shoulder as an example, radiographic projection was conducted in a 180° horizontal plane. Radiographic images were taken every 5°

than the average lower value for the lower boundary, for example if the average value was 8 we chose 10; and we chose the first multiple of five less than the average higher value for the higher boundary, for example if the average value was 8 we chose 5 (Fig. 5).

Results

As each screw was positioned one by one to penetrate the humeral head in each shoulder, the same radiographic process was performed as described above, and screw penetrations could be identified on the images (Fig. 6).

After calculating the average minimum and maximum sensitive angles of all six shoulders, the optimal range of viewing angles to visualize penetration of every head screw was identified. Taking No. 1 screw as an example, the viewing angles ranged from – 35° to 20° in the horizontal plane (Fig. 5a) and – 5° to 45° in the coronal plane (Fig. 5b). All viewing angle ranges are collated in Fig. 7. In the coronal plane, the angles in the range between 0° and 10° were able to visualize all screws except No. 8 and 9. Furthermore, penetration of screws No. 8 and 9 could not be identified on any axillary view, but could be identified in the horizontal plane only. In this study, we maintained the body and arm in a fixed position, therefore theoretically, our angle data could be transferred to another type of fluoroscope in which we could rotate the arm or move it without moving the c-arm. The internal and external rotation of the arm in anteroposterior projections is equal to the rotation of the c-arm in the horizontal plane, and the transferred data are presented in Fig. 8.

Discussion

The PHILOS plate is a widely-used implant for fixing proximal humeral fractures; it is designed to position divergent screws in the humeral head in order to increase screw purchase; however, its unique design makes it difficult to identify the screws' position during surgery. Screw penetration is found to occur frequently during surgery as well as at follow-up, resulting in damage to the glenoid fossa caused by the screw tip and causing the patient to suffer severe pain [14–18]. Screw penetration of PHILOS plate is the primary object of our study, and our results concerning the optimal viewing angle ranges for intraoperative fluoroscopy to detect screw penetration lead the way for surgeons. Traditional standard anteroposterior and lateral fluoroscopy may miss penetration of at least 3 screws (No. 5, 8 and 9), while for three orthogonal views, in the trauma-series of x-rays (true glenoid anteroposterior, trans-scapular lateral and axillary views), penetration of screw No. 8 can still be missed. This may be the reason why screw penetration remains the most frequent complication. Penetration of screws No. 8 and 9 could not be identified on our axillary

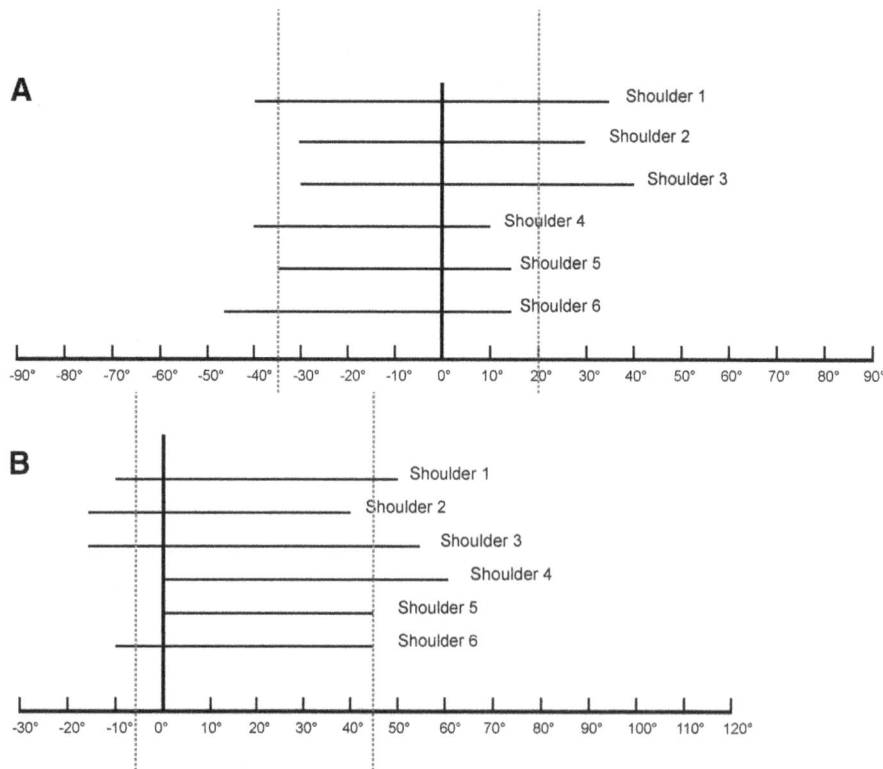

Fig. 5 For each shoulder, the range of sensitive angles of the No. 1 screw is presented by a solid black line, and the two dotted red lines present the average minimum and maximum sensitive angles of the 6 shoulders. **a** Horizontal plane; **b** Coronal plane

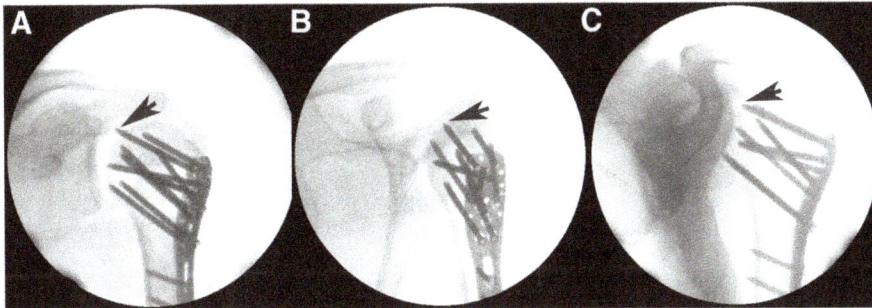

Fig. 6 Three images present three different viewing angles in the horizontal plane for the No. 1 screw in shoulder 1. Screw penetrations can be identified in three viewing angles, **a** 0°; **b** 40°; **c** -35°

views; this may be because these two screws are positioned on the lower part of the spherical head, so that the superior part may easily hide the 1 mm cut out and our view angles are limited between – 30°and 90°.

Some instances of penetration found at follow-up may have happened during surgery and have been missed because of inadequate fluoroscopy. In a study by Charalambous et al. [5], 4 of 25 patients were found to have screw penetration at follow-up, and subsequent review of the intra-operative radiographs showed that the penetration was missed intra-operatively in one case.

Thanasas et al. [19] highlighted the use of intraoperative fluoroscopy and recommended fluoroscopy in at least two different planes to avoid screw penetration. However, in their study, little information is available about which angles or planes have a high sensitivity for detecting screw penetration during surgery. Spross et al. [12] conducted a study to test some widely-used radiographic projections for detecting screw penetration, and found that anteroposterior and outlet radiographs, especially in internal rotation, may miss almost half the instances of screw penetration, while the standard axillary view (30°

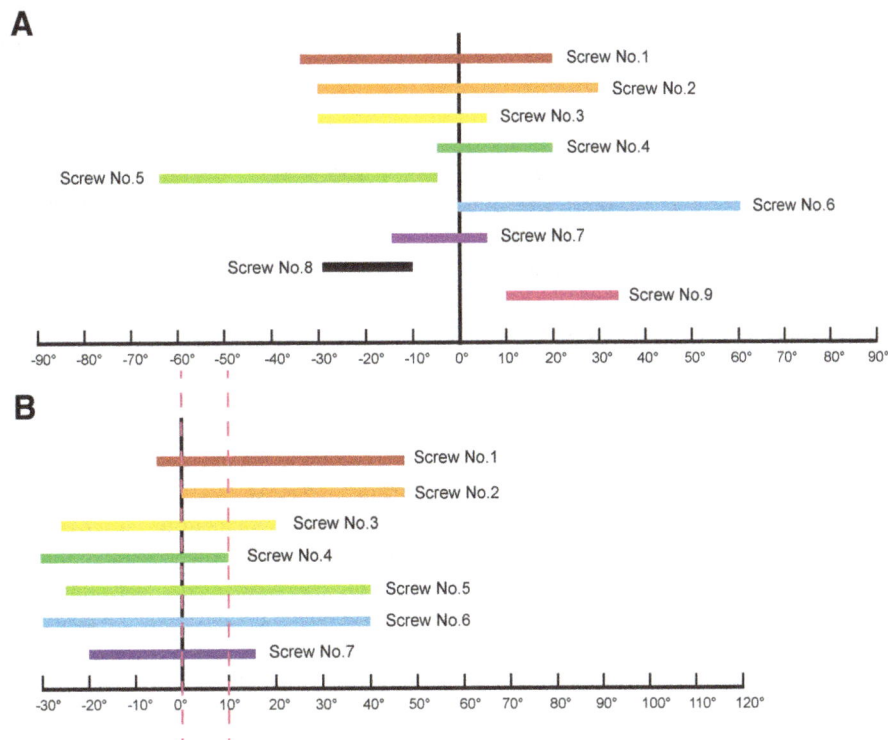

Fig. 7 The optimal viewing angles for each screw are indicated in the diagram by colored bands. **a** Horizontal plane; **b** Coronal plane. The angles between the two dotted red lines provide sensitive visualization of all seven screws

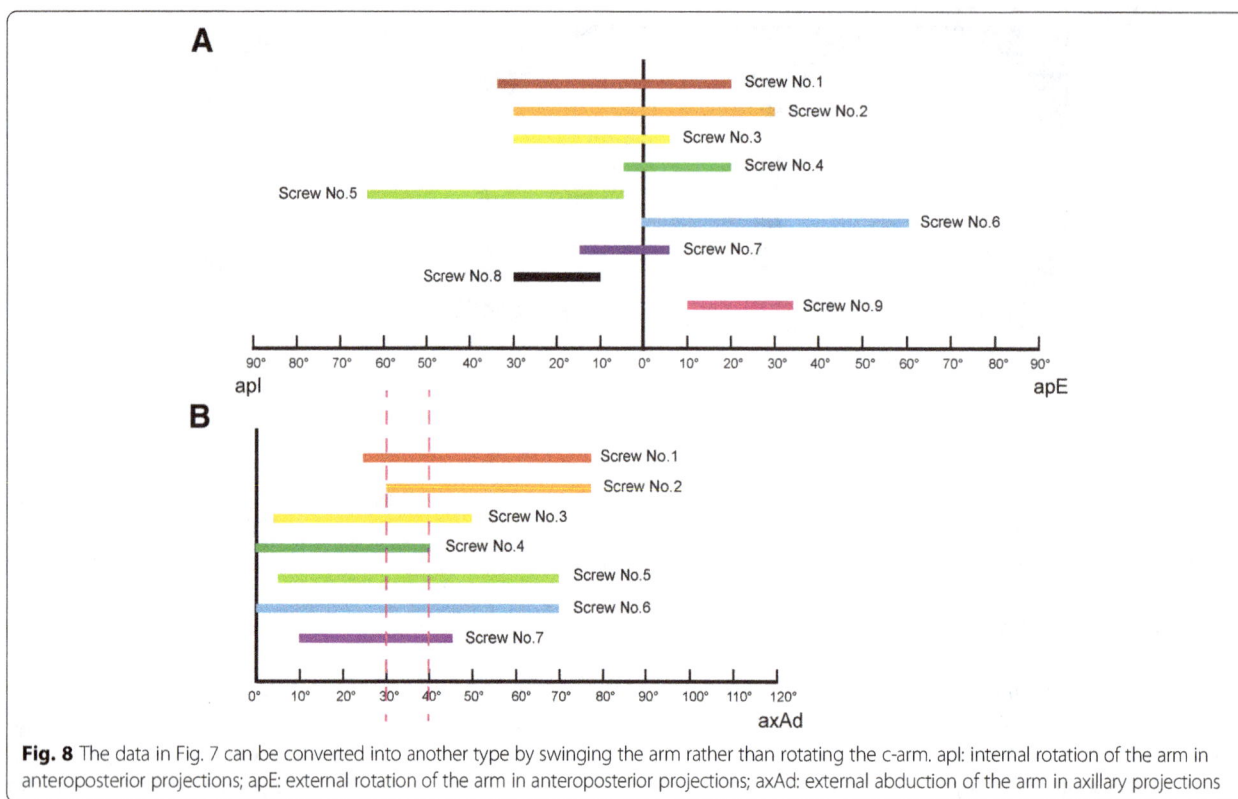

Fig. 8 The data in Fig. 7 can be converted into another type by swinging the arm rather than rotating the c-arm. apI: internal rotation of the arm in anteroposterior projections; apE: external rotation of the arm in anteroposterior projections; axAd: external abduction of the arm in axillary projections

abduction) presented the highest sensitivity in a single radiographic projection.

According to our data, the standard axillary view with the arm at 30° abduction should be recommended, and the angles in the range between 0° and 10° (abduction 30–40°) show the same high sensitivity. In the horizontal plane, at least two different projections should be used to detect screws No. 8 and 9, one in the range between – 30° and – 10°, another between 10° and 35°, which equate to internal rotation of the arm 10–30° and external rotation of 10–35°. In addition, we found that the standard lateral view was not able to identify any screw penetration, which may be because 1 mm is too short to be detected. We recommend that our results should be used intraoperatively to reduce the rate of primary screw penetration rather than at follow-up. This is because, on the one hand, a large proportion of secondary screw penetrations are secondary to severe humeral head deformities, such as varus and necrosis, so that the optimal angles for these heads would be different from our data, while on the other hand, it may be impractical to perform fluoroscopy using such accurate angles at each follow-up.

In the process of carrying out this study, we chose to rotate the c-arm rather than rotate the arm (internal and external rotation), because it is easier and more precise to control the angle according to the angle indexes on the c-arm, and it is also more practical during surgery.

Based on our results, we can conclude that the sensitivity of every radiographic projection, for anteroposterior and outlet radiographs, means that penetration of three screws may be missed, while the result of a standard axillary view is similar to that found in the study by Spross et al., showing that it is sensitive to all screws but No. 8 and 9. So we recommend 0°–10° axillary view with the arm at 30° abduction combined with two horizontal angles in the range of – 30° to – 10° and 10° to 35° as a good combination; however, this is not the only one which can achieve 100% sensitivity, because the standard 0° axillary view with the arm at 30° abduction is used in many places and is easy to remember.

There are some limitations to this research. Firstly, the protocol was designed based on healthy shoulders with no history of bone diseases, so we simulated an anatomical reduction model. Although for some fractures it is difficult to obtain the absolute anatomical reduction [20], we believe a slight deformity can be acceptable under the angle ranges. Secondly, there are wide variations in the length of the screw tip clinically cut out of the head; we set all screws cut out of the head to 1 mm, so shorter penetrations can still be missed under these views. Finally, we studied only one kind of plate. Although it is used commonly, the screws on this plate are divergently positioned in every section of the humeral head, so its unique design means that our data may be unsuitable for application to other implants.

Conclusion

In conclusion, after studying the viewing angles of every proximal screw on PHILOS plate-fixed proximal humeral fractures, we obtained an optimal viewing angle range for every screw. Consequently, we recommend 0°–10° axillary view with the arm at 30° abduction, while another two horizontal angles in the range of − 30° to − 10° and 10° to 35° should be included. Our results will be helpful for avoiding screw penetration during surgery.

Abbreviation
PHILOS: Proximal Humerus Internal Locking System

Funding
This study was supported by Three-year Project for Enhancing Clinical and Innovative Competence of Municipal Hospitals (16CR3042A).

Authors' contributions
QW and YL designed and carried out the subject; MZ and YZ wrote the article; LW and YC reviewed and edited the article. All authors read and approved the final manuscript.

Competing interests
The authors declare that they have no competing interests.

References
1. Helwig P, Bahrs C, Epple B, Oehm J, Eingartner C, Weise K. Does fixed-angle plate osteosynthesis solve the problems of a fractured proximal humerus? Acta Orthop. 2009;80:92–6. https://doi.org/10.1080/17453670902807417.
2. Ricchetti ET, Warrender WJ, Abboud JA. Use of locking plates in the treatment of proximal humerus fractures. J Shoulder Elbow Surg. 2010;19: 66–75.
3. Yang H, Li Z, Zhou F, Wang D, Zhong B. A prospective clinical study of proximal humerus fractures treated with a locking proximal humerus plate. J Orthop Trauma. 2011;25(1):11–7. https://doi.org/10.1097/BOT. 0b013e3181d2d04c.
4. Clavert P, Adam P, Bevort A, Bonnomet F, Kempf JF. Pitfalls and complications with locking plate for proximal humerus fracture. J Shoulder Elb Surg. 2010;19(4):489–94. https://doi.org/10.1016/j.jse.2009.09.005.
5. Charalambous CP, Siddique I, Valluripalli K, Kovacevic M, Panose P, Srinivasan M, et al. Proximal humeral internal locking system (PHILOS) for the treatment of proximal humeral fractures. Arch Orthop Trauma Surg. 2007;127(3):205–10. https://doi.org/10.1007/s00402-006-0256-9.
6. Erasmo R, Guerra G, Guerra L. Fractures and fracture-dislocations of the proximal humerus: a retrospective analysis of 82 cases treated with the Philos((R)) locking plate. Injury. 2014;45(Suppl 6):S43–8. https://doi.org/10. 1016/j.injury.2014.10.022.
7. Fazal MA, Haddad FS. Philos plate fixation for displaced proximal humeral fractures. J Orthop Surg. 2009;17(1):15–8. https://doi.org/10.1177/ 230949900901700104.
8. Koukakis A, Apostolou CD, Taneja T, Korres DS, Amini A. Fixation of proximal humerus fractures using the PHILOS plate: early experience. Clin Orthop Relat Res. 2006;442:115–20.
9. Egol KA, Ong CC, Walsh M, Jazrawi LM, Tejwani NC, Zuckerman JD. Early complications in proximal humerus fractures (OTA types 11) treated with locked plates. J Orthop Trauma. 2008;22(3):159–64. https://doi.org/10.1097/ BOT.0b013e318169ef2a.
10. Gardner MJ, Weil Y, Barker JU, Kelly BT, Helfet DL, Lorich DG. The importance of medial support in locked plating of proximal humerus fractures. J Orthop Trauma. 2007;21(3):185–91. https://doi.org/10.1097/BOT. 0b013e3180333094.
11. Roderer G, Erhardt J, Kuster M, Vegt P, Bahrs C, Kinzl L, et al. Second generation locked plating of proximal humerus fractures--a prospective multicentre observational study. Int Orthop. 2011;35(3):425–32. https://doi. org/10.1007/s00264-010-1015-7.
12. Spross C, Jost B, Rahm S, Winklhofer S, Erhardt J, Benninger E. How many radiographs are needed to detect angular stable head screw cut outs of the proximal humerus - a cadaver study. Injury. 2014;45:1557–63. https://doi.org/ 10.1016/j.injury.2014.05.025.
13. Theopold J, Weihs K, Marquass B, Josten C, Hepp P. Detection of primary screw perforation in locking plate osteosynthesis of proximal humerus fracture by intra-operative 3D fluoroscopy. Arch Orthop Trauma Surg. 2017; 137:1491–8. https://doi.org/10.1007/s00402-017-2763-2.
14. Theopold J, Weihs K, Feja C, Marquass B, Josten C, Hepp P. Detection of articular perforations of the proximal humerus fracture using a mobile 3D image intensifier - a cadaver study. BMC Med Imaging. 2017;17:47. https:// doi.org/10.1186/s12880-017-0201-0.
15. Boesmueller S, Wech M, Gregori M, Domaszewski F, Bukaty A, Fialka C, et al. Risk factors for humeral head necrosis and non-union after plating in proximal humeral fractures. Injury. 2016;47(2):350–5. https://doi.org/10.1016/ j.injury.2015.10.001.
16. Egol KA, Sugi MT, Ong CC, Montero N, Davidovitch R, Zuckerman JD. Fracture site augmentation with calcium phosphate cement reduces screw penetration after open reduction-internal fixation of proximal humeral fractures. J Shoulder Elb Surg. 2012;21(6):741–8. https://doi.org/10.1016/j.jse. 2011.09.017.
17. Fankhauser F, Boldin C, Schippinger G, Haunschmid C, Szyszkowitz R. A new locking plate for unstable fractures of the proximal humerus. Clin Orthop Relat Res. 2005;430:176–81.
18. Wang Q, Zhu Y, Liu Y, Wang L, Chen Y. Correlation between classification and secondary screw penetration in proximal humeral fractures. PLoS One. 2017;12(9):e0183164. https://doi.org/10.1371/journal.pone.0183164.
19. Thanasas C, Kontakis G, Angoules A, Limb D, Giannoudis P. Treatment of proximal humerus fractures with locking plates: a systematic review. J Shoulder Elb Surg. 2009;18(6):837–44. https://doi.org/10.1016/j.jse.2009.06.004.
20. Schnetzke M, Bockmeyer J, Porschke F, Studier-Fischer S, Grutzner PA, Guehring T. Quality of reduction influences outcome after locked-plate fixation of proximal humeral type-C fractures. J Bone Joint Surg Am. 2016; 98(21):1777–85. https://doi.org/10.2106/JBJS.16.00112.

8

Descriptive epidemiology and outcomes of bone sarcomas in adolescent and young adult patients in Japan

Takashi Fukushima[1,2], Koichi Ogura[3,4], Toru Akiyama[1*] ⑩, Katsushi Takeshita[2] and Akira Kawai[3]

Abstract

Background: There have been fewer improvements in the clinical outcomes of adolescent and young adult (AYA) patients with cancer than for children and older adults, possibly because fewer studies focus on patients in this age group. The aims of this study were (1) to determine survival rates of bone sarcoma among AYAs in Japan (for comparison with other age groups), and (2) to establish whether belonging to the AYA age group at diagnosis was correlated with poor cancer survival in Japan.

Methods: A total of 3457 patients diagnosed with bone sarcoma (1930 male and 1527 female) were identified from 63,931 records in the Bone and Soft Tissue Tumor (BSTT) registry, a nationwide Japanese database, from 2006 to 2013. The histologic subtypes of bone sarcoma were osteosarcoma, chondrosarcoma, and Ewing sarcoma. The primary endpoints for prognosis were the occurrence of tumor-related death. We compared the epidemiological features of AYAs with other age groups. The cancer survival rates were calculated using the Kaplan-Meier method. Cox proportional hazards models were used to analyze the prognostic factors for cancer survival.

Results: The majority of AYA had osteosarcoma 631 (56.2%), while 198 (17.6%) had chondrosarcoma. The frequency of bone sarcoma occurrence was highest among AYA patients, who accounted for a marked proportion of patients with each type of sarcoma. With the exception of sarcoma type, AYA patients did not significantly differ from patients in other age groups for any of the investigated clinicopathological parameters. Cancer survival of AYA patients was significantly higher than in the elderly. Univariate and multivariate analyses revealed that AYA status was not a predictor of poor cancer survival. However, older age (≥65 years) was a predictor of poor cancer survival in patients with overall bone sarcoma, osteosarcoma, chondrosarcoma.

Conclusion: This epidemiological study is the first to investigate AYA patients with bone sarcoma using the nationwide BSTT Registry. We found that cancer survival of AYA patients was significantly higher than that of the elderly. AYA status was not a predictor of poor cancer survival in Japan.

Keywords: Bone sarcoma, Adolescent and young adult, Cancer survival, Japan, Database

Background

There have been significant advances in the early detection and treatment of cancer, which have led to improvements in overall survival rates in general patient populations over several decades [1]. However, the clinical outcomes of adolescent and young adult (AYA) patients, defined as those between the ages of 15 to 39, with cancer

have not improved [1–4]. One explanation for this is that, to date, little attention and few resources have been devoted to studying the incidence, biology, and treatment outcomes in AYA patients with cancer [5].

AYA patients with cancer are predominantly afflicted by lymphoma, melanoma, testicular cancer, sarcoma, thyroid cancer, leukemia, and breast cancer [5]. Sarcomas comprise up to 6% of total malignancies in AYAs and represent one of the most common types of cancer in this population [5]. However, sarcoma is generally a rare disease, and its estimated total crude incidence rate

* Correspondence: toruakiyama827@jichi.ac.jp
[1]Department of Orthopaedic Surgery, Saitama Medical Center, Jichi Medical University, Saitama, Japan
Full list of author information is available at the end of the article

in Europe is 5.6 per 100,000 individuals per year [6]. A few previous studies have investigated the clinical outcomes of AYAs with bone sarcoma using nationwide or large databases with sufficient numbers of patients. However, most previous studies were based on data derived from small numbers of cases, and those with larger sample sizes have only analyzed a few disease-related factors [7–11].

In Japan, no studies on the epidemiology and clinical outcomes of AYA patients with sarcoma compared with patients diagnosed at other ages have been conducted because of the lack of a suitable database. In 2014, the Bone and Soft Tissue Tumor (BSTT) registry—a nationwide organ-specific cancer registry for bone and soft tissue tumors in Japan—became available for the purposes of clinical research, enabling a large-scale nationwide epidemiological investigation of AYA patients with sarcoma.

The aims of the present study were: 1) to determine survival rates of bone sarcoma among AYAs in Japan (for comparison with other age groups), and 2) to establish whether belonging to the AYA age group at diagnosis was correlated with poor cancer survival in Japan.

Methods
Data source
The BSTT Registry is a nationwide patient data collection system for organ-specific bone and soft tissue tumors that was launched in the 1950s by the Japanese Orthopaedic Association (JOA). All JOA-certified hospitals of musculoskeletal oncology (89 facilities) are required to participate in the registry; hence, almost all musculoskeletal malignant tumor cases treated by Japanese orthopedic surgeons are registered.

Detailed data of patients with primary bone and soft tissue tumors (both benign and malignant) and metastatic bone tumors treated at the participating hospitals are collected annually. The BSTT registry survey of patients diagnosed from January 1 to December 31 of the previous year are conducted annually in May. The survey includes basic demographic data of the patient, as well as information on the tumor, surgery, and treatment other than surgery. The next survey is conducted 2, 5, and 10 years after the initial registration at prognosis. The data for patients with bone and soft tissue sarcomas (not for patients with benign and metastatic bone tumors) are collected. It includes information on several outcomes at the time of the latest follow-up.

The BSTT Registry is similar to the Surveillance, Epidemiology, and End Results Program database in the United States; however, it has some additional advantages in that data are provided by the treating physicians themselves, and include histologic findings, treatment modalities, and surgical, functional, and oncologic outcomes.

The Musculoskeletal Tumor Committee of the JOA approved the use of the BSTT Registry for the purposes of clinical research in 2014 [12].

Study approval was obtained from the Institutional Review Board of the JOA.

Data extraction
The focus of this study was only bone sarcomas recorded in the BSTT Registry for patients diagnosed between 2006 and 2013. Data on 3457 patients with primary bone sarcoma were extracted from the database that encompassed 63,931 patients. Of these, 521, 1123, 982, and 831 were patients aged ≤14 years (children), 15–39 years (AYAs), 40–64 years (adults), and ≥ 65 years (elderly), respectively. The analyzed data included the year of registration; demographic characteristics; tumor size, location, grade, and histological characteristics; TNM and Enneking stages; treatment details (surgical vs. non-surgical); and prognosis at the last follow-up visit (no evidence of disease, alive with disease, dead of disease, or dead of other causes). Patients who were registered less than 2 years from the study enrollment date were excluded. Data on 2651 patients with primary bone sarcoma were extracted from the database. Cases with insufficient data were excluded.

Statistical analyses and study size
The primary endpoint was the occurrence of tumor-related deaths. The cancer survival time was defined as the period from the date of diagnosis to the tumor-related death. Patients without tumor-related deaths, or patients who died due to other causes, were censored at their last follow-up visit. The cancer survival rates for overall bone sarcoma (all types), osteosarcoma, chondrosarcoma, and Ewing sarcoma were calculated using the Kaplan-Meier method. Cox proportional hazards models were used to analyze the prognostic factors for cancer survival. The variables selected for the analysis were previously reported to be related to cancer survival [13–16]. Control variables for multivariate analysis were indicated by "reference", including AYA, males, low grade, ≤8 cm, upper extremity, salvaged and negative. The level of significance was set at $P < 0.05$.

IBM SPSS version 19.0 software (IBM SPSS, Armonk, NY, USA) was used for all statistical analyses. The study size was dictated by the total number of patients with bone sarcoma in the BSTT database during the study period.

Results
The study included 3457 patients with bone sarcoma (1930 male and 1527 female) who were registered in the BSTT database from 2006 to 2013. Table 1 shows characteristics of bone sarcomas in AYAs by age at diagnosis

Table 1 Characteristics of bone sarcomas in AYAs by age at diagnosis and relevant clinical factor

	Overall		AYA (15-39 years)		Child (−14 years)		Adult (40-64 years)		Elderly (65- years)		P value
	N	%	N	%	N	%	N	%	N	%	
Total	3457		1123	32.5%	521	15.1%	982	28.4%	831	24.0%	
Histologic subtype											< 0.001
Osteosarcoma	1497	43.3%	631	56.2%	405	77.7%	278	28.3%	183	22.0%	
Chondrosarcoma	885	25.6%	198	17.6%	8	1.5%	376	38.3%	303	36.5%	
Ewing's sarcoma	260	7.5%	139	12.4%	92	17.7%	28	2.9%	1	0.1%	
Bone MFH	205	5.9%	22	2.0%	2	0.4%	82	8.4%	99	11.9%	
Chordoma	253	7.3%	16	1.4%	2	0.4%	88	9.0%	147	17.7%	
HG sarcoma(others)	214	6.2%	52	4.6%	4	0.8%	85	8.7%	73	8.8%	
LG sarcoma(others)	143	4.1%	65	5.8%	8	1.5%	45	4.6%	25	3.0%	
Sex											0.028
Male	1930	55.8%	656	58.4%	278	53.4%	561	57.1%	435	52.3%	
Female	1527	44.2%	467	41.6%	243	46.6%	421	42.9%	396	47.7%	
Tumor size (cm), mean [SD]	9.1 [4.9]		8.8 [4.5]		10.3 [4.8]		8.9 [5.1]		9.0 [5.1]		< 0.001
≤8 cm	1655	47.9%	538	47.9%	193	37.0%	510	51.9%	414	49.8%	
> 8 cm and ≤ 16 cm	1299	37.6%	432	38.5%	246	47.2%	322	32.8%	299	36.0%	
> 16 cm	243	7.0%	61	5.4%	50	9.6%	67	6.8%	65	7.8%	
Unknown	260	7.5%	92	8.2%	32	6.1%	83	8.5%	53	6.4%	
Tumor location											< 0.001
Upper extremity	349	10.1%	134	11.9%	40	7.7%	105	10.7%	70	8.4%	
Lower extremity	1689	48.9%	629	56.0%	395	75.8%	399	40.6%	266	32.0%	
Trunk	1276	36.9%	303	27.0%	72	13.8%	437	44.5%	464	55.8%	
Head and neck	35	1.0%	18	1.6%	2	0.4%	10	1.0%	5	0.6%	
Multiple disease	108	3.1%	39	3.5%	12	2.3%	31	3.2%	26	3.1%	
Surgery	2473	71.5%	868	77.3%	430	82.5%	713	72.6%	462	55.6%	< 0.001
Chemotherapy	1765	51.1%	769	68.5%	474	91.0%	374	38.1%	148	17.8%	< 0.001
Radiotherapy	724	20.9%	188	16.7%	81	15.5%	206	21.0%	249	30.0%	< 0.001

SD standard deviation, *AYA* adolescent and young adult, *MFH* malignant fibrous histiocytoma, *HG sarcoma* High grade sarcoma, *LG sarcoma* Low grade sarcoma

and relevant clinical factors. The frequency of bone sarcoma occurrence was highest in AYA patients, who accounted for a marked proportion of patients with each type of sarcoma. Except for this, no categories were notably more or less prevalent in the AYA patient groups when compared with the same categories in other age groups. The majority of AYA had osteosarcoma 631 (56.2%), while 198 (17.6%) had chondrosarcoma. Among children, osteosarcoma was the most common 405 (77.7%), while 92 (17.7%) had Ewing sarcoma. Chondrosarcoma was the most common among adults 376 (38.3%), while 278 (28.3%) had osteosarcoma. Finally, among elderly, chondrosarcoma was the most common 303 (36.5%), while 183 (22.0%) had osteosarcoma. The incidences of osteosarcoma and Ewing sarcoma decreased with age, while the incidences of chondrosarcoma increased with age.

Figure 1a–d shows the cancer survival curves for patients with overall bone sarcoma (all types), as well as in those with osteosarcoma, chondrosarcoma, and Ewing sarcoma. There were no elderly patients with Ewing sarcoma. The cancer survival rate of AYA patients with osteosarcoma tended to be similar to that of children, but was better than those of adult and elderly patients. The cancer survival rate of AYA patients with chondrosarcoma tended to be similar to those of adults and was better than that of elderly patients. The cancer survival rates of children, AYA, and adult patients with Ewing sarcoma exhibited distinct tendencies, while the cancer survival rates of patients with Ewing sarcoma worsened with advancing age.

Table 2 shows the 5-year cancer survival statistics by age and sarcoma type. AYA patients with overall bone sarcoma did not exhibit worse cancer survival rates;

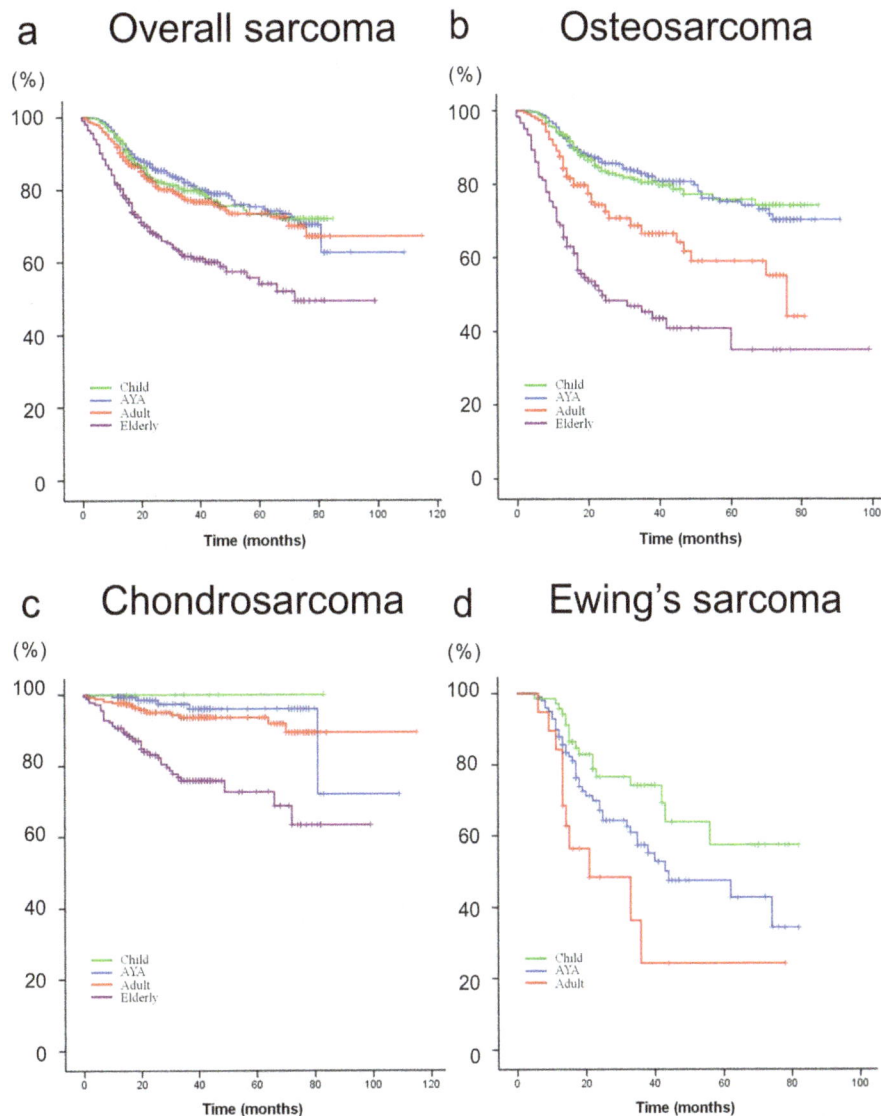

Fig. 1 a-d Kaplan-Meier survival curves showing disease-specific survival for overall sarcoma (**a**), osteosarcoma (**b**), chondrosarcoma (**c**), and Ewing sarcoma (**d**), stratified by age. Child: ≤14 years, adolescent and young adult (AYA): 15–39 years, adult: 40–64 years, and elderly: ≥65 years. No elderly patients were included in **d** as no elderly patients were diagnosed with Ewing sarcoma

Table 2 Five-year survival statistics by age and sarcoma type

	All sarcomas		Osteosarcoma		Chondrosarcoma		Ewing sarcoma	
	N	5-year survival (%)	N	5-year survival (%)	N	5-year survival (%)	N	5-year survival (%)
Overall	2651	71.3%	1124	68.4%	603	88.0%	187	49.0%
Age at diagnosis								
AYA	912	75.3%	483	75.2%	150	96.0%	98	47.5%
Child	431	73.8%	327	75.7%	7	100.0%	70	57.5%
Adult	741	74.2%	192	59.0%	264	93.6%	19	24.2%
Elderly	567	58.5%	122	35.0%	182	72.7%	NA	

AYA adolescent and young adult

however, the cancer survival was inversely correlated with age. The same tendencies were observed for each of osteosarcoma, chondrosarcoma, and Ewing sarcoma.

Table 3 shows univariate and multivariate analyses of prognostic factors of cancer survival by sarcoma type.

Overall, the prognostic factors associated with poor cancer survival in patients with overall bone sarcoma were age ≥ 65 years (hazard ratio [HR]: 3.74; 95% confidence interval [CI]: 2.66–5.28; $P < 0.001$), high tumor grade (HR: 3.77; 95% CI: 1.93–7.37; $P < 0.001$), tumor size >

Table 3 Univariate and multivariate analyses of prognostic factors of cancer survival by sarcoma type

	All sarcomas		Osteosarcoma		Chondrosarcoma		Ewing sarcoma	
	Univariate HR (95% CI)	Multivariate HR (95% CI)	Univariate HR (95% CI)	Multivariate HR (95% CI)	Univariate HR (95% CI)	Multivariate HR (95% CI)	Univariate HR (95% CI)	Multivariate HR (95% CI)
Age at diagnosis								
AYA	Reference	Reference	Reference	Reference	Reference	Reference	Reference	Reference
Child	1.04 (0.79–1.36)	0.83 (0.59–1.18)	1.02 (0.73–1.42)	1.00 (0.70–1.43)			0.57 (0.33–1.00)	0.35 (0.15–0.83)
Adult	1.14 (0.92–1.43)	1.61 (1.16–2.24)	1.99 (1.42–2.78)	1.58 (1.11–2.24)	1.82 (0.66–5.02)	1.77 (0.63–4.94)	1.92 (0.98–3.74)	1.97 (0.69–5.65)
Elderly	1.99 (1.61–2.46)	3.74 (2.66–5.28)	4.35 (3.14–6.02)	3.26 (2.29–4.64)	7.38 (2.91–18.75)	6.13 (2.38–15.75)	NA	NA
Sex								
Male	Reference	Reference	Reference	Reference	Reference	Reference	Reference	Reference
Female	0.93 (0.79–1.10)	0.85 (0.68–1.06)	1.01 (0.80–1.29)	0.96 (0.75–1.23)	1.07 (0.64–1.78)	1.20 (0.70–2.06)	0.96 (0.60–1.55)	1.08 (0.53–2.19)
Histologic grade								
Low	Reference	Reference			Reference	Reference		
High	6.63 (4.71–9.34)	3.77 (1.93–7.37)			4.73 (2.75–8.14)	3.27 (1.84–5.83)		
Tumor size								
≤8 cm	Reference	Reference	Reference	Reference	Reference	Reference	Reference	Reference
> 8 cm and ≤ 16 cm	1.84 (1.53–2.21)	1.26 (0.99–1.62)	1.74 (1.32–2.30)	1.63 (1.23–2.16)	2.79 (1.55–5.02)	2.03 (1.12–3.70)	0.86 (0.51–1.44)	0.55 (0.25–1.23)
> 16 cm	2.92 (2.21–3.87)	2.20 (1.52–3.19)	2.65 (1.74–4.030)	2.84 (1.86–4.35)	4.81 (2.30–10.07)	3.06 (1.40–6.68)	3.00 (1.41–6.37)	2.39 (0.87–6.57)
Tumor location								
Upper extremity	Reference	Reference	Reference	Reference	Reference	Reference	Reference	Reference
Lower extremity	1.64 (1.14–2.37)	1.41 (0.94–2.12)	1.30 (0.79–2.14)	1.19 (0.72–1.98)	2.65 (0.78–9.04)	2.30 (0.66–8.03)	1.37 (0.52–3.61)	1.63 (0.51–5.22)
Trunk	2.48 (1.72–3.59)	1.43 (0.91–2.23)	4.43 (2.63–7.46)	2.64 (1.53–4.56)	4.40 (1.36–14.25)	3.62 (1.08–12.15)	1.01 (0.40–2.55)	1.19 (0.36–3.91)
Head and neck	1.93 (0.75–4.95)	0.82 (0.19–3.51)	1.35 (0.40–4.60)	1.73 (0.50–6.04)			1.78 (0.21–15.34)	5.16 (0.53–50.02)
Multiple disease	5.99 (3.68–9.74)	2.60 (1.17–5.78)						
Limb salvage								
Salvaged	Reference	Reference	Reference	Reference	Reference		Reference	
Amputated	2.15 (1.72–2.70)	2.98 (2.28–3.89)	2.47 (1.83–3.33)	2.80 (2.05–3.83)	1.56 (0.62–3.96)		2.01 (0.80–5.07)	
Surgical margin								
Negative (wide or marginal)	Reference	Reference	Reference		Reference		Reference	Reference
Positive (intralesional)	1.14 (0.81–1.60)	1.78 (1.21–2.62)	1.26 (0.52–3.07)		0.68 (0.26–1.76)		3.67 (1.60–8.40)	5.28 (1.90–14.62)

AYA adolescent and young adult, *HR* Hazard ratio, *CI* confidence interval

16 cm (HR: 2.20; 95% CI: 1.52–3.19; $P < 0.001$), and positive surgical margins (HR: 1.78; 95% CI: 1.21–2.62; $P = 0.004$) (Table 3).

The results of univariate and multivariate analysis of prognostic factors for cancer survival in patients with osteosarcoma are shown in Table 3. Upon multivariate analysis, the negative prognostic factors included age 40–64 years (HR: 1.58; 95% CI: 1.11–2.24; $P < 0.001$), age ≥ 65 years (HR: 3.26; 95% CI: 2.29–4.64; $P < 0.001$), tumor size > 16 cm (HR: 2.84; 95% CI: 1.86–4.35; $P < 0.001$), and tumor location on the trunk (HR: 2.64; 95% CI: 1.53–4.56; $P < 0.001$) (Table 3). AYA patients had a similar HR to children and did not exhibit an increased risk of tumor-related death compared with the other age groups.

Likewise, the prognostic factors associated with poor cancer survival in patients with chondrosarcoma were age ≥ 65 years (HR: 6.13; 95% CI: 2.38–15.75; $P < 0.001$), tumor size > 16 cm (HR: 3.06; 95% CI: 1.40–6.68; $P = 0.005$), and tumor location on the trunk (HR: 3.62; 95% CI: 1.08–12.15; $P = 0.038$) (Table 3). Being in the AYA age group did not increase the risk of tumor-related deaths compared with the child and adult groups; furthermore, the risk of tumor-related deaths in AYA patients was lower than that in the elderly group.

Lastly, the sole prognostic factor associated with poor cancer survival in patients with Ewing sarcoma was a positive surgical margin (HR: 5.28; 95% CI: 1.90–14.62; $P = 0.001$). AYA patients had an increased risk of tumor-related deaths compared with children (HR: 0.35; 95% CI: 0.15–0.83; $P = 0.016$), but not with adults. None of the patients with Ewing sarcoma in our study were ≥ 65 years of age (Table 3).

Discussion

There have been fewer improvements in the clinical outcomes of AYA patients with cancer than for children and older adults, possibly because fewer studies focus on patients in this age group. Our study revealed the outcomes of AYA patients with bone sarcomas. We found that the AYA age group was not an independent poor prognostic factor for bone sarcoma overall, or for osteosarcoma, chondrosarcoma, or Ewing sarcoma individually. This was in contrast to other cancers, such as those of the breast and colon [17]. The cancer survival rate in AYA patients with bone sarcoma was similar to that of children and adults, and was more favorable than that of elderly patients. However, there have been no significant improvements in the overall 5-year survival rates for patients with bone sarcoma over the past few decades, unlike other cancers [10]. It is possible that this finding is the same in Japan. There have been significant improvements in the overall 5-year relative survival rates for patients with other cancers because of established effective

chemotherapy and molecular targeted drugs [18, 19]. It is possible that AYA patients do not stand out because there have been no improvements in the overall 5-year relative survival rates for other age groups.

In addition, insurance rates are significantly lower in AYA patients [20]. AYA cancer survivors without health insurance do not receive cancer-related medical care, while those with insurance do [21]. In Japan, every Japanese person belongs to the public medical insurance that bears 70–90% of the treatment costs. Japan has a national bail out system for officially acknowledged people in need, which covers almost 100% of the actual treatment costs. It is possible that cancer survival rates of AYA patients did not differ from patients in other age groups because patients of all ages received equal medical treatment. To our knowledge, this study is the first to investigate bone sarcomas based on age groups, including AYAs, and their clinical outcomes [22, 23].

Previous epidemiological analyses conducted in Australia and the United States showed that the cancer survival rates of AYA patients with osteosarcoma were significantly worse than those of children [10, 11]. However, our study showed that Japanese AYA patients with osteosarcoma had cancer survival rates that were statistically equivalent to those in children. The standard chemotherapy for osteosarcoma is methotrexate, doxorubicin, and cisplatin (MAP). Although the use of chemotherapy children and AYA patients was high, it was infrequently used in adult patients (data not shown). This likely explains why the cancer survival rates of AYA patients with osteosarcoma were better than those in adult and elderly patients. One other possible reason is that in Japan, one of the inclusion criteria for many clinical trials regarding osteosarcoma is patients aged ≤ 40 years [24–26]. AYA patients with osteosarcoma receive the same therapy as children. Tumor size is one of prognostic factors associated with poor survival among those with osteosarcoma [27]. In this study, there were few differences in the mean tumor size between AYA and adult patients (Additional file 1). Although children had the best osteosarcoma outcomes, the mean tumor size in children was the largest. For chondrosarcoma in particular, we found no other published studies with which to compare our results. The cancer survival rates of elderly patients with chondrosarcoma in our study were inferior to those of other age groups. One possible reason for this might be that elderly patients cannot be treated using surgery as a result of their advanced age. The proportions of patients who underwent surgery in the various age groups were as follows: children, 85.7%; AYA, 86.0%; adults, 87.1%; elderly, 73.1% (data not shown).

Tumor size is also a prognostic factor in Ewing sarcoma [28]. In this study, there were no significant differences in the mean tumor size between the age groups.

One possible reason for this might be the distinct biological features of Ewing sarcoma in different age groups. It was reported that a gain in chromosome 1q and a loss in chromosome 16q were each associated with significantly worse outcomes; these mutations were more common in patients' ≥15 years of age than in children [29]. Hence, the biology of Ewing sarcoma in AYA patients appears to be distinct from that in children [29]. In our study the frequency of Ewing sarcoma in AYA patients in Japan was lower than that in Australia and the United States [9, 11]. This is the reason why Caucasian populations are much more frequently affected, while there are low rates of the disease in East Asian and African populations [30].

The other independent risk factors for poor cancer survival in patients with bone sarcoma, as revealed in our study, are similar to those in previous studies of similar types of sarcoma. Consistent with our study, previous studies also reported that older age, large tumor size, high grade, and positive surgical margins were major factors that adversely influenced prognoses [28, 31–33].

Our study had several limitations. First, the BSTT Registry was computerized in 2006, and no long-term observations of over 10-years were possible. Second, there were many patients for whom functional outcomes were not recorded in the BSTT Registry; these would have been useful to evaluate. Third, AYA cancer survivors experience adverse effects on their quality of life that persist beyond cancer diagnosis and treatment, including issues with infertility, body image, difficulty establishing relationships, and many other aspects of physical and social functioning [18]. There are no data with which to evaluate such parameters in the BSTT Registry. Forth, due to the extremely low incidence rate, the number of children with chondrosarcoma and elderly with Ewing sarcoma was insufficient. However, despite these limitations, our findings provide detailed information on the epidemiology of bone sarcoma among AYAs in Japan.

Conclusions

Our study is the first to provide data on the descriptive epidemiology and clinical outcomes of AYA patients with bone sarcomas using a nationwide, large-scale database. We found that, contrary to expectations, cancer survival rates of AYA patients with bone sarcomas were not inferior to those of other age groups in Japan.

Abbreviations
AYA: Adolescent and young adult; BSTT: Bone and soft tissue tumor (registry); CI: Confidence interval; HR: Hazard ratio

Acknowledgments
We would like to thank all the subjects who volunteered for this study.

Authors' contributions
TF, KO, TA and AK contributed to the conception and design of the study. TF, KO, TA and KT contributed to the analysis, and all authors contributed to the interpretation of the results. TF drafted the article; all authors revised it critically and approved the final version submitted for publication. All authors read and approved the final manuscript.

Competing interests
The authors declare that they have no competing interests.

Author details
[1]Department of Orthopaedic Surgery, Saitama Medical Center, Jichi Medical University, Saitama, Japan. [2]Department of Orthopaedic Surgery, Jichi Medical University, Tochigi, Japan. [3]Department of Musculoskeletal Oncology, National Cancer Center Hospital, Tokyo, Japan. [4]Department of Orthopaedic Surgery, Faculty of Medicine, The University of Tokyo, Tokyo, Japan.

References
1. Potosky AL, Harlan LC, Albritton K, Cress RD, Friedman DL, Hamilton AS, et al. Use of appropriate initial treatment among adolescents and young adults with cancer. J Natl Cancer Inst. 2014;106(11). https://doi.org/10.1093/jnci/dju300. Print 2014 Nov.
2. Albritton K, Bleyer WA. The management of cancer in the older adolescent. Eur J Cancer. 2003;39(18):2584–99.
3. Bleyer A, Budd T, Montello M. Adolescents and young adults with cancer: the scope of the problem and criticality of clinical trials. Cancer. 2006;107(7 Suppl):1645–55.
4. Thomas DM, Albritton KH, Ferrari A. Adolescent and young adult oncology: an emerging field. J Clin Oncol. 2010;28(32):4781–2.
5. Children's Oncology Group, SEER Program (National Cancer Institute (U.S.)). Cancer epidemiology in older adolescents and young adults 15 to 29 years of age : including SEER incidence and survival, 1975–2000. Bethesda: U.S. Dept. of Health and Human Services, National Institutes of Health, National Cancer Institute; 2006. x, 205 p. p.
6. Stiller CA, Trama A, Serraino D, Rossi S, Navarro C, Chirlaque MD, et al. Descriptive epidemiology of sarcomas in Europe: report from the RARECARE project. Eur J Cancer. 2013;49(3):684–95.
7. Eleuterio SJ, Senerchia AA, Almeida MT, Da Costa CM, Lustosa D, Calheiros LM, et al. Osteosarcoma in patients younger than 12 years old without metastases have similar prognosis as adolescent and young adults. Pediatr Blood Cancer. 2015;62(7):1209–13.
8. Haggar FA, Preen DB, Pereira G, Holman CD, Einarsdottir K. Cancer incidence and mortality trends in Australian adolescents and young adults, 1982-2007. BMC Cancer. 2012;12:151.
9. Herzog CE. Overview of sarcomas in the adolescent and young adult population. J Pediatr Hematol Oncol. 2005;27(4):215–8.
10. Keegan TH, Ries LA, Barr RD, Geiger AM, Dahlke DV, Pollock BH, et al. Comparison of cancer survival trends in the United States of adolescents and young adults with those in children and older adults. Cancer. 2016; 122(7):1009–16.
11. Khamly KK, Thursfield VJ, Fay M, Desai J, Toner GC, Choong PF, et al. Gender-specific activity of chemotherapy correlates with outcomes in chemosensitive cancers of young adulthood. Int J Cancer. 2009;125(2):426–31.
12. Ogura K, Higashi T, Kawai A. Statistics of bone sarcoma in Japan: report from the bone and soft tissue tumor registry in Japan. J Orthop Sci. 2017; 22(1):133–43.
13. Balamuth NJ, Womer RB. Ewing's sarcoma. Lancet Oncol. 2010;11(2):184–92.
14. Grier HE, Krailo MD, Tarbell NJ, Link MP, Fryer CJ, Pritchard DJ, et al. Addition of ifosfamide and etoposide to standard chemotherapy for Ewing's sarcoma and primitive neuroectodermal tumor of bone. N Engl J Med. 2003;348(8): 694–701.
15. Bielack SS, Kempf-Bielack B, Delling G, Exner GU, Flege S, Helmke K, et al. Prognostic factors in high-grade osteosarcoma of the extremities or trunk: an analysis of 1,702 patients treated on neoadjuvant cooperative osteosarcoma study group protocols. J Clin Oncol. 2002;20(3):776–90.

16. Giuffrida AY, Burgueno JE, Koniaris LG, Gutierrez JC, Duncan R, Scully SP. Chondrosarcoma in the United States (1973 to 2003): an analysis of 2890 cases from the SEER database. J Bone Joint Surg Am. 2009;91(5):1063–72.

17. Tricoli JV, Seibel NL, Blair DG, Albritton K, Hayes-Lattin B. Unique characteristics of adolescent and young adult acute lymphoblastic leukemia, breast cancer, and colon cancer. J Natl Cancer Inst. 2011;103(8):628–35.

18. Pfreundschuh M, Trumper L, Osterborg A, Pettengell R, Trneny M, Imrie K, et al. CHOP-like chemotherapy plus rituximab versus CHOP-like chemotherapy alone in young patients with good-prognosis diffuse large-B-cell lymphoma: a randomised controlled trial by the MabThera international trial (MInT) group. Lancet Oncol. 2006;7(5):379–91.

19. Roy L, Guilhot J, Krahnke T, Guerci-Bresler A, Druker BJ, Larson RA, et al. Survival advantage from imatinib compared with the combination interferon-alpha plus cytarabine in chronic-phase chronic myelogenous leukemia: historical comparison between two phase 3 trials. Blood. 2006; 108(5):1478–84.

20. Adams SH, Newacheck PW, Park MJ, Brindis CD, Irwin CE Jr. Health insurance across vulnerable ages: patterns and disparities from adolescence to the early 30s. Pediatrics. 2007;119(5):e1033–9.

21. Keegan TH, Tao L, DeRouen MC, Wu XC, Prasad P, Lynch CF, et al. Medical care in adolescents and young adult cancer survivors: what are the biggest access-related barriers? J Cancer Surviv. 2014;8(2):282–92.

22. Akiyama T, Saita K, Chikuda H, Horiguchi H, Fushimi K, Yasunaga H. Mortality and morbidity following surgery for primary malignant musculoskeletal tumors in the pelvis and limbs: a retrospective analysis using the Japanese diagnosis procedure combination database. J Cancer Ther. 2016;07(04):303–10.

23. Ogura K, Yasunaga H, Horiguchi H, Ohe K, Shinoda Y, Tanaka S, et al. Impact of hospital volume on postoperative complications and in-hospital mortality after musculoskeletal tumor surgery: analysis of a national administrative database. J Bone Joint Surg Am. 2013;95(18):1684–91.

24. Ferrari S, Ruggieri P, Cefalo G, Tamburini A, Capanna R, Fagioli F, et al. Neoadjuvant chemotherapy with methotrexate, cisplatin, and doxorubicin with or without ifosfamide in nonmetastatic osteosarcoma of the extremity: an Italian sarcoma group trial ISG/OS-1. J Clin Oncol. 2012;30(17):2112–8.

25. Kudawara I, Aoki Y, Ueda T, Araki N, Naka N, Nakanishi H, et al. Neoadjuvant and adjuvant chemotherapy with high-dose ifosfamide, doxorubicin, cisplatin and high-dose methotrexate in non-metastatic osteosarcoma of the extremities: a phase II trial in Japan. J Chemother. 2013;25(1):41–8.

26. Whelan JS, Bielack SS, Marina N, Smeland S, Jovic G, Hook JM, et al. EURAMOS-1, an international randomised study for osteosarcoma: results from pre-randomisation treatment. Ann Oncol. 2015;26(2):407–14.

27. Bieling P, Rehan N, Winkler P, Helmke K, Maas R, Fuchs N, et al. Tumor size and prognosis in aggressively treated osteosarcoma. J Clin Oncol. 1996; 14(3):848–58.

28. Duchman KR, Gao Y, Miller BJ. Prognostic factors for survival in patients with Ewing's sarcoma using the surveillance, epidemiology, and end results (SEER) program database. Cancer Epidemiol. 2015;39(2):189–95.

29. Bleyer A, Barr R, Hayes-Lattin B, Thomas D, Ellis C, Anderson B, et al. The distinctive biology of cancer in adolescents and young adults. Nat Rev Cancer. 2008;8(4):288–98.

30. Worch J, Matthay KK, Neuhaus J, Goldsby R, DuBois SG. Ethnic and racial differences in patients with Ewing sarcoma. Cancer. 2010;116(4):983–8.

31. Bertrand TE, Cruz A, Binitie O, Cheong D, Letson GD. Do surgical margins affect local recurrence and survival in extremity, nonmetastatic, high-grade osteosarcoma? Clin Orthop Relat Res. 2016;474(3):677–83.

32. Buchner M, Bernd L, Zahlten-Hinguranage A, Sabo D. Primary malignant tumours of bone and soft tissue in the elderly. Eur J Surg Oncol. 2004; 30(8):877–83.

33. Duchman KR, Gao Y, Miller BJ. Prognostic factors for survival in patients with high-grade osteosarcoma using the surveillance, epidemiology, and end results (SEER) program database. Cancer Epidemiol. 2015;39(4):593–9.

9

Bone shape mediates the relationship between sex and incident knee osteoarthritis

Barton L. Wise[1,2,6*] (iD), Jingbo Niu[3], Yuqing Zhang[3], Felix Liu[4], Joyce Pang[5], John A. Lynch[4] and Nancy E. Lane[1]

Abstract

Background: Knee bone shape differs between men and women and the incidence of knee osteoarthritis (OA) is higher in women than in men. Therefore, the purpose of the present study was to determine whether the observed difference in the incidence of knee radiographic OA (ROA) between men and women is mediated by bone shape.

Methods: We randomly sampled 304 knees from the OAI with incident ROA (i.e., development of Kellgren/ Lawrence grade $\geq$ 2 by month 48) and 304 knees without incident ROA. We characterized distal femur and proximal tibia shape on baseline radiographs using Statistical Shape Modeling. If a specific bone shape was associated with the risk of incident ROA, marginal structural models were generated to assess the mediation effect of that bone shape on the relation of sex and risk of incident knee ROA adjusting for baseline covariates.

Results: Case and control participants were similar by age, sex and race, but case knees were from higher body mass index (BMI) participants (29.4 vs. 27.0; $p < 0.001$). Women had 49% increased odds of incident knee ROA compared with men (adjusted odds ratio (OR) = 1.49, 95% Confidence Interval (C.I.): 1.04, 2.12). There was an inconsistent mediation effect for tibial mode 2 between sex and incident knee ROA, with an indirect effect OR of 0. 96 (95% C.I.: 0.91–1.00) and a direct effect OR of 1.56 (95% C.I.: 1.08–2.27), suggesting a protective effect for this mode. Similar findings were also observed for the mediation effect of tibia mode 10 and femur mode 4. These shape modes primarily involved differences in the angular relation of the heads to the shafts of the femur and tibia.

Conclusions: Distal femur and proximal tibia bone shapes partially and inconsistently mediated the relationship between sex and incident knee OA. Women had a higher risk of incident ROA, and specific bone shapes modestly protected them from even higher risk of ROA. The clinical significance of these findings warrant further investigation.

Keywords: Knee, Osteoarthritis, Bone shape, Sex, Statistical shape modeling, Radiography

Background

Osteoarthritis (OA) is the most common form of arthritis, with at least 27 million US adults diagnosed with OA in 2008 [1]. The radiographic appearance of the joint degeneration of knee OA is characterized by a loss of the joint space or loss of articular cartilage in the medial compartment and/or the lateral compartment of

the joint. The majority of knee OA is characterized by medial compartment joint space loss, and the radiographic observation of lost joint space width has been confirmed by magnetic resonance imaging that demonstrates loss of cartilage.

Women have a higher prevalence of OA, different patterns of OA in the knee, and an increased risk of total knee arthroplasty due to OA compared with men [2–4] and the explanation for these differences by sex are incompletely explained. Women also have smaller cartilage volume in the knee and this appears to be independent of two known risk factors for knee OA, bone size and

* Correspondence: blwise@ucdavis.edu
[1]Department of Internal Medicine, University of California, Davis School of Medicine, Sacramento, CA, USA
[2]Department of Orthopaedic Surgery, University of California, Davis School of Medicine, Sacramento, CA, USA
Full list of author information is available at the end of the article

body mass [5–7]. A number of factors have been identified that increase the risk of tibio-femoral radiographic OA including obesity, age, female sex, number of childbirths, and African American race, several of which are sex related [8, 9]. Body mass index (BMI) is related to severity of OA in varus alignment but not in valgus alignment [10] and is thus dependent on specifics of malalignment in the knee, which differ by sex. Thus, despite a significant body of research in the epidemiology of knee OA as noted above, comprehensive understanding of the factors that account for the difference in prevalence of knee OA by sex remain unclear.

Our research group and others have reported that knee bone shape differs between men and women without knee OA [7, 11, 12]. However, recently investigators have used Statistical Shape Modeling (SSM) in both two and three dimensions and determined that specific shapes are associated with incident knee OA [13, 14]. Based on these new findings, the aims of this study were to determine whether knee bone shape is associated with risk of knee OA, and to what extent the difference in the incidence of knee radiographic OA (ROA) between men and women is mediated by bone shape.

Methods

Study Subjects

Subjects were drawn from the NIH funded cohort the Osteoarthritis Initiative (OAI) which enrolled 4796 participants at baseline who had knee OA or were at high risk of the condition and were aged 45–79, in 4 clinical centers and with a coordinating Center at University of California, San Francisco (more information is available online at https://oai.epi-ucsf.org/datarelease/). Approval for the overall OAI project was given by the institutional review boards at each OAI center, and this project (373289–1) was determined at the IRB at University of California, Davis to be "not human subjects research as defined by Department of Health and Human Services".

Subjects for the current study were eligible if they had no rheumatoid arthritis, osteonecrosis, or amputation and still had the patella present. Knees were excluded that had been replaced at baseline. In order to be included, knees had to have radiographs available at baseline, 12 month, 24 month, 36 month and 48 month visits. Included knees could not have radiographic knee OA (ROA) at baseline, defined as Kellgren/Lawrence (KL) grade < 2. Cases were knees with incident ROA, defined as KL grade ≥ 2 by the 48 month visit, randomly selected from the universe of such knees within the OAI. Control knees had KL grade < 2 at the 48 month visit, and were frequency matched by age and clinic site to the case knees [11, 15].

Assessment of bone shape

Bilateral weight-bearing fixed flexion posterior-anterior radiographs were obtained using a plexiglass fixed-frame positioning device at the baseline, 12-month, 24-month, 36-month, and 48-month visits for all subjects. The methods for the SSM methods applied in this study have been previously described [11, 16]. Prior to the shape modeling, all radiographs were reviewed for image quality and sufficient anatomical coverage in the film, and films that had bone edges that extended beyond the border of the radiograph or where poor penetration prevented identification of the edge of the knee were excluded. One reader (JP) outlined the distal end of the femur and proximal tibia using a standardized semi-automatic algorithm on digitized baseline AP radiographs for all knees. Separate shapes were defined for the femur and tibia. SSM were derived for the femur (with 41 points) and the tibia (40 points). Composite femoral and tibial shapes from only the participants analyzed in this study were compiled to generate reference models then used for measuring modes of variation of shape from these references. Mean shape and modes (variations of bone shape) sufficient to explain 95% of total shape variance in this population were derived using principal components analysis; each mode of variation was independent of the other modes of variation. We checked for correlation between modes and found very weak correlation, indicating that the modes were independent of each other. Correlation between modes ranged from − 0.0172 to 0.0218, or the absolute value of correlation between modes ranged from 0.000001– 0.0218. We recorded mode scores as the number of standard deviations of that particular mode that the individual knee was away from the mean value for the bone shape mode (constrained to a maximum of ±3 standard deviations in any one mode), and we refer to that as the "standardized score of bone shape".

Reliability

Intra-rater reliability was evaluated by repeating measurements in 342 randomly selected subjects and observing the point placement within 2 mm and within 3 mm of the prior knee shape points. The reader was blinded to reliability status and read the repeated radiographs with 5 months of time in-between readings. Intra-rater reliability for the distal femur and proximal tibia were 96.8% and 92.3%, respectively, for point placement within 2 mm and 98.8% and 96.9% for point placement within 3 mm. These results closely parallel reliability results reported in the literature for this type of SSM assessment [17].

Assessment of incident radiographic knee OA

Knee X-rays were read for Kellgren/Lawrence (KL) grade (0–4) by two experienced readers [15]. The OAI knee radiograph reading data version 0.8 was used in the analysis. Knees were scored for all five visit X-rays concurrently. Baseline visit X-rays were known to readers, but the order of follow-up X-rays was blinded. Readers were blinded to existing clinical or radiological data. Disagreements were adjudicated by an expert panel. Cross-sectional KL grade scores had a kappa of 0.7.

Assessment of covariates

Information on age, race, clinic site, history of knee injury, and history of knee surgery were collected by questionnaire at the baseline visit of the OAI study. Body mass index (BMI) was calculated using height and weight measurements taken at the baseline visit and applying the appropriate equation to obtain units of kg/m^2 [18].

Statistical analysis

First the relation of sex to the risk of incident radiographic knee OA was evaluated using logistic regression model adjusting for age, race, clinic site, history of knee

injury and of knee surgery, and BMI. Next, the association of sex with measurement of each bone shape was determined using the linear regression model. Lastly, the relation of each bone shape measurement to the risk of incident radiographic knee OA was evaluated using a logistic regression model adjusting for age, race, clinic site, history of knee injury and of knee surgery, and BMI. Finally, the total effect of sex on risk of incident radiographic knee OA was partitioned into indirect effect (i.e., the effect of sex on incident OA via a specific bone shape; an effect mediated via the effect of sex on bone shape) and direct effect (not mediated through bone shape) using marginal structural models (MSM) [19]. MSM was conducted under a counterfactual framework. In the MSM, sex was an exposure variable, bone shape measurement was the mediator, status of knee OA was an outcome variable, and age, race, clinic site, history of knee injury, history of knee surgery and BMI were covariates. Results are reported as odds ratios (OR) per standard deviation increase in the standardized score

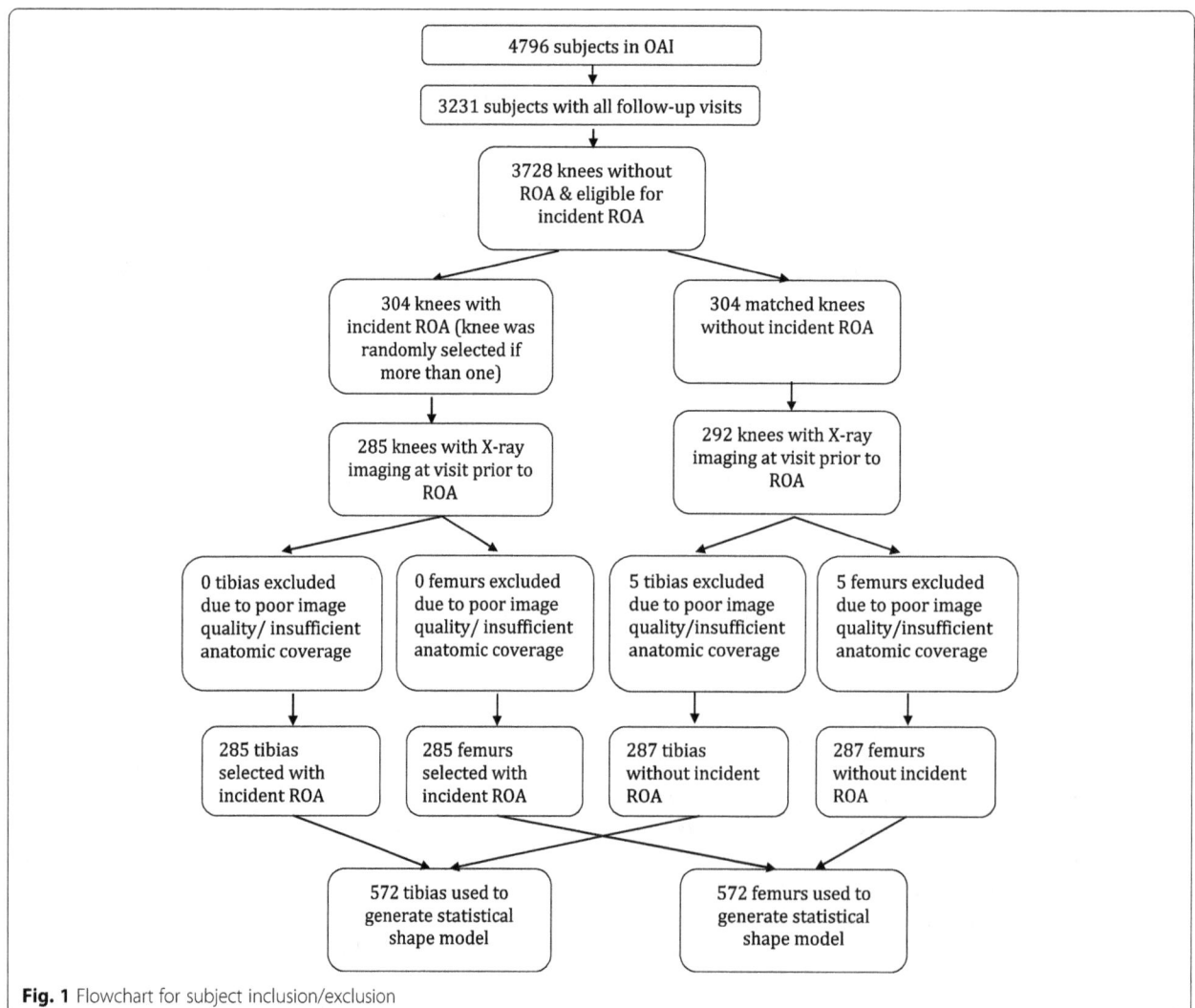

Fig. 1 Flowchart for subject inclusion/exclusion

of bone shape. SAS v9.2 (SAS, Inc., Cary, North Carolina) was used to complete statistical analyses.

Results

This study included 304 cases of incident knee OA and the same number of controls without radiographic knee OA (see Fig. 1). The percentage of white and mean age in cases were similar to those in controls; however, the proportion of women in cases (65.1%) was slightly higher than that in controls (59.9), and average BMI was greater in cases than that in controls (see Tables 1 and 2). Fifty-eight persons contributed two knees in the study, 21 with cases in both knees, 26 with controls in both knees, and the others with one knee as case and the other knee as control.

OAI subjects as a whole with K/L 0–1 at baseline were 60.3 years old (SD = 9.2) with BMI 27.8 kg/m^2 (SD = 4.5). 56.2% of them were women, 84.1% were Whites or Caucasian, and 86.3% had college or above college education. The cases/controls in our study were thus slightly more likely to be women and slightly less likely to be Whites or Caucasian. These differences might be due to the fact that they were selected from subjects who came back for the 48-month visit.

Compared with men, women had a higher risk of developing incident knee OA (adjusted OR = 1.49, 95% C.I.: 1.04, 2.12). On average, males who developed incident disease did so 2.08 years after baseline. On average, females who developed incident disease did so 2.11 years after baseline. Of 13 modes of bone shape of tibia and 13 modes of the femur examined (see Fig. 2), statistically

significant differences were found between men and women among control knees in modes 2, 3, 8, 10 and 11 in the tibia and modes 1, 4, 5, 8, 12 and 13 in the femur (See Table 3).

As shown in Table 3, six modes of bone shape were associated with incident radiographic knee OA after adjusting for age, race, clinic site, history of knee injury and knee surgery and BMI: high values of mode 2 and mode 9 at the tibia were associated with an increased risk of incident knee radiographic OA; however, high values of mode 10 and mode 12 at tibia and mode 4 and mode 10 at femur were associated with a lower risk of knee ROA.

The results of mediation analyses are presented in Table 4. Tibial modes 2 and 10 and femoral mode 4 were found to mediate the relation between sex and ncident knee OA. While the direct effect of sex on risk of knee ROA was greater than 1, indicating that women had a higher risk of knee ROA not including the effect of the specific bone shape mode, the indirect effect of

Table 1 Participant characteristics

Characteristics	Case knees (N = 304)	Control knees (N = 304)	p-value
Baseline age, mean (SD)	60.2 (8.6)	60.2 (8.5)	0.798
Baseline BMI, mean (SD)	29.4 (4.9)	27.0 (4.7)	<.0001
Sex			0.178
Men	106 (34.9%)	123 (40.5%)	
Women	198 (65.1%)	181 (59.5%)	
Race			0.639
Whites or Caucasian	241 (79.3%)	247 (81.3%)	
Black or African American	53 (17.4%)	52 (17.1%)	
Asian	6 (2.0%)	2 (0.7%)	
Other	4 (1.3%)	3 (1.0%)	
Education			0.984
High school or less	33 (11.1%)	36 (11.9%)	
College	140 (47.1%)	138 (45.7%)	
Above college	124 (41.8%)	128 (42.4%)	
Baseline KL grade			
1	162 (53.3%)	45 (14.8%)	<.0001

Table 2 Tibia and femur bone shape characteristics

Bone shape mode	Case knees mean (SD)	Control knees mean (SD)
tibia, mode 1	0.004 (0.955)	−0.077 (0.986)
tibia, mode 2	0.073 (1.018)	−0.032 (0.972)
tibia, mode 3	0.048 (1.009)	0.047 (1.007)
tibia, mode 4	−0.034 (0.972)	−0.017 (0.966)
tibia, mode 5	0.094 (0.980)	−0.058 (0.970)
tibia, mode 6	−0.042 (1.036)	0.015 (0.9765)
tibia, mode 7	−0.005 (1.021)	−0.042 (0.983)
tibia, mode 8	−0.036 (0.965)	0.043 (1.022)
tibia, mode 9	0.070 (0.978)	−0.069 (1.055)
tibia, mode 10	−0.049 (1.024)	0.067 (1.024)
tibia, mode 11	0.050 (1.019)	−0.007 (0.987)
tibia, mode 12	−0.057 (0.994)	−0.010 (1.056)
tibia, mode 13	−0.051 (0.944)	0.076 (1.017)
femur, mode 1	0.057 (1.031)	−0.033 (1.006)
femur, mode 2	−0.047 (1.027)	0.054 (0.917)
femur, mode 3	−0.057 (1.033)	−0.095 (0.999)
femur, mode 4	−0.064 (0.993)	0.088 (0.956)
femur, mode 5	−0.067 (1.043)	−0.009 (0.932)
femur, mode 6	0.048 (1.028)	−0.021 (0.975)
femur, mode 7	0.025 (1.022)	−0.013 (0.994)
femur, mode 8	−0.014 (0.983)	−0.023 (0.983)
femur, mode 9	−0.004 (0.987)	0.080 (0.964)
femur, mode 10	−0.094 (1.001)	0.060 (0.968)
femur, mode 11	−0.058 (1.027)	0.020 (0.975)
femur, mode 12	−0.035 (1.020)	0.017 (0.940)
femur, mode 13	0.001 (1.027)	0.036 (0.960)

sex on risk of knee ROA in each significant mode was smaller than 1, suggesting that effect of being a woman on bone shape modestly protected them from developing incident knee ROA.

Discussion

This study confirmed that bone shape in both the tibia and femur differ by sex and that knee bone shape is associated with incident knee ROA. In addition, we made a novel observation that some distal femur and proximal tibia shapes appear to protect women from developing knee OA.

In this study, women had a 49% increased odds of incident ROA compared with men. Our results are in the same range as other reports of sex differences in incident ROA. Felson et al. reported that women had an 80% increased odds of incident ROA in the Framingham group over approximately 9 years, while Muraki et al. reported women had a 58–60% increased odds (depending on K/L grade) of incident ROA over 3.3 years in a Japanese cohort [20, 21]. These study results provide face validity for the current study.

We previously found that femoral mode 4, which mediated the relation of sex with incident knee OA in the current study, was also found to have a borderline significance for difference by sex among persons without OA

[11]. Similarly, tibial mode 2 was found to be a mediator for incident knee OA in the current study and represents the same type of shape difference as tibial mode 3 in the prior study of persons without knee ROA, and was found to be significantly different between women and men there. Tibial mode 10 in the present study is similar to tibial mode 10 in the prior study, which was borderline for significant difference by sex. All of these modes that confirm prior related study findings of difference by sex support the validity of our current findings.

The most interesting finding of the current study is that all 3 identified mediating bone shapes exerted a protective effect between sex and incident OA, although the effect size is relatively modest in each case and this size is small enough that there remains some inferential uncertainty as to their meaning. This was an unanticipated finding as bone shape in normal knees is primarily determined by genetics, including chromosomal sex determination [6, 22–26], but the genetic determination of a factor such as bone shape is present prior to exposure to deleterious factors that cause OA, such as pregnancies [9], hormonal effects [27], and joint injuries [28]. Given that these risk factors for OA are common and have existed throughout human evolution, it is likely that natural selection and the evolutionary process would result over time in the appearance of genetic

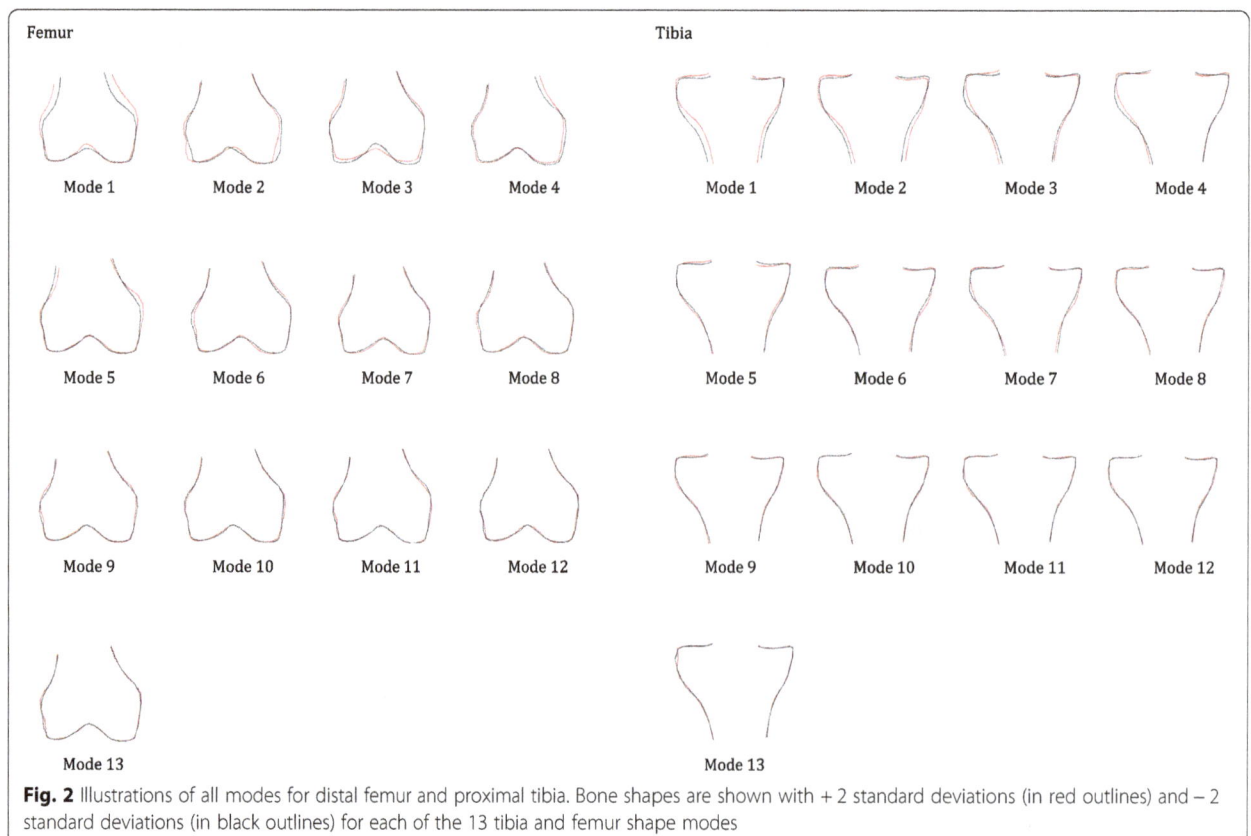

Fig. 2 Illustrations of all modes for distal femur and proximal tibia. Bone shapes are shown with + 2 standard deviations (in red outlines) and − 2 standard deviations (in black outlines) for each of the 13 tibia and femur shape modes

factors (such as bone shape) that could mitigate or protect against risks for OA.

It is not possible to say definitively what elements of the shape difference explain the finding of a protective effect for women without further work. Nonetheless, we did observe that femoral mode 4 primarily involves differences in the relative angle of the condyles to the shaft, with a concomitant alteration of the relative elevation of the articular surface of the medial and lateral condyles. Tibial modes 2 and 10 also appear to involve alterations in the relation of the shaft to the head, again with coincident inverse differences in the relative elevation of the medial versus lateral tibial plateau. With the exception of tibial mode 5, none of the other modes display these types of inverse differences in articular surface elevations. These observations lead us

to hypothesize that with activity, knee shape causes force to be offloaded in a compartment-specific manner that may produce the protective effect.

Several prior studies have reported differences in knee bone shape between women and men using a variety of radiographic and measurement approaches [6, 7, 29–31], and each of these studies has reported that men have larger femoral condyle width than women as one of their primary findings. This basic shape difference corresponds with femoral mode 1 in the current study, which was not found to mediate the relationship between sex and incident OA. Other studies have also reported 33–42% greater cartilage volume in men than in women [32], similar to the larger size condyles, but there has been controversy over whether baseline cartilage volume is associated with incident OA [33, 34], and this

Table 3 Bone shape mode and sex, incident knee ROA

Mode	Association of mode and incident knee ROA		Mode among knees without incident ROA, by gender	
	OR (95% C.I.)*	p-value	Men Mean (SD)	Women Mean (SD)
tibia, mode 1	1.12(0.97,1.29)	0.130	−0.06 (0.93)	−0.11 (1.02)
tibia, mode 2	1.18(1.03,1.37)	0.021	0.20 (1.00)	−0.23 (0.94)**
tibia, mode 3	0.99(0.87,1.13)	0.868	−0.25 (1.05)	0.22 (0.92)**
tibia, mode 4	0.95(0.83,1.09)	0.496	0.001 (0.93)	−0.03 (1.00)
tibia, mode 5	1.12(0.97,1.28)	0.117	0.02 (0.94)	−0.13 (0.97)
tibia, mode 6	0.94(0.82,1.08)	0.400	−0.07 (1.06)	0.05 (0.91)
tibia, mode 7	1.06(0.92,1.22)	0.445	−0.17 (1.05)	0.03 (0.93)
tibia, mode 8	0.94(0.82,1.08)	0.387	0.30 (0.89)	−0.13 (0.07)**
tibia, mode 9	1.15(1.00,1.32)	0.042	−0.06 (1.11)	−0.09 (1.00)
tibia, mode 10	0.79(0.67,0.93)	0.006	−0.21 (0.98)	0.25 (0.98)**
tibia, mode 11	1.04(0.90,1.19)	0.598	0.27 (1.03)	−0.20 (0.91)**
tibia, mode 12	0.86(0.75,0.99)	0.031	−0.004 (1.08)	0.06 (1.04)
tibia, mode 13	0.94(0.82,1.08)	0.381	0.05 (1.01)	0.09 (1.02)
femur, mode 1	1.05(0.90,1.21)	0.552	−0.54 (0.92)	0.30 (0.91)**
femur, mode 2	1.00(0.88,1.15)	0.943	−0.04 (0.86)	0.10 (0.95)
femur, mode 3	1.11(0.96,1.29)	0.170	−0.13 (1.01)	−0.07 (1.02)
femur, mode 4	0.85(0.73,0.98)	0.025	−0.21 (1.00)	0.30 (0.89)**
femur, mode 5	0.95(0.83,1.09)	0.468	0.16 (0.95)	−0.12 (0.91)**
femur, mode 6	1.11(0.97,1.27)	0.147	−0.15 (1.00)	0.02 (0.95)
femur, mode 7	1.01(0.88,1.15)	0.912	0.08 (0.98)	−0.08 (1.01)
femur, mode 8	0.93(0.81,1.08)	0.339	−0.21 (1.01)	0.10 (0.95)**
femur, mode 9	1.01(0.88,1.16)	0.899	0.11 (0.97)	0.02 (0.96)
femur, mode 10	0.81(0.70,0.94)	0.005	−0.09 (0.98)	0.21 (0.95)
femur, mode 11	0.93(0.81,1.06)	0.276	0.04 (0.91)	0.01 (1.01)
femur, mode 12	0.95(0.83,1.08)	0.423	−0.12 (0.83)	0.14 (0.98)**
femur, mode 13	0.94(0.81,1.09)	0.380	0.14 (1.01)	−0.08 (0.90)**

Total effect of sex (women vs. men): OR (95% CI)*= 1.49 (1.04, 2.12)
*Adjusting for age, BMI, race, clinic site, knee injury and surgery
**p-value < 0.05

Table 4 Mediation analysis results, including indirect and direct effect for each mode

Mediator effect of mode on sex and incident knee ROA	Indirect effect		Direct effect	
	OR (95% C.I.)*	p-value	OR (95% C.I.)*	p-value
tibia, mode 1	1.00(0.99,1.00)	0.322	1.50(1.03,2.16)	0.033
tibia, mode 2	0.96(0.91,1.00)	0.043	1.56(1.08,2.27)	0.019
tibia, mode 3	0.99(0.97,1.02)	0.642	1.49(1.03,2.16)	0.033
tibia, mode 4	1.00(1.00,1.00)	0.724	1.49(1.03,2.15)	0.035
tibia, mode 5	0.99(0.99,1.00)	0.207	1.49(1.03,2.16)	0.034
tibia, mode 6	0.99(0.98,1.01)	0.576	1.50(1.04,2.18)	0.030
tibia, mode 7	1.00(0.99,1.02)	0.560	1.48(1.02,2.13)	0.038
tibia, mode 8	1.01(0.99,1.03)	0.533	1.46(1.01,2.12)	0.042
tibia, mode 9	0.99(0.99,1.00)	0.119	1.50(1.04,2.17)	0.032
tibia, mode 10	0.96(0.92,1.00)	0.034	1.53(1.05,2.21)	0.025
tibia, mode 11	0.98(0.94,1.02)	0.246	1.53(1.06,2.22)	0.024
tibia, mode 12	0.99(0.99,1.00)	0.145	1.50(1.04,2.17)	0.032
tibia, mode 13	1.00(1.00,1.00)	0.244	1.49(1.03,2.15)	0.035
femur, mode 1	1.03(0.95,1.12)	0.441	1.44(0.98,2.09)	0.061
femur, mode 2	1.00(0.99,1.01)	0.779	1.47(1.01,2.12)	0.042
femur, mode 3	1.01(0.99,1.03)	0.266	1.45(1.00,2.10)	0.049
femur, mode 4	0.97(0.94,1.00)	0.045	1.50(1.03,2.17)	0.034
femur, mode 5	1.01(0.98,1.04)	0.647	1.47(1.01,2.13)	0.043
femur, mode 6	1.00(1.00,1.00)	0.265	1.46(1.01,2.12)	0.043
femur, mode 7	1.00(0.98,1.01)	0.741	1.47(1.01,2.12)	0.042
femur, mode 8	0.98(0.95,1.02)	0.340	1.50(1.03,2.18)	0.032
femur, mode 9	1.00(1.00,1.00)	0.970	1.46(1.01,2.12)	0.043
femur, mode 10	0.97(0.94,1.00)	0.061	1.50(1.03,2.17)	0.034
femur, mode 11	1.01(1.00,1.01)	0.226	1.46(1.01,2.11)	0.046
femur, mode 12	0.99(0.97,1.01)	0.412	1.47(1.02,2.13)	0.040
femur, mode 13	1.01(0.99,1.02)	0.406	1.46(1.01,2.11)	0.046

Total effect of sex (women vs. men): OR (95% CI)*= 1.49 (1.04, 2.12)
*Adjusting for age, race, clinic site, knee injury and surgery, and BMI
**p-value < 0.05

is complicated by the fact that women may lose cartilage with age more rapidly than men [35]. Thus, the relationship between sex and bone/cartilage size and incident OA are unclear and complex, and the fact that we found no mediating effect for femoral mode 1 suggests that simple condylar size differences are not responsible for the relationship between sex and incident OA. The current study's report of differences in the relation of the head to the shaft of both femur and tibia as being a mediating factor has not been reported before and identifies a new and potentially fruitful avenue for investigation.

Other joints also display complex relationships between bone shape and OA. In the hip joint, it has long been known that shape abnormalities are associated with radiographic OA [36, 37], and more recently SSM

techniques have been employed to establish shapes that are associated with OA [38, 39], but in these studies there has been no examination of differences by sex, let alone shape-related mediation of the association of sex with hip OA. However, the multiple reports of shapes and shape modes predating incident OA establish the concept that genetic variants in bone shape alter the mechanical milieu in a joint and its predisposition to OA. A prior report of differences in the shape of the proximal femur found specific shape modes in the hip were associated with compartment-specific knee osteoarthritis, but that there was no interaction by sex [16]; because shape differences in the hip might affect the knee through alterations of femur shaft biomechanics, the current finding of differences in head orientation to shaft in the femur mediating sex-OA associations is of even greater interest, and suggest the possibility that protective knee bone shapes may have arisen in opposition to mechanical forces that develop at a distance in the bones.

We did not perform sensitivity analyses in the current study. Confounding on the association between sex and knee ROA, sex and bone shape, bone shape and knee ROA all can bias the direct and indirect effect estimates. This makes sensitivity analyses in mediation analysis complex. To make things simple, we calculated E-value for the total, direct and indirect effect based on confounding on the association between sex and knee ROA. E-value is a recently developed measure of the minimum strength of association, on the risk ratio scale, that an unmeasured confounder would need to have with both the treatment and the outcome to fully explain away a specific treatment–outcome association, conditional on the measured covariates [40]. The total effect of sex on incident knee OA was 1.49, and the E-value was 2.34, i.e., the total effect could be explained away by an unmeasured confounder that was associated with both the sex and incident knee OA by a risk ratio of 2.34 fold each or larger. The direct and indirect effect of sex on incident knee OA, for example through tibia mode 2, were 1.56 and 0.96, and the corresponding E-values were 2.49 and 1.25, respectively. However, we do not know of any genetic factor(s) with an RR ≥ 1.25 [41]; thus it is unlikely there is a confounding factor of this size or larger.

The current study has several strengths. We used the OAI cohort, in which radiograph acquisition and reading are standardized and reliable, and in which clinical and demographic characteristics are reliably collected at each time point. Furthermore, the OAI is diverse and representative of populations of both whites and African Americans and thus this study can be considered to be generalizable to persons at risk of knee OA in United States. Lastly, the internal inter- and intra-rater reliability numbers for the SSM for the current study are very good.

The study also has a few limitations. Positioning of study subjects for radiographs could influence the SSM findings which could lead to a misclassification bias; this is despite the extensive efforts made to standardize positioning, beam angle and other elements of radiograph acquisition. The SSM process itself includes a component that is operator dependent which may introduce human error with the potential for unknown effects on derived bone shapes. Final knee alignment data for the entire cohort (including most of the selected knees in this study) was not available at the time of this analysis, so adjustment for this was not possible. Finally, there may have been early OA in the knees chosen even at baseline which was not radiographically observable, but which still might have biased our findings.

Conclusions

In summary, femoral and tibial knee shapes differ by sex and are associated with incident knee ROA. The shapes of the distal femur and proximal tibia partially and inconsistently mediate the relationship between sex and incident knee OA. Although women had increased risk of incident ROA, their bone shape modestly protects them from having even higher risk.

Abbreviations
95% C.I.: 95% confidence interval; BMI: Body mass index; KL: Kellgren/Lawrence; MSM: Marginal structural model; OA: Osteoarthritis; OAI: Osteoarthritis Initiative; OR: Odds ratio; ROA: Radiographic osteoarthritis; SSM: Statistical Shape Modeling

Acknowledgments
The authors thank the participants in the Osteoarthritis Initiative.

Funding
This work was supported by the following funding sources: the Center for Musculoskeletal Health at University of California, Davis School of Medicine; Nancy Lane support by NIH K24 AR048841; Barton Wise and Nancy Lane support by NIH P50 AR060752; NIH P50 AR063043; and the Endowed Chair for Aging at University of California, Davis School of Medicine. The Osteoarthritis Initiative (OAI) is a public–private partnership comprised of 5 contracts (N01-AR-2-2258, N01-AR-2-2259, N01-AR-2-2260, N01-AR-2-2261, and N01-AR-2-2262) funded by the NIH, a branch of the Department of Health and Human Services, and conducted by the OAI Study Investigators. Private funding partners include Pfizer, Novartis Pharmaceuticals, Merck Research Laboratories, and Glaxo-SmithKline. Private sector funding for the OAI is managed by the Foundation for the NIH.

Authors' contributions
Conception and design: BLW, JAL, YZ, NEL. Analysis and interpretation of data: BLW, FL, JAL, JN, YZ, NEL. Drafting of the article: BLW, JN, YZ, NEL. Critical revision of the article for important intellectual content: BLW, FL, JP, JAL, JN, YZ, NEL. Final approval of the article: BLW, FL, LK, JAL, JN, YZ, NEL. Collection and assembly of data: BLW, FL, JP, JAL. Obtaining funding: BLW, NEL. All authors read and approved the final manuscript.

Competing interests
Dr. Wise had an unrelated research analysis contract with Pfizer, Inc., over five years ago. The other authors declare that they have no competing interests.

Author details
[1]Department of Internal Medicine, University of California, Davis School of Medicine, Sacramento, CA, USA. [2]Department of Orthopaedic Surgery, University of California, Davis School of Medicine, Sacramento, CA, USA. [3]Boston University School of Medicine, Boston, MA, USA. [4]Department of Epidemiology and Biostatistics, University of California, San Francisco, San Francisco, CA, USA. [5]University of New Mexico School of Medicine, Albuquerque, NM, USA. [6]Center for Musculoskeletal Health, Departments of Orthopaedic Surgery and Internal Medicine, University of California, Davis School of Medicine, 4625 2nd Avenue, Suite 2002, Sacramento, CA 95817, USA.

References
1. Lawrence RC, Felson DT, Helmick CG, Arnold LM, Choi H, Deyo RA, et al. Estimates of the prevalence of arthritis and other rheumatic conditions in the United States. Part II. Arthritis Rheum. 2008;58:26–35.
2. Skousgaard SG, Skytthe A, Moller S, Overgaard S, Brandt LP. Sex differences in risk and heritability estimates on primary knee osteoarthritis leading to total knee arthroplasty: a nationwide population based follow up study in Danish twins. Arthritis Res Ther. 2016;18:46.

3. Srikanth VK, Fryer JL, Zhai G, Winzenberg TM, Hosmer D, Jones G. A meta-analysis of sex differences prevalence, incidence and severity of osteoarthritis. Osteoarthr Cartil. 2005;13:769–81.

4. Wise BL, Niu J, Yang M, Lane NE, Harvey W, Felson DT, et al. Patterns of compartment involvement in tibiofemoral osteoarthritis in men and women and in whites and African Americans. Arthritis Care Res (Hoboken). 2012;64:847–52.

5. Cicuttini F, Forbes A, Morris K, Darling S, Bailey M, Stuckey S. Gender differences in knee cartilage volume as measured by magnetic resonance imaging. Osteoarthr Cartil. 1999;7:265–71.

6. Mahfouz M, Abdel Fatah EE, Bowers LS, Scuderi G. Three-dimensional morphology of the knee reveals ethnic differences. Clin Orthop Relat Res. 2012;470:172–85.

7. Bellemans J, Carpentier K, Vandenneucker H, Vanlauwe J, Victor J. The John Insall award both Morphotype and gender influence the shape of the knee in patients undergoing TKA. Clin Orthop Relat Res. 2010;468:29–36.

8. Felson DT, Lawrence RC, Dieppe PA, Hirsch R, Helmick CG, Jordan JM, et al. Osteoarthritis: new insights. Part 1: the disease and its risk factors. Ann Intern Med. 2000;133:635–46.

9. Wise BL, Niu J, Zhang Y, Felson DT, Bradley LA, Segal N, et al. The association of parity with osteoarthritis and knee replacement in the multicenter osteoarthritis study. Osteoarthr Cartil. 2013;21:1849–54.

10. Sharma L, Lou C, Cahue S, Dunlop DD. The mechanism of the effect of obesity in knee osteoarthritis: the mediating role of malalignment. Arthritis Rheum. 2000;43:568–75.

11. Wise BL, Liu F, Kritikos L, Lynch JA, Parimi N, Zhang Y, et al. The association of distal femur and proximal tibia shape with sex: the osteoarthritis initiative. Semin Arthritis Rheum. 2016;46:20–6.

12. Lonner JH, Jasko JG, Thomas BS. Anthropomorphic differences between the distal femora of men and women. Clin Orthop Relat Res. 2008;466:2724–9.

13. Haverkamp DJ, Schiphof D, Bierma-Zeinstra SM, Weinans H, Waarsing JH. Variation in joint shape of osteoarthritic knees. Arthritis Rheum. 2011;63(11):3401-7.

14. Neogi T, Bowes MA, Niu J, De Souza KM, Vincent GR, Goggins J, et al. Magnetic resonance imaging-based three-dimensional bone shape of the knee predicts onset of knee osteoarthritis: data from the osteoarthritis initiative. Arthritis Rheum. 2013;65:2048–58.

15. Kellgren JH, Lawrence JS. Radiological assessment of osteo-arthrosis. Ann Rheum Dis. 1957;16:494–502.

16. Wise BL, Kritikos L, Lynch JA, Liu F, Parimi N, Tileston KL, et al. Proximal femur shape differs between subjects with lateral and medial knee osteoarthritis and controls: the osteoarthritis initiative. Osteoarthr Cartil. 2014;22:2067–73.

17. Lynch JA, Parimi N, Chaganti RK, Nevitt MC, Lane NE, Study of Osteoporotic Fractures Research G. The association of proximal femoral shape and incident radiographic hip OA in elderly women. Osteoarthr Cartil. 2009;17:1313–8.

18. Deurenberg P, Weststrate JA, Seidell JC. Body mass index as a measure of body fatness: age- and sex-specific prediction formulas. Br J Nutr. 1991;65:105–14.

19. Lange T, Vansteelandt S, Bekaert M. A simple unified approach for estimating natural direct and indirect effects. Am J Epidemiol. 2012;176:190–5.

20. Felson DT, Zhang Y, Hannan MT, Naimark A, Weissman B, Aliabadi P, et al. Risk factors for incident radiographic knee osteoarthritis in the elderly: the Framingham study. Arthritis Rheum. 1997;40:728–33.

21. Muraki S, Akune T, Oka H, Ishimoto Y, Nagata K, Yoshida M, et al. Incidence and risk factors for radiographic knee osteoarthritis and knee pain in Japanese men and women: a longitudinal population-based cohort study. Arthritis Rheum. 2012;64:1447–56.

22. Zhai G, Ding C, Stankovich J, Cicuttini F, Jones G. The genetic contribution to longitudinal changes in knee structure and muscle strength: a sibpair study. Arthritis Rheum. 2005;52:2830 4.

23. Zhai G, Stankovich J, Ding C, Scott F, Cicuttini F, Jones G. The genetic contribution to muscle strength, knee pain, cartilage volume, bone size, and radiographic osteoarthritis: a sibpair study. Arthritis Rheum. 2004;50:805–10.

24. Yue B, Varadarajan KM, Ai S, Tang T, Rubash HE, Li G. Differences of knee anthropometry between Chinese and white men and women. J Arthroplast. 2011;26:124–30.

25. Zengin A, Pye SR, Cook MJ, Adams JE, Wu FC, O'Neill TW, et al. Ethnic differences in bone geometry between white, black and South Asian men in the UK. Bone. 2016;91:180–5.

26. Christians JK, de Zwaan DR, Fung SH. Pregnancy associated plasma protein A2 (PAPP-A2) affects bone size and shape and contributes to natural variation in postnatal growth in mice. PLoS One. 2013;8:e56260.

27. Liu B, Balkwill A, Cooper C, Roddam A, Brown A, Beral V, et al. Reproductive history, hormonal factors and the incidence of hip and knee replacement for osteoarthritis in middle-aged women. Ann Rheum Dis. 2009;68:1165–70.

28. Felson DT. Osteoarthritis as a disease of mechanics. Osteoarthr Cartil. 2013;21:10–5.

29. Yan M, Wang J, Wang Y, Zhang J, Yue B, Zeng Y. Gender-based differences in the dimensions of the femoral trochlea and condyles in the Chinese population: correlation to the risk of femoral component overhang. Knee. 2014;21:252–6.

30. Yang B, Yu JK, Zheng ZZ, Lu ZH, Zhang JY. Comparative study of sex differences in distal femur morphology in osteoarthritic knees in a Chinese population. PLoS One. 2014;9:e89394.

31. Yue B, Varadarajan KM, Ai S, Tang T, Rubash HE, Li G. Gender differences in the knees of Chinese population. Knee Surg Sports Traumatol Arthrosc. 2011;19:80–8.

32. Ding C, Cicuttini F, Scott F, Glisson M, Jones G. Sex differences in knee cartilage volume in adults: role of body and bone size, age and physical activity. Rheumatology (Oxford). 2003;42:1317–23.

33. Ding C, Cicuttini F, Blizzard L, Jones G. Genetic mechanisms of knee osteoarthritis: a population-based longitudinal study. Arthritis Res Ther. 2006;8:R8.

34. Jones G, Ding C, Scott F, Cicuttini F. Genetic mechanisms of knee osteoarthritis: a population based case-control study. Ann Rheum Dis. 2004;63:1255–9.

35. Ding C, Cicuttini F, Blizzard L, Scott F, Jones G. A longitudinal study of the effect of sex and age on rate of change in knee cartilage volume in adults. Rheumatology (Oxford). 2007;46:273–9.

36. Harris WH. Etiology of osteoarthritis of the hip. Clin Orthop Relat Res. 1986;213:20-33.

37. Murray RO. The aetiology of primary osteoarthritis of the hip. Br J Radiol. 1965;38:810–24.

38. Gregory JS, Waarsing JH, Day J, Pols HA, Reijman M, Weinans H, et al. Early identification of radiographic osteoarthritis of the hip using an active shape model to quantify changes in bone morphometric features: can hip shape tell us anything about the progression of osteoarthritis? Arthritis Rheum. 2007;56:3634–43.

39. Waarsing JH, Rozendaal RM, Verhaar JA, Bierma-Zeinstra SM, Weinans H. A statistical model of shape and density of the proximal femur in relation to radiological and clinical OA of the hip. Osteoarthr Cartil. 2010;18:787–94.

40. VanderWeele TJ, Ding P. Sensitivity analysis in observational research: introducing the E-value. Ann Intern Med. 2017;167:268–74.

41. Rodriguez-Fontenla C, Calaza M, Evangelou E, Valdes AM, Arden N, Blanco FJ, et al. Assessment of osteoarthritis candidate genes in a meta-analysis of nine genome-wide association studies. Arthritis Rheumatol. 2014;66:940–9.

10

Clinical and radiographic outcomes of cervical disc arthroplasty with Prestige-LP Disc: a minimum 6-year follow-up study

Junfeng Zeng[1], Hao Liu[1*], Xin Rong[1], Beiyu Wang[1], Yi Yang[1], Xinlin Gao[1], Tingkui Wu[1] and Ying Hong[2]

Abstract

Background: Cervical disc arthroplasty (CDA) has been considered as an alternative to cervical arthrodesis in the treatment of cervical degenerative disc diseases (CDDD). The aim of this study was to assess the long-term clinical and radiographic outcomes of CDA with Prestige-LP Disc.

Methods: A total of 61 patients who underwent single- or two-level CDA with Prestige-LP Disc were retrospectively investigated at a minimum of 6-year follow-up. Clinical assessments included visual analogue scale (VAS) for neck and arm pain, Neck Disability Index (NDI), and Japanese Orthopedic Association (JOA) score. Radiological evaluations included range of motion (ROM) of the index and adjacent levels, segmental angle, cervical sagittal alignment, heterotopic ossification (HO) and adjacent segment degeneration (ASD).

Results: Significant and maintained improvement in VAS for neck and arm, NDI and JOA were observed after a mean follow-up of 82.3 months ($p < 0.001$). The preoperative ROM of the index level was 9.7°, which was maintained at 2-and 4-year follow-up (9.3°, $p = 0.597$; 9.0°, $p = 0.297$), but was decreased to 8.0° at final follow-up ($p = 0.019$). Mobility was maintained in 80.5% (62/77) of the implanted prostheses at final follow-up. ROM of the superior and inferior adjacent segments, cervical sagittal alignment and cervical angel were all maintained. The incidence of HO was 42.9% at final follow-up, but it did not influence the clinical outcome. Radiographic ASD were detected in 29.5% of the patients. However, the incidence of symptomatic ASD was only 6.6%.

Conclusion: Cervical disc arthroplasty with Prestige-LP Disc demonstrated a maintained and satisfactory clinical outcome at a minimal of 6-year follow-up, with majority of the prostheses remained mobile. Cervical disc arthroplasty with Prestige-LP Dis can be considered as an effective surgical method in treating CDDD.

Keywords: Cervical disc arthroplasty, Prestige-LP Disc, Cervical degenerative disc disease, Heterotopic ossification, Adjacent segment degeneration

Background

Anterior cervical discectomy and fusion (ACDF) has been considered as golden standard surgical procedure in the treatment of cervical degenerative disc disease (CDDD). However, biomechanical study suggested that fusion of the operated level may increase the stress at the adjacent level [1], and accelerate the degeneration of adjacent segment. In the 10-year postoperative follow-up study, Hilibrand et al. [2] reported that the incidence of

symptomatic adjacent segment degeneration (ASD) was 2.9% per year after the cervical fusion surgery, and 25.6% of the patients developed symptomatic ASD within 10 years postoperatively.

Cervical disc arthroplasty (CDA) has been established as an alternative to ACDF for treating CDDD over the past decade. Previous studies have demonstrated that CDA achieved equivalent clinical outcome compared with ACDF [3–8]. Cervical disc arthroplasty was developed to maintain motion at the operated segment and theoretically slow down or avoid the occurrence of ASD. However, long-term clinical results and functional sustainability still need to be proven. Moreover, heterotopic

* Correspondence: liuhaosurgery@126.com
[1]Department of Orthopedics, West China Hospital, Sichuan University, 37 Guoxue Lane, Chengdu 610041, Sichuan, China
Full list of author information is available at the end of the article

ossification (HO) was reported to increase with the follow-up time [9], which may affect the mobility of the device.

Prestige-LP Disc (Medtronic, Memphis, TN, USA) was one of the artificial cervical discs approved by the Food and Drug Administration (FDA) for treating single- and two-level CDDD. The short- and mid-term results of Prestige LP Disc were satisfactory in previous studies [10–12]. To date, long-term clinical and radiographic follow-up results of Prestige-LP Disc were seldom reported, except for two FDA trails [5, 6]. The purpose of this study was to evaluate the clinical and radiographic outcomes of CDA with Prestige-LP Disc in treating single- and two-level CDDD at minimum 6-year follow-up in a single center.

Methods
Study design
The retrospective study was approved by the Ethical Committee of West China Hospital of Sichuan University, and informed consent was obtained from all of the patients. There were 78 consecutive patients underwent single- or two- level CDA with Prestige-LP Disc for the treatment of CDDD between January 2008 and July 2011 in our institution. A total of 61 patients who had completed at least 6-years follow-up were included in this study. The other 17 patients were excluded for incomplete data or lost to follow-up. Clinical and radiographic data were routinely collected preoperatively, postoperatively at 1 week and 3, 6, 12, 24, months, and biennially up to minimum of 72 months.

The inclusion criterion was patients with single- or two-level CDDD between C3 to C7 causing radiculopathy or myelopathy that did not respond to at least 6 weeks of non-operative treatment. Exclusion criteria for this study included: radiographic signs of cervical instability or severe facet joint degeneration, ossification of the posterior longitudinal ligament, prior cervical spine surgery, osteoporosis (T-score ≤ -2.5), ankylosing spondylitis, rheumatoid arthritis, tumor, trauma, infection, and metabolic bone diseases.

Prosthesis description
The Prestige-LP cervical disc is an unconstrained ball-in-trough articulation composed of titanium ceramic composite. This prosthesis serves to maintain segmental cervical motion and disc space height. The metal-on-metal prosthesis contains dual serrated kneels which are attached to vertebral bodies through impaction for fixation. The prosthesis has various combinations of depth and height for accommodating the intervertebral disc space.

Surgical procedure
All surgeries were performed by a single senior surgeon using a standard Smith-Robinson approach. A right side transverse skin incision was made at the index level. After thorough exposure, the anterior longitudinal ligament and diseased disc were completely removed, along with the posterior longitudinal ligament and osteophytes if present. After the discectomy and decompression was completed, a high-speed burr was used to carefully prepare the endplate in a flat and parallel fashion. A sized Implant Trial was used to confirm the size of the prepared disc space. Rail Cutter Guide and Bit were used to drill the fixation channels in the endplate. Prestige-LP Disc corresponding to the trial was inserted into the vertebral body. The same procedure was performed at the other level in patient with two-level CDDD. Lastly, lateral and anterior-posterior fluoroscopies were taken to ensure proper placement.

Outcome assessment
Clinical outcomes were assessed by visual analogue scale (VAS), Neck Disability Index (NDI), and Japanese Orthopedic Association (JOA) score. The VAS scores were used to evaluate the neck and arm pain. The NDI scores were used to assess the function of neck. The JOA scores were used to assess the neurological status.

Radiological examinations consisted of anteroposterior and lateral radiographs, as well as dynamic lateral radiographs. Range of motion (ROM) of the index and adjacent levels were determined on the dynamic lateral radiographs at maximum flexion and extension by measuring the disc space angle. An ROM of less than 2° was defined as failure to maintain the mobility of prosthesis [9]. Segmental angle was defined as the Cob angle of the index level which was measured on the lateral radiograph. Cervical sagittal alignment was measured by the C2–7 angle. The grade of HO was assessed according to McAfee classification [13]. Radiological evidence of ASD was defined on the lateral radiograph by any presence of the following findings: (1) new or enlarged ossification of the anterior longitudinal ligament; (2) a new or increased narrowing of the disc space > 30%; and (3) new anterior enlarged osteophyte formation [14, 15]. The radiographic assessments were conducted by two independent orthopedic surgeons.

Statistical analysis
Statistical analysis was conducted using SPSS 22.0 (SPSS Inc., Chicago, Illinois, USA). The two-tailed paired t test was used to compare pre- and postoperative results. Results between independent groups were compared using Mann-Whitney U test. Statistical significance is defined as $p < 0.05$.

Results

Patient characteristics

This study included 61 patients with a mean follow-up of 82.3 months (range, 72–108 months). There were 28 male and 33 female patients, with a mean age of 44.1 years (range, 26–62 years). A single-level CDA was performed in 45 cases and two-level CDA was performed in 16 cases. A total of 77 Prestige-LP Discs were implanted from C3/4 to C6/7 as demonstrated in Table 1.

Clinical outcomes

A statistically significant improvement in VAS, NDI and JOA scores was observed at every evaluation period (Fig. 1). The mean VAS score for neck and arm was significantly decreased from 6.0 ± 2.2 and 6.2 ± 2.5 preoperatively to 2.0 ± 1.4 ($p < 0.001$) and 1.9 ± 1.4 ($p < 0.001$) at final follow-up, respectively. The average preoperative NDI score was 33.9 ± 10.1, which was significantly decreased to 12.9 ± 5.4 ($p < 0.001$) at final follow-up. The NDI scores revealed a mean improvement of 21 points at final follow-up. The overall NDI success rate was 83.6% (at least 15 points improvement based on the FDA criteria). Likewise, the mean JOA score significantly increased from 10.7 ± 1.9 preoperatively to 14.5 ± 1.4 ($p < 0.001$) at final follow-up.

Radiological outcomes

Radiological outcomes regarding cervical alignment and ROM are presented in Table 2. The average preoperative cervical sagittal alignment and cervical angle were

Table 1 Characteristics of patients

Characteristics	
No. of patients	61
Gender	
Male	28 (45.9%)
Female	33 (54.1%)
Age (years)	44.1 ± 6.7
Follow-up (months)	82.3 ± 9.6
Diagnosis	
Radiculopathy	31 (50.8%)
Myelopathy	17 (27.9%)
Radiculopathy & Myelopathy	13 (21.3%)
Single-level surgery	45 (73.8%)
Two-level surgery	16 (26.2%)
Level of surgery	
C3/4	1 (1.3%)
C4/5	13 (16.9%)
C5/6	39 (50.6%)
C6/7	24 (31.2%)
Total number of implants	77

$10.5 \pm 9.3°$ and $3.1 \pm 2.2°$, which were maintained at $11.0 \pm 9.7°$ and $2.9 \pm 3.6°$ at final follow-up ($p = 0.658$ and $p = 0.591$), respectively. The mean ROM of the index level was $9.7 \pm 4.7°$ preoperatively and was maintained at $9.3 \pm 5.8°$ and $9.0 \pm 5.1°$ at 2- and 4-year follow-up ($p = 0.597$ and $p = 0.297$), while it was significantly decreased to $8.0 \pm 5.6°$ at final follow-up ($p = 0.019$). Mobility of the prosthesis was maintained in 80.5% (62/77) of the operated segments at final follow-up (Fig. 2). There were no significant differences in ROM of superior and inferior levels between pre-operation and final follow-up ($p = 0.434$ and $p = 0.463$) (Table 2).

According to the McAfee classification, the incidence of HO was 23.4% (18/77) and 42.9% (33/77) at 2-year and final follow-up, respectively (Table 3). There were 10 levels (13.0%) with grade 3 HO, and 8 (10.4%) with grade 4 at final follow-up (Fig. 3). The mean ROM for HO group was significant lower than that of non-HO group at final-follow-up (9.5° vs 5.9°, $p = 0.001$). However, no significant differences were seen in VAS for neck and arm, NDI and JOA scores between HO group and non-HO group ($p = 0.349$, $p = 0.750$, $p = 0.407$, and $p = 0.917$).

In addition, radiological evidence of ASD was observed in 29.5% (18/61) of the patients at final follow-up. The ASD at inferior level was detected in 18 cases, and 3 cases with ASD at superior level. Symptomatic ASD was found in 4 patients (6.6%). Three patients complained neck pain and one patients complained arm pain. All four patients were successfully treated by conservative treatment. No patients required a revision surgery. No prosthesis dislocation or failure was seen in all the 77 implanted prosthesis.

Discussion

Cervical disc arthroplasty has been accepted as an alternative surgical method for treating CDDD. Previous clinical studies have demonstrated satisfactory short- and mid-term results of CDA with Prestige-LP Disc [10–12]. In our present study, favorable and stable clinical outcome was seen at a minimal of 6-year follow-up. Clinical outcome parameters, including VAS for neck and arm, NDI, and JOA scores, were all significantly improved and maintained at all postoperative evaluation periods compared with those of preoperatively. Similar results were seen in other long-term studies with various types of cervical artificial disc [5–9]. We found an NDI success rate of 83.6%, which was also comparable to the NDI success rate of 86.1% [5] and 87.0% [6] in the two FDA studies. The reported incidence of prosthesis dislocation after CDA varied from 3.1 to 19.6% [9, 16, 17]. No serious adverse events including prosthesis dislocation or failure were occurred in the present study. Our study confirmed that CDA with Prestige-LP Disc can

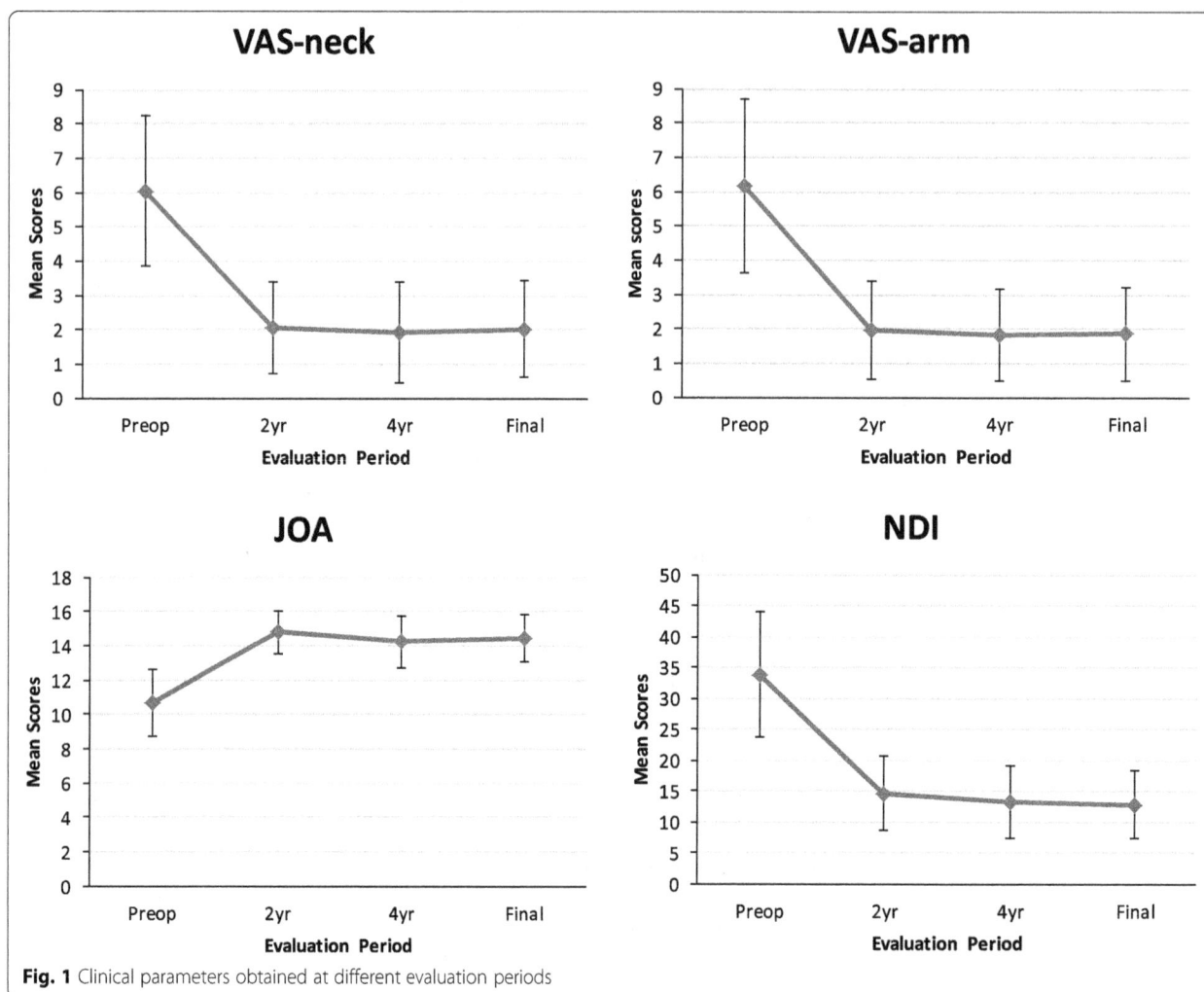

Fig. 1 Clinical parameters obtained at different evaluation periods

yield satisfactory long-term clinical outcome in treating CDDD.

As cervical disc arthroplasty was designed to preserve motion at the operated level and avoid hypermobility of the adjacent segments, long-term functionality is particularly important. Our study demonstrated that 80.5% of the prosthesis maintained mobile and the mean ROM of the operated level was 8.0° after a mean follow-up of 82.3 months. In addition, cervical sagittal alignment and cervical angle were well maintained. Similarly, Gornet et al.

reported a mean operated segmental ROM of 6.78° after single-level Prestige-LP Discs implantation at 84-month follow-up [5]. Lanman et al. reported both the ROM at superior and inferior operated level was above 6° after two-level Prestige-LP disc arthroplasty at 84-month follow-up [6]. Dejaegher et al. reported that 81% of the Bryan cervical disc remained mobile with a mean ROM of 8.6° at 8-year follow-up [7]. In addition, in a 15-year follow-up study of Bryan disc arthroplasty, Pointillart et al. reported that 68.2% (15/22) of the prosthesis maintained

Table 2 Pre- and post-operative mean cervical alignment and range of motion

	Preoperative	2-year FU	4-year FU	Final FU
Cervical sagittal alignment(°)	10.5 ± 9.3	11.5 ± 9.1	11.4 ± 10.3	11.0 ± 9.7
Segmental angle(°)	3.1 ± 2.2	3.0 ± 3.0	2.8 ± 3.3	2.9 ± 3.6
ROM of operated level(°)	9.7 ± 4.7	9.3 ± 5.8	9.0 ± 5.1	8.0 ± 5.6*
ROM of superior level(°)	10.2 ± 5.1	9.9 ± 5.2	10. 1 ± 5.2	9.5 ± 5.7
ROM of inferior level(°)	10.0 ± 4.3	9.4 ± 3.7	8.8 ± 4.6	9.4 ± 4.7

FU follow-up, *ROM* range of motion
*P < 0.05, compared with preoperative

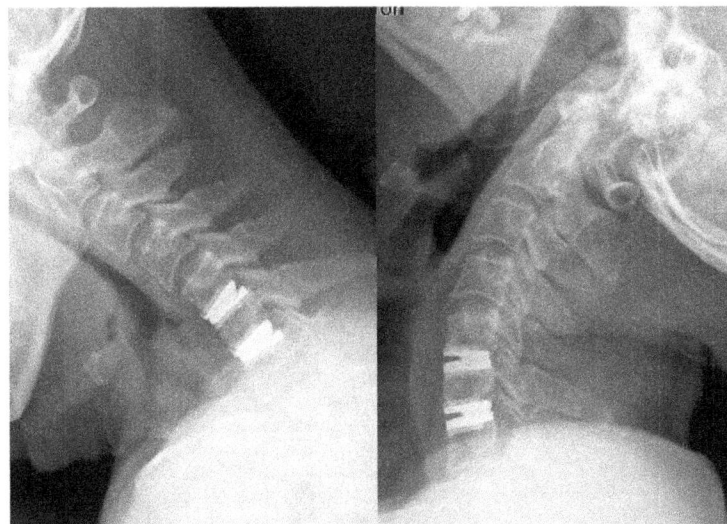

Fig. 2 Lateral flexion and extension radiographs showing satisfactory prosthesis mobility at C5/6 and C6/ 7 at 89 months after surgery

mobile with an average of 9° at final follow-up [18]. Previous studies demonstrated that both CDA and ACDF had gained good long-term clinical outcome, and most of the cervical discs remained satisfactory segmental mobility [5, 6, 19]. Furthermore, our study shown maintained ROM at the superior and inferior levels, which means no hypermobility were occurred at adjacent segments. Our data confirmed that Prestige-LP Disc arthroplasty has the potential to maintain long-term mobility at the operated level and avoid hypermobility of adjacent segments.

Heterotopic ossification is well-known occurrence after cervical disc arthroplasty. We noted that 23.4% of the prosthesis developed HO at 2-year follow-up. The incidence of HO was 42.9% at final follow-up. Our study revealed that HO rate was increased with the prolongation of follow-up time. The incidence of HO ranged from 7.7 to 90% at 6–10 years follow-up time with different types of prosthesis in other studies [8, 9, 20, 21]. The progression of HO was also reported in previous studies [8, 9, 22]. According to McAfee classification [13], HO of grade 3 and 4 can damage the ROM of the treated level. We found HO-group had lower ROM than that of non-HO group at final follow-up. However, HO did not influence clinical outcome in the present study.

Table 3 Grades of heterotopic ossification at 2-year and final-follow-up

Grade of HO	2-year follow-up	Final follow-up
0	59 (76.6%)	44 (57.1%)
1	6 (7.8%)	7 (9.1%)
2	4 (5.2%)	8 (10.4%)
3	6 (7.8%)	10 (13.0%)
4	2 (2.6%)	8 (10.4%)

The formation of HO after CDA and its effect on clinical outcome still need further studies.

It is still controversial that ASD is due to cervical fusion or simply the natural degeneration of cervical spine. Kong et al. reported that the prevalence of radiographic ASD following cervical spine surgery was 28.28% in a Meta-analysis [23]. In a 10-year follow-up of asymptomatic volunteers and patients underwent cervical fusion, Matsumoto et al. found that both ACDF patients and healthy subjects shown progression of disc degeneration, but ACDF patients had higher incidence of progression of degeneration at adjacent segments than healthy subjects [24]. Lee et al. investigated the natural history of cervical degeneration and ASD of patient underwent cervical fusion in a systematic review [25]. Similarly, they concluded that ASD may occur at a higher rate than natural cervical degeneration, and biomechanical effect of fusion may accelerate pathologic changes at adjacent segments. Previous biomechanical study also demonstrated that fusion may increase the stress at the adjacent segments, and accelerate its degeneration [1].

Cervical disc arthroplasty aims to maintain the segmental motion and then theoretically reduce or slow down the occurrence of ASD. Lower incidence of ASD were reported in other long-term studies when compared CDA with ACDF [3, 4, 26]. We found a radiographic ASD in 29.5% of the patients at final follow-up. However, only 6.6% of the patients developed symptomatic ASD. Zhao et al. reported the rate of radiographic ASD was 47.6% at 10-year follow-up after Bryan cervical disc arthroplasty [21]. Quan et al. noted 19% of patients had radiographic ASD after 8-year follow-up of Bryan disc [9]. Mehren et al. found 35.7% of the patients developed radiographic ASD at 10-year follow-up of Prodisc

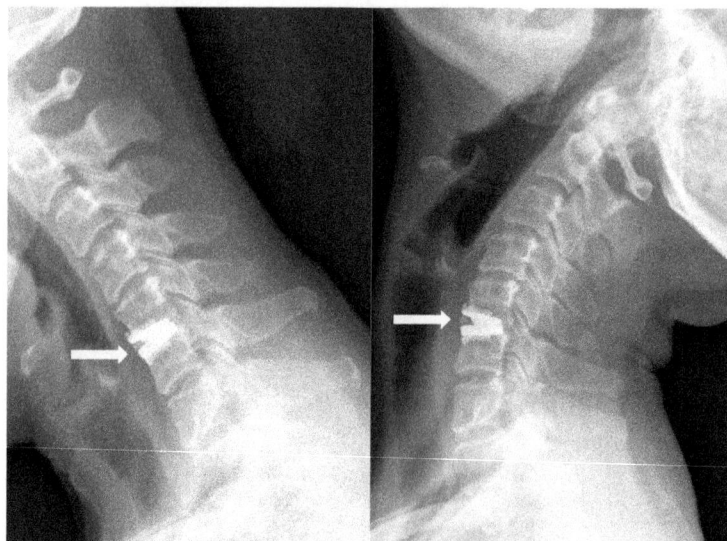

Fig. 3 Lateral flexion and extension radiographs showing heterotopic ossification at C5/6 at 72 months after surgery

C disc [8]. Whether ASD can be reduced by CDA remains to be investigated. Because HO damaged the mobility of cervical disc, the correlation between HO and ASD is of particular importance in future studies.

Our study has some limitations. Firstly, this was a retrospective study and lack of a control group. For this reason, we cannot directly compare the result with ACDF. Secondly, the sample was relatively small compared to the previous FDA studies [5, 6]. However, all of the surgeries in our study were performed by a single senior surgeon in a single center. Lastly, it is challenging to precisely evaluate the degeneration of adjacent segments without postoperative MRI imaging of cervical spine. However, we still can adequately assess ASD according to above mentioned radiographic criterion. Future randomized control trials were needed to further evaluate the functional and clinical results of CDA.

Conclusion
Cervical disc arthroplasty with Prestige-LP Disc demonstrated maintained and significant improvement in all measured clinical parameters at a minimum 6-year follow-up. Radiological evaluations shown 80.5% of the prostheses maintained mobility with a mean ROM of 8.0°. Though the incidence of HO was 42.9%, HO did not influence the clinical outcome. Hypermobility were not occurred at the adjacent segments and a low incidence of symptomatic ASD was detected. Cervical disc arthroplasty with Prestige-LP Dis can be regarded an effective surgical method in treating CDDD.

Abbreviations
ACDF: Anterior cervical discectomy and fusion; ASD: Adjacent segment degeneration; CDA: Cervical disc arthroplasty; CDDD: Cervical degenerative disc diseases; HO: Heterotopic ossification; JOA: Japanese Orthopedic Association; NDI: Neck Disability Index; ROM: Range of motion; VAS: Visual analogue scale

Acknowledgements
We thank the patients enrolled in this study.

Authors' contributions
JFZ performed the data collection and analysis and participated in manuscript writing. HL, BYW, and YY participated in the study design and coordination and helped to draft the manuscript. XLG and TKW performed statistical analysis. HL, BYW, YH, and XR performed the operations. All authors read and approved the final manuscript.

Competing interests
The authors declare that they have no competing interests.

Author details
[1]Department of Orthopedics, West China Hospital, Sichuan University, 37 Guoxue Lane, Chengdu 610041, Sichuan, China. [2]Department of Operation Room, West China Hospital, Sichuan University, Chengdu 610041, Sichuan, China.

References
1. Eck JC, Humphreys SC, Lim TH, Jeong ST, Kim JG, Hodges SD, An HS. Biomechanical study on the effect of cervical spine fusion on adjacent-level intradiscal pressure and segmental motion. Spine. 2002;27(22):2431–4.
2. Hilibrand AS, Carlson GD, Palumbo MA, Jones PK, Bohlman HH. Radiculopathy and myelopathy at segments adjacent to the site of a previous anterior cervical arthrodesis. J Bone Joint Surg Am. 1999; 81(4):519–28.
3. Burkus JK, Traynelis VC, Haid RW Jr, Mummaneni PV. Clinical and radiographic analysis of an artificial cervical disc: 7-year follow-up from the Prestige prospective randomized controlled clinical trial: clinical article. J Neurosurg Spine. 2014;21(4):516–28.
4. Hisey MS, Zigler JE, Jackson R, Nunley PD, Bae HW, Kim KD, Ohnmeiss DD. Prospective, Randomized Comparison of One-level Mobi-C Cervical Total Disc Replacement vs. Anterior Cervical Discectomy and Fusion: Results at 5-year Follow-up. Int J Spine Surg. 2016;10:10.
5. Gornet MF, Burkus JK, Shaffrey ME, Nian H, Harrell FE Jr. Cervical disc arthroplasty with Prestige LP disc versus anterior cervical discectomy and fusion: seven-year outcomes. Int J Spine Surg. 2016;10:24.
6. Lanman TH, Burkus JK, Dryer RG, Gornet MF, McConnell J, Hodges SD. Long-term clinical and radiographic outcomes of the Prestige LP artificial cervical disc replacement at 2 levels: results from a prospective randomized controlled clinical trial. J Neurosurg Spine. 2017;27:7–19.

7. Dejaegher J, Walraevens J, van Loon J, Van Calenbergh F, Demaerel P, Goffin J. 10-year follow-up after implantation of the Bryan cervical disc prosthesis. Eur Spine J. 2017;26(4):1191–8.

8. Mehren C, Heider F, Siepe CJ, Zillner B, Kothe R, Korge A, Mayer HM. Clinical and radiological outcome at 10 years of follow-up after total cervical disc replacement. Eur Spine J. 2017;26(9):2441–9.

9. Quan GM, Vital JM, Hansen S, Pointillart V. Eight-year clinical and radiological follow-up of the Bryan cervical disc arthroplasty. Spine. 2011; 36(8):639–46.

10. Gornet MF, Burkus JK, Shaffrey ME, Argires PJ, Nian H, Harrell FE Jr. Cervical disc arthroplasty with PRESTIGE LP disc versus anterior cervical discectomy and fusion: a prospective, multicenter investigational device exemption study. J Neurosurg Spine. 2015;23:558–73.

11. Gornet MF, Lanman TH, Burkus JK, Hodges SD, McConnell JR, Dryer RF, Copay AG, Nian H, Harrell FE Jr. Cervical disc arthroplasty with the Prestige LP disc versus anterior cervical discectomy and fusion, at 2 levels: results of a prospective, multicenter randomized controlled clinical trial at 24 months. J Neurosurg Spine. 2017;26:653–667.

12. Peng CW, Yue WM, Basit A, Guo CM, Tow BP, Chen JL, Nidu M, Yeo W, Tan SB. Intermediate results of the Prestige LP cervical disc replacement: clinical and radiological analysis with minimum two-year follow-up. Spine. 2011; 36(2):E105–11.

13. McAfee PC, Cunningham BW, Devine J, Williams E, Yu-Yahiro J. Classification of heterotopic ossification (HO) in artificial disk replacement. J Spinal Disord Tech. 2003;16(4):384–9.

14. Robertson JT, Papadopoulos SM, Traynelis VC. Assessment of adjacent-segment disease in patients treated with cervical fusion or arthroplasty: a prospective 2-year study. J Neurosurg Spine. 2005;3(6):417–23.

15. Lee SE, Jahng TA, Kim HJ. Correlation between cervical lordosis and adjacent segment pathology after anterior cervical spinal surgery. Eur Spine J. 2015;24(12):2899–909.

16. Lei T, Tong T, Miao D, Gao X, Xu J, Zhang D, Shen Y. Anterior migration after Bryan cervical disc arthroplasty: the relationship between hyperlordosis and its impact on clinical outcomes. World Neurosurg. 2017;101:534–539.

17. Ozbek Z, Ozkara E, Arslantas A. Implant migration in cervical disk arthroplasty. World Neurosurg. 2017;97:390–7.

18. Pointillart V, Castelain JE, Coudert P, Cawley DT, Gille O, Vital JM. Outcomes of the Bryan cervical disc replacement: fifteen year follow-up. Int Orthop. 2018;42(4):851–7.

19. Sasso WR, Smucker JD, Sasso MP, Sasso RC. Long-term clinical outcomes of cervical disc arthroplasty: a prospective, randomized, Controlled Trial. Spine. 2017;42(4):209–16.

20. Pimenta L, Oliveira L, Coutinho E, Marchi L. Bone formation in cervical Total disk replacement (CTDR) up to the 6-year follow-up: experience from 272 levels. Neurosurg Q. 2013;23(1):1–6.

21. Zhao Y, Zhang Y, Sun Y, Pan S, Zhou F, Liu Z. Application of cervical arthroplasty with Bryan cervical disc. Spine. 2016;41(2):111–5.

22. Yi S, Oh J, Choi G, Kim TY, Shin HC, Kim KN, Kim KS, Yoon DH. The fate of heterotopic ossification associated with cervical artificial disc replacement. Spine. 2014;39(25):2078–83.

23. Kong L, Cao J, Wang L, Shen Y. Prevalence of adjacent segment disease following cervical spine surgery: a PRISMA-compliant systematic review and meta-analysis. Medicine. 2016;95(27):e4171.

24. Matsumoto M, Okada E, Ichihara D, Watanabe K, Chiba K, Toyama Y, Fujiwara H, Momoshima S, Nishiwaki Y, Iwanami A, et al. Anterior cervical decompression and fusion accelerates adjacent segment degeneration: comparison with asymptomatic volunteers in a ten-year magnetic resonance imaging follow-up study. Spine. 2010;35(1):36–43.

25. Lee MJ, Dettori JR, Standaert CJ, Brodt ED, Chapman JR. The natural history of degeneration of the lumbar and cervical spines: a systematic review. Spine. 2012;37(22 Suppl):S18–30.

26. Lei T, Liu Y, Wang H, Xu J, Ma Q, Wang L, Shen Y. Clinical and radiological analysis of Bryan cervical disc arthroplasty: eight-year follow-up results compared with anterior cervical discectomy and fusion. Int Orthop. 2016; 40(6):1197–203.

11

Immediate and short-term effects of kinesiotaping on muscular activity, mobility, strength and pain after rotator cuff surgery: a crossover clinical trial

Fabienne Reynard[1]* , Philippe Vuistiner[2], Bertrand Léger[2] and Michel Konzelmann[3]

Abstract

Background: Kinesiotape (KT) is widely used in musculoskeletal rehabilitation as an adjuvant to treatment, but minimal evidence supports its use. The aim of this study is to determine the immediate and short-term effects of shoulder KT on muscular activity, mobility, strength and pain after rotator cuff surgery.

Methods: Thirty-nine subjects who underwent shoulder rotator cuff surgery were tested 6 and 12 weeks post-surgery, without tape, with KT and with a sham tape (ST). KT and ST were applied in a randomized order. For each condition, the muscular activity of the upper trapezius, three parts of the deltoid and the infraspinatus were measured during shoulder flexion, and range of motion (ROM) and pain intensity were assessed. At 12 weeks, the isometric strength at 90° of shoulder flexion, related muscular activity and pain intensity were also measured. Subjects maintained the last tape that was applied for three days and recorded the pain intensity at waking up and during the day.

Results: Modifications in muscle activity were observed with KT and with ST. Major changes in terms of decreased recruitment of the upper trapezius were observed with KT ($P < 0.001$). KT and ST also increased flexion ROM at 6 weeks ($P = 0.004$), but the differences with the no tape condition were insufficient to be clinically important. No other differences between conditions were found.

Conclusions: Shoulder taping has the potential to decrease over-activity of the upper trapezius, but no clinical benefits of KT on ROM, strength or pain were noted in a population of subjects who underwent rotator cuff surgery.

Keywords: Athletic tape, Electromyography, Rehabilitation, Musculoskeletal disorder, Shoulder

Background

Rotator cuff injury is a common source of complaint that leads to pain and decreased function. Symptomatic tears are often repaired surgically. After surgery, physical therapy is necessary to restore shoulder function. Beginning with passive shoulder joint mobility exercises, the treatment becomes more active after 6 weeks, with emphasis on active-assisted to active motion, shoulder proprioception training and sub-maximal isometric exercises. During this phase, resistance work is avoided. From week 13, progressive strengthening is possible, with proprioception and coordination tasks [1].

Rehabilitation protocols often recommend the application of kinesiotape (KT) to decrease pain and enhance motion control. KT is an elastic acrylic adhesive tape, that supports and stabilizes muscles and joints without restricting the range of motion (ROM). The application of KT over manually stretched structures causes the skin to form convolutions that lift the skin. The theory behind this method is that the convolutions facilitate the regeneration of injured tissues by increasing the interstitial space, which allows for increased lymphatic and

* Correspondence: Fabienne.Reynard@crr-suva.ch
[1]Department of Physiotherapy, Clinique romande de réadaptation Suva, Sion, Switzerland
Full list of author information is available at the end of the article

venous fluid flow. The decrease in pressure between the skin and the underlying connective tissues decompresses subcutaneous nociceptors, leading to decreased pain [2]. Other proposed benefits are 1) on muscular function, by modifying the recruitment activity patterns of the treated muscles and by increasing the strength of weakened muscles; 2) on joint function, by facilitating realignment; and 3) on sensory function, by improving joint position sense and kinaesthetic awareness [2, 3]. Indications for the use of KT are numerous, but scientific evidence remains scarce, with less evidence in favour of KT found with increasing methodological quality of the studies [4–12].

For shoulder pathologies, KT has been used in ten studies between 2007 and 2017 [13–22]. All the studies concerned shoulder impingement syndrome. KT was either compared with sham tape (ST) [13, 16–18, 20, 22], exercises [14, 15], or nonsteroidal anti-inflammatory drugs and sub-acromial corticosteroid injections [19, 21]. Different outcomes were used: questionnaires on upper extremity function and quality of life, pain, ROM and strength. Only one study used electromyography (EMG) to assess muscle activity [13]. The efficacy of KT in shoulder pathologies concern essentially pain [14, 15, 17–19], pain-free ROM [16, 19] and scapular ROM [13]. Improvements were modest in all of these studies and were limited to some spatial and temporal components. To the best of our knowledge, the effects of KT have never been studied after shoulder surgery.

Methods

Aim
The aim of this study was to investigate the immediate and short-term effects of KT on shoulder muscle activity, mobility, strength and pain in a population of subjects who underwent rotator cuff surgery. Our hypotheses were that KT would not improve muscle function, mobility, strength or pain in a clinically meaningful way.

Study design
A controlled crossover study with three treatment arms - no tape (NT) vs KT vs ST - was conducted between January 2013 and October 2016 at the Clinique romande de réadaptation Suva in Sion (Switzerland). A computer block ($n = 8$) randomization process with sealed opaque envelopes was performed to determine the order of passage of the two taping procedures. The physiotherapist who applied the tape was not blinded, but he did not participate in outcome assessment. The main investigator (first author) who collected the data was blinded, as the subjects wore long-sleeved shirts that hid the tape, and the tape was applied behind a folding screen. All subjects provided written informed consent, and all their rights were protected. The study was approved by the

regional medical ethics committee (Commission Cantonale Valaisanne d'Ethique Médicale, CCVEM n° 026/12 Sion, Switzerland).

Subjects
Four local orthopaedic surgeons specializing in shoulder surgery conducted the subject recruitment. The inclusion criteria were as follows: adult subjects who had surgery less than 6 weeks prior after a shoulder rotator cuff tear. The exclusion criteria were as follows: re-tear of the rotator cuff, associated neurological lesion, or concomitant cervical or elbow lesion.

The sample size was calculated a priori using STATA Version 13.1 software (StataCorp, College Station, TX, USA). Based on the data of muscular activity from the study by Hsu et al. [13] and considering a statistical power of 80% and a Type I error of 0.05, a need for at least 36 subjects was necessary to highlight group differences. We enrolled 39 subjects.

Taping procedure
A trained physiotherapist applied the two different tapes, a therapeutic KT and an ST, on each subject, as shown in Fig. 1. For KT, elastic beige 5-cm width Leukotape®K (BSN Medical, Hamburg, Germany) was used. It was applied according to the Kase model [2]. The first strip, a Y-strip, was applied with 10 to 15% tension over the deltoid muscle from its origin to insertion, with the first tail along the anterior deltoid while the arm was externally rotated and horizontally abducted. The second tail was applied along the posterior deltoid with the arm horizontally adducted and internally rotated. A second strip, an I-strip, was applied for mechanical correction transversely in the sagittal plane over the acromioclavicular joint with downward pressure applied to the KT, with the arm held along the side.

For the sham condition, rigid Leukotape®Classic (BSN medical, Hamburg, Germany) was used. A 5-cm strip was applied transversely under the deltoid tuberosity with no tension and with no direct influence on shoulder area.

The subjects were informed that two different taping techniques were applied, but they were not given any further details about the taping procedure and effects.

Testing procedure
Subjects were assessed on two occasions: 6 and 12 weeks after repair (Fig. 2). Each time, they first answered the French version of the quick Disabilities of the Arm, Shoulder and Hand (DASH) questionnaire in order to assess their physical function and symptoms. This 11-item questionnaire is valid, reliable and responsive in shoulder disorders [23, 24]. They also estimated their pain intensity at rest using a 100-mm visual analogue scale (VAS).

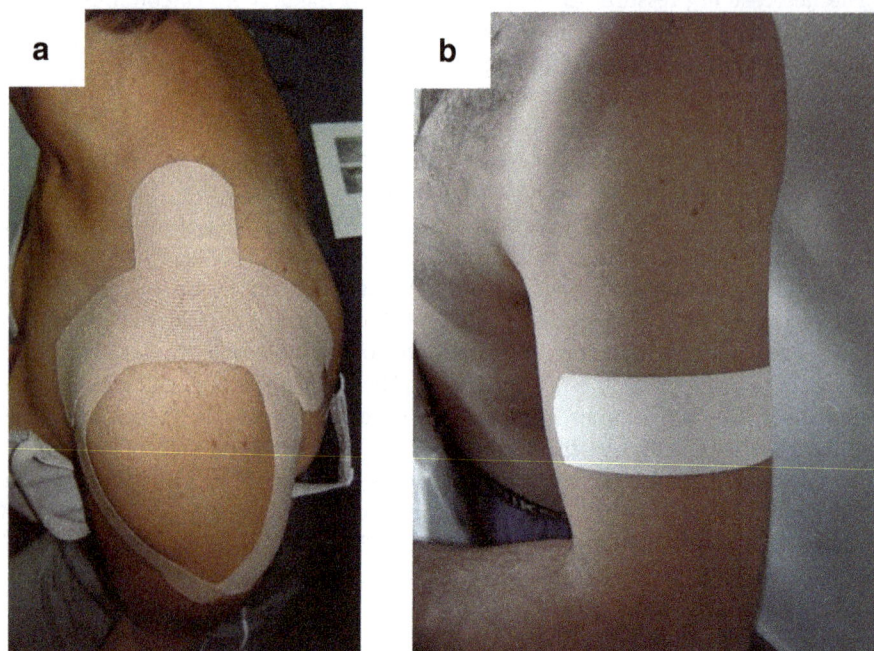

Fig. 1 Tape application. **a** Therapeutic kinesiotape application with a Y-strip surrounding the deltoid muscle and an I-strip over the acromioclavicular joint. **b** Sham tape applied under the deltoid tuberosity

A baseline measurement was then performed without any tape, corresponding to the NT condition. The subjects were seated in a chair without resting on the backrest, with their arms beside their body. Shoulder rotation was neutral, with the elbow extended and the forearm in neutral position. The subjects had to lift their arms in the sagittal plane as high as possible, hold the position for 5 s and then return to the initial position. The movement was repeated once after 1 min of rest.

During the second session at 12 weeks postoperatively, a maximal voluntary isometric contraction (MVIC) measurement was also performed. Measurements were made at 90° of shoulder flexion, neutral rotation, with the elbow extended, the forearm pronated and the fist closed. The strap of the dynamometer was applied at the level of the wrist [25]. The subjects were asked to generate maximal force over a 5-s period. After 1 min of rest, a second trial was performed. The whole session was videotaped for further analysis. At the end of the testing sessions, the subjects were instructed not to remove for 72 h the last tape that was applied.

The sequence always began with the NT condition. Then, the two tapes were applied in a randomized order, and the subjects underwent the same assessment procedures. Group allocation in the KT vs ST group corresponded to the last type of tape the subject had applied, and the tape was worn for three consecutive days.

Outcome measures

Our primary outcome concerned the activities of important shoulder muscles, i.e., the upper trapezius, the anterior, middle and posterior parts of the deltoid and the infraspinatus. An EMG signal was recorded by a wireless surface EMG system (TeleMyo™ Direct Transmission System; Noraxon, Scottsdale/ US). This system has a baseline noise < 1 µV root mean square, an input impedance > 100 MΩ, a common mode rejection ratio > 100 db and a gain of 400. All EMG signals were recorded at a sampling rate of 1500 Hz with 16 bit-resolution. Prior to electrode application, the skin was prepared according to the SENIAM recommendations [26]. Self-adhesive bipolar silver/silver chloride surface electrodes with 1.75 cm inter-electrode distance (Noraxon Dual Electrodes, Noraxon, Scottsdale/US) were placed in accordance with the SENIAM guidelines [26] and the Criswell [27] proposition (Table 1).

Muscular activities were recorded and processed with the Myoresearch XP Master Edition 1.08.38 software. For data analysis, EMG signal was bandpass filtered from 10 Hz to 500 Hz using a first order high-pass Butterworth filter at 10 Hz and a low-pass eighth order Butterworth filter at 500 Hz, and the root-mean-square was calculated using a 50-ms moving window. To allow comparison of the EMG signal among different individuals, the data were normalized to a reference voluntary contraction (RVC). This normalization method was used

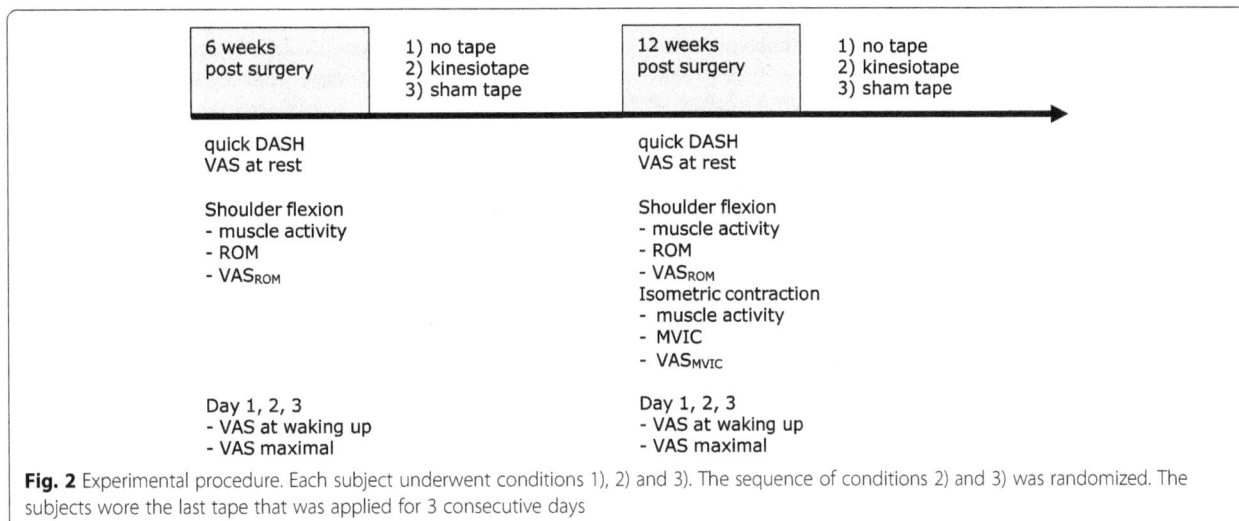

Fig. 2 Experimental procedure. Each subject underwent conditions 1), 2) and 3). The sequence of conditions 2) and 3) was randomized. The subjects wore the last tape that was applied for 3 consecutive days

to avoid the appearance of pain that a maximum voluntary contraction would have produced in this group of subjects. The RVC method has demonstrated good reliability [28, 29]. The reference contraction was performed at the beginning of the testing procedure without tape in a seated position with the shoulder abducted at 45° in the scapular plane and the elbow flexed at 90°. The position was maintained for 5 s. After discarding the first and last second and applying the same filtering procedure as described above, normalization processing was performed using a 3-s moving window for the peak of the RVC.

The mean amplitude EMG signal, expressed as a percentage of the RVC, was used to assess muscle activity during isometric conditions at the end range for the mobility test and at 90° for the strength test. As we could not standardize the movement velocity, which is dependent on ROM and pain limitations, the dynamic values of the mobility test, in concentric and eccentric mode, were discarded. As each measure was repeated twice, the mean of both trials was used for analysis. We used a 15% change in muscle activity as the smallest meaningful difference [30].

In terms of secondary outcomes, we investigated active ROM, strength and pain. ROM was measured a posteriori using a video-based motion analysis system (Dartfish 7 ProSuite 7.0 software; Dartfish, Switzerland). The mean of the two trials was recorded. We defined a meaningful clinical change of a 14° difference [31].

Shoulder strength was assessed with MVIC measurements. These measurements were performed with the Isobex 3.0 isometric dynamometer (Medical Device Solutions AG, Oberburg, Switzerland; sampling frequency of 10 Hz, min-max of 0–40 kg, accuracy of 0.1 kg, and measurement threshold of 1.0 kg). The validity of this instrument has been shown in different studies [25, 32, 33]. The mean of the two trials was recorded. To our knowledge, there is no defined minimal clinical change for shoulder flexion isometric strength.

Shoulder pain intensity was assessed with a 100-mm VAS at the end-point of ROM (VAS_{ROM}) and after isometric force assessment (VAS_{MVIC}). This measurement is known for its excellent reliability [34]. The assessment took place after the two trials of mobility and strength. During the 3 days the subjects had to wear the tape, each day they recorded the pain intensity at waking

Table 1 Electrode placement

Muscles	Electrode placement (location and orientation)
upper trapezius	50% on the line from the acromion to the spine on vertebra C7, in the direction of the line from the acromion to the spine on vertebra C7
anterior part of deltoid	at one finger width distal and anterior to the acromion, in the direction of the line between the acromion and the thumb
middle part of deltoid	line from the acromion to the lateral epicondyle of the elbow, at the greatest bulge of the muscle, in the direction of the line between the acromion and the hand
posterior part of deltoid	two fingerbreadths behind the angle of the acromion, in the direction of the line between the acromion and the little finger
infraspinatus	approximatively 4 cm below the spine of the scapula, over the infraspinatus fossa on the lateral aspect of the muscle, parallel to the spine of the scapula

up ($VAS_{waking\ up}$) and at the most painful moment during the day (VAS_{max}) in a logbook. The activity that was being performed at this time was also noted. For pain intensity, a 20-mm difference was considered a meaningful change [35, 36].

Statistical analysis

Comparisons between the baseline characteristics of the two groups were computed using nonparametric Mood's median tests for continuous variables or the chi-squared test for categorical variables.

The outcome variables measured during the mobility and strength tests were compared between the three conditions. For the VAS outcomes during the 3 days after tape application, comparisons were performed between KT and ST alone. As the distributions of the outcome variables were not normal, nonparametric tests comparing the medians (sign tests of matched pairs) were performed. All analyses were conducted using Stata 13.1 software.

As multiple comparisons were performed, the level of statistical significance was set at $P < 0.017$ (0.05/3) for the comparisons between the three tape conditions (comparison of NT vs KT, NT vs ST, and KT vs ST). For comparison between the KT group and the ST group alone, the level of significance was set at $P < 0.05$.

Results

Subjects

Of the 39 subjects enrolled, 26 underwent both testing sessions. Two subjects were assessed only at 6 weeks, as

one subject (group ST) had an allergic reaction to the tape and the other (group KT) thereafter developed a complex regional pain syndrome. Eleven subjects were enrolled only at the 12-week assessment, as their surgeons did not recommend active shoulder mobilization in flexion with the elbow extended at 6 weeks (Fig. 3). The subject characteristics are described in Table 2. There were no significant differences between the groups in terms of gender, age, weight, height, arm tested and the number of tendons repaired ($P > 0.05$). There were also no significant differences in quick DASH and VAS scores at rest between the two groups at 6 and at 12 weeks ($P > 0.05$).

In the 39 surgeries, the supraspinatus was repaired 32 times, the subscapularis 18 times and the infraspinatus 10 times. In 69% of cases, the procedure was completed by an acromioplasty.

The first evaluation was performed an average of 44.2 ± 1.8 days after surgery, and the second was performed 86.0 ± 1.7 days after surgery.

Muscular activity

Figure 4 summarizes results of the EMG signals. At 6 weeks during active forward flexion, the muscular activity was greater in the KT than in the NT condition for the posterior deltoid (median difference of 7%, $P = 0.013$) and for the infraspinatus (+ 11%, $P = 0.004$). In the ST condition, the muscular activity was also greater than in the NT condition for the posterior deltoid (+ 8%, $P = 0.001$) and the infraspinatus (+ 8%, $P = 0.001$), as well as for the upper trapezius (+ 16%, $P = 0.013$). On the

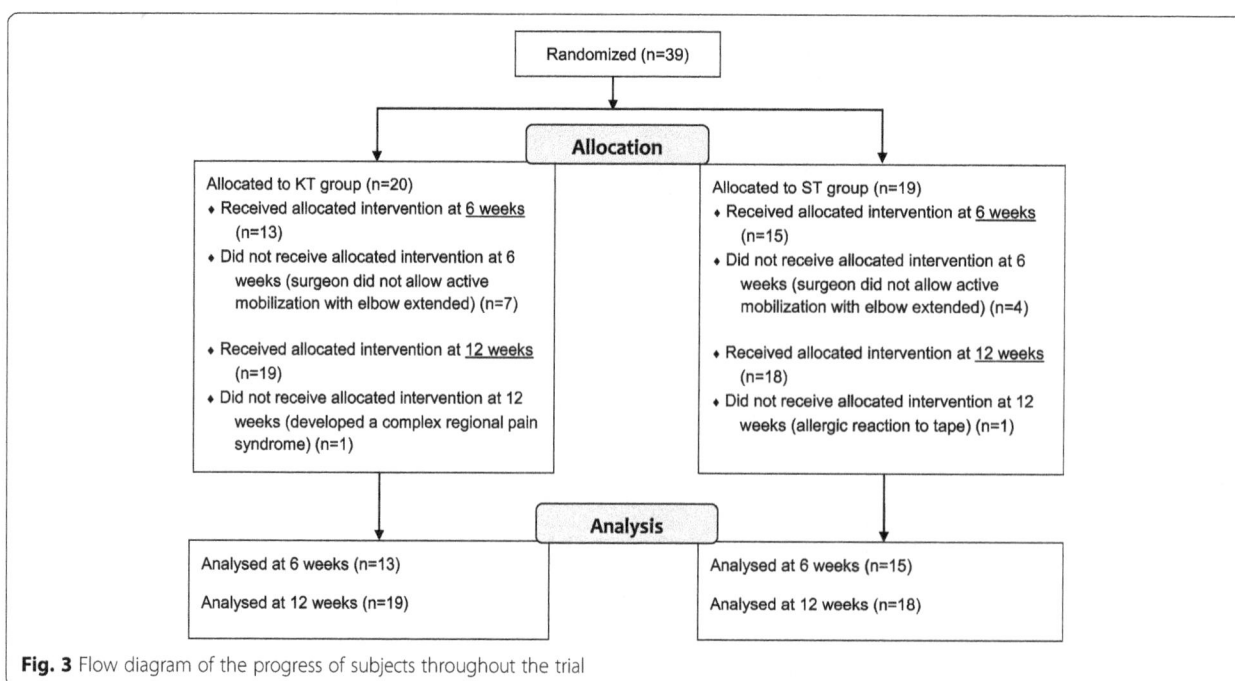

Fig. 3 Flow diagram of the progress of subjects throughout the trial

Table 2 Subject characteristics

	KT group (n = 20)	ST group (n = 19)
Subjects assessed (n)		
Only at 6 weeks	1	1
Only at 12 weeks	7	4
At 6 and 12 weeks	12	14
Gender (n)		
Men/women	16/4	14/5
Age, y	59 (9)	60 (10)
Height, m	1.75 (0.08)	1.72 (0.13)
Weight, kg	87.5 (13.5)	78 (35)
Arm tested (n)		
Dominant/non-dominant	12/8	13/6
Number of tendon repair (n)		
1	13	10
2	3	8
3	4	1
Quick DASH		
6 weeks	64 (25)	52 (22)
12 weeks	41 (16)	41 (16)
VAS at rest		
6 weeks	4 (18)	8 (15)
12 weeks	2 (19)	7 (17)

Data are expressed as number (n) or median (interquartile range)

other hand, the activity was lower for the anterior deltoid (– 9%, $P = 0.004$). No difference was found between KT and ST.

At 12 weeks, the muscular activity was greater in the KT than in the NT condition for the middle and posterior deltoid (+ 13% and + 26%, respectively; $P = 0.001$). The ST and NT conditions showed similar results for these two portions of the deltoid (+ 21% and + 33%, respectively; $P = 0.001$). The anterior deltoid also showed increased activation in the ST condition (+ 9%, $P = 0.004$). Comparing the KT and ST conditions, a decreased activity of the upper trapezius was observed with KT (– 31%, $P = 0.001$).

In the strength test, significant differences were found for the upper trapezius, with a decreased activity in the KT condition compared with the NT (– 21%, $P = 0.016$) and the ST (– 19%, $P = 0.001$) conditions. The posterior deltoid showed lower activity in the KT condition than in the ST condition (– 1%, $P = 0.008$), but this difference was negligible.

ROM

At 6 weeks, active shoulder flexion was statistically greater in the KT condition (P = 0.004) and in the ST condition (P = 0.004) than in the NT condition. However,

the magnitude of the median difference was lower, as defined by the minimum clinically important change, with differences of 5.9° and 5.6°. There was no difference between the KT and ST conditions ($P = 0.04$). At 12 weeks, no difference was observed (Table 3).

Strength

At 12 weeks post-surgery, 7 subjects, 3 in the KT group and 4 in the ST group, could not reach 90° elevation, and the strength test could not be performed. For the remaining subjects, no statistically significant differences were found between the three conditions (Table 3).

Pain

There were no significant differences in pain values between NT, KT and ST at end-point of active ROM at 6 and at 12 weeks. Pain after MVIC measurements was also similar between conditions (Table 3). Moreover, there were no significant differences either in pain upon awakening or during activity between the KT and ST groups (Table 4). During this follow-up period, activities that triggered the most pain were comparable between the groups and between the two sessions. Physical therapy and home exercise programmes were usually associated with maximal pain, followed by rest, basic activities of daily life and finally more strenuous activities requiring some strength.

Discussion

In this study, we explored the immediate and short-term effects of shoulder KT on muscular activity, mobility, strength and pain. KT was compared to ST and to NT at 6 and 12 weeks after rotator cuff surgery. These two points in time are key instances in the rehabilitation process, corresponding to the time when rotator cuff loading can be initiated and, at 12 weeks, when initial strengthening can begin. Indeed, at 6 weeks, the remodelling phase has begun, and the collagen network can handle gentle stress; at 12 weeks, the repaired rotator cuff tissue is relatively mature, and tendon-to-bone healing should be able to endure the initiation of strengthening exercises [37].

As expected, we did not find any clinical benefits of KT on ROM, strength or pain. On the other hand, some beneficial effects were observed on muscular activity. Fifteen statistically significant changes among the different muscle groups were observed, but only seven of them were of clinical interest. Furthermore, we failed to demonstrate a clear pattern of changes. Indeed, in the two mobility tests, compared with NT, only the activity of the posterior deltoid was increased at 6 and 12 weeks with KT and with ST, but at 6 weeks the difference was not considered clinically important. As the function of the posterior deltoid is to control flexion by eccentric

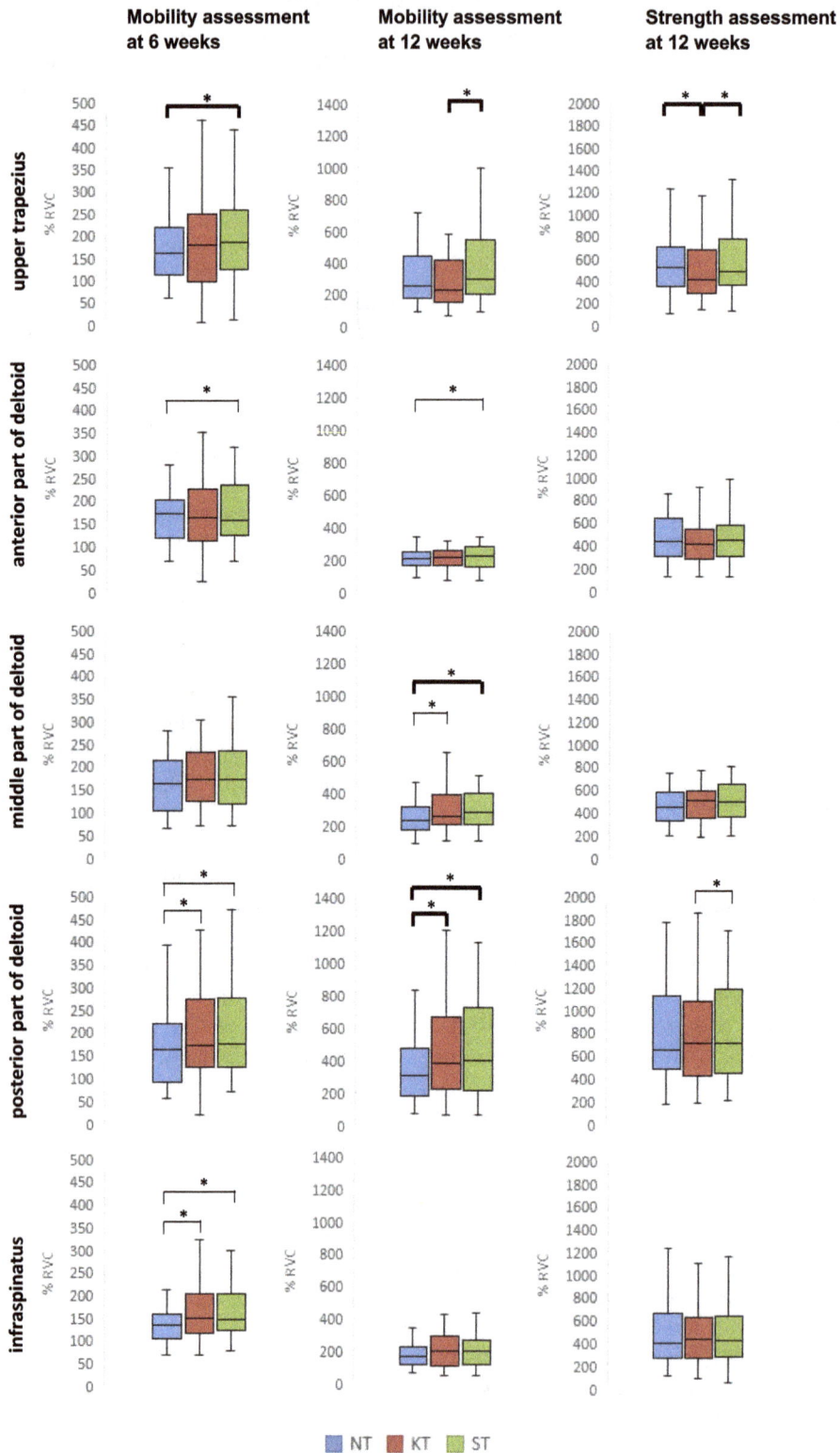

Fig. 4 Descriptive statistics of muscle activity. Electromyographic activity of the upper trapezius, the anterior, middle and posterior parts of deltoid and the infraspinatus muscles was recorded. The spread of the data among the subjects is presented with boxplots (median and quartiles). Data are normalized to the reference voluntary contraction (RVC). *significant difference. In bold: statistically and clinically significant difference

Table 3 Range of motion (ROM), strength (MVIC) and pain (VAS) at 6 and 12 weeks post-surgery

	6 weeks			12 weeks		
	NT	KT	ST	NT	KT	ST
ROM	53.1(36.9)	59.0(40.4)	58.7(35.9)	104.5(68.3)	106.2(47.2)	110.0(53.9)
P-value	a) 0.004*	b) 0.004*	c) 0.04	a) 0.90	b) 0.30	c) 0.30
VAS_{ROM}	20.5(34.5)	21(30)	23.5(31)	13(20)	9(16)	9(19)
P-value	a) 0.20	b) 0.20	c) 0.70	a) 1	b) 0.40	c) 1
MVIC	–	–	–	1.75(1.70)	1.78(1.45)	1.73(1.4)
P-value				a) 0.09	b) 0.90	c) 0.20
VAS_{MVIC}	–	–	–	16(31)	11(24)	16(31)
P-value				a) 1	b) 0.50	c) 1

Data are expressed as median (interquartile range)
*significant difference
a): NT vs KT; b): NT vs ST; c): KT vs ST.

contraction and to stabilize the shoulder downward and inward [38], this increased activity may improve the coordination of this movement, without having an impact on mobility or pain sensation. Unfortunately, for methodological reasons, we could not analyse the ascending and lowering phases of the flexion movement, which might have given us a better understanding of our disparate results. As we found similar results with KT and with ST for several muscles, we could not determine a beneficial effect of KT. However, it should be noted that compared with ST, the upper trapezius activity at 12 weeks was significantly decreased with KT. The same finding was observed during the strength test, as well as a decreased activity of the upper trapezius compared with NT. This result is consistent with the results of Hsu et al. [13] who also found an inhibition of muscle activity of the upper trapezius with KT. As upper trapezius activity is often increased in shoulder pathology [39–41], its inhibition by KT is of clinical interest. In healthy participants, Lin et al. [42] found also a decreased activity of this muscle with KT as well as a decreased activity of the anterior deltoid, which we did not observe. They stated that the decreased muscular activity was related to proprioceptive feedback and neuromuscular control.

In terms of shoulder mobility, we obtained different findings depending on the period of the session. No difference was noted at 12 weeks, whereas at 6 weeks post-surgery, the KT and ST conditions demonstrated increased flexion amplitude compared with the NT condition. The median difference was less than 6° in both situations, which was not considered clinically important. However, we were surprised to obtain similar effects for KT and ST. This finding suggests that a placebo effect is present and that the slight increase in mobility cannot be considered to be caused by the properties of the KT. Placebo response is known to affect motor performance as well as pain [43]. However, it seems unusual that in our case it affected only ROM and not the pain component. It could also be that the tactile stimulation of the rigid ST, although it was not directly applied to the shoulder area, provided a supportive sensation that facilitated the flexion movement. Among the other studies, only Thelen et al. [16], who compared therapeutic and sham tape application, found an effect of KT on pain-free shoulder mobility in abduction at day one, with an increase of 19°; however, the effect was only transitory. Moreover, no effect of KT was observed for shoulder flexion.

Third, the isometric strength test showed similar performance between conditions, with a maximal median difference of 50 g. The study by Keenan et al. [22] was in accordance with our findings, with no change in

Table 4 Pain intensity (VAS) during the follow-up period at 6 and 12 weeks post-surgery

		6 weeks			12 weeks		
		KT	ST	P-value	KT	ST	P-value
$VAS_{waking\ up}$	Day 1	13 (17)	7 (13)	1	6 (13)	8 (12)	0.70
	Day 2	15 (17)	20 (22)	0.70	5 (15)	9 (15)	0.30
	Day 3	16 (24)	20 (17)	0.70	4 (17)	8 (17)	0.80
VAS_{max}	Day 1	28 (22)	26 (24)	0.70	18 (39)	27 (38)	0.70
	Day 2	32.5 (41)	39 (29)	0.80	12 (37)	20 (36)	0.10
	Day 3	27 (35)	34 (38)	0.70	8 (28)	15 (37)	0.20

Data are expressed as median (interquartile range)

isokinetic shoulder rotation strength immediately after KT application. On the other hand, Simsek et al. [18] observed an improvement in shoulder lateral rotation strength 12 days post-tape application, but no difference was observed at 5 days or in other movement directions. In terms of scapular performance, Hsu et al. [13] found no strength differences between KT and ST on the lower trapezius strength. Different studies on knee pathologies have also had mixed results [44–47]. Moreover, the results of the meta-analysis by Csapo and Alegre [48] that evaluated healthy individuals indicated that the potential to increase muscle strength by applying KT was negligible.

Finally, in terms of pain intensity, Lim and Tay [5] proposed various neurophysiological and mechanical mechanisms to explain pain reduction with KT; for example, by the inhibition of the transmission of nociceptive signals, stimulation of the descending pain inhibitory mechanisms, decongestive properties, or by pressure reduction of the subcutaneous nociceptors. However, our results do not allow us to corroborate any of these hypotheses. Indeed, we found no differences among the three conditions at the end range of flexion, during the isometric strength test, or during the follow-up period. Various authors have also studied the immediate or short-term (1 week or less) effects of KT on pain with a population of subjects with shoulder dysfunction [15–18]. Thelen et al. [16] found no effect of KT on pain when assessed immediately or at 3 and 6 days post-application. On the other hand, Shakeri et al. [17] observed decreased pain intensity during movement immediately after KT application. However, the difference between KT and ST was 1.4 points on a 10-point scale, which was not a result that could be considered clinically significant. Moreover, this effect vanished afterwards. Other authors reported decreased pain during activity in the short-term with KT compared with placebo tape [18] or with a physical therapy programme [15]. However, our results do not allow us to recommend the use of KT for the objective of pain reduction.

Our population, which is representative of the usual population undergoing shoulder rotator cuff surgery [49, 50], makes it possible to generalize and apply our results without selection bias. However, this trial has some limitations that need to be addressed. First, at 6 weeks, we did not have the desired number of subjects, as one surgeon thought that it was too early in the rehabilitation process to perform active flexion movements with a large lever arm. Therefore, a larger sample size would be necessary to confirm our results. Another limitation is due to the randomization of the conditions. Indeed, we only randomized the KT and ST conditions, as the protocol always started with NT. This may be the reason why the EMG signals and ROM findings were similar between KT and ST, while they were significantly different from NT. It can be hypothesized that initially the patient mobilizes his arm cautiously and thus gains confidence for the next trial. Third, the normalization procedure for the EMG data was used only in one position for all 5 muscles, so muscle fibre recruitment was unequal between muscles. Moreover, for some subjects, this reference position was effortless to maintain (sub-maximal contraction), whereas it was strenuous (maximal contraction) for others, making the activity level very variable from one person to another. This may influence the results obtained for muscle activity. Finally, we were mainly interested in the immediate effects of KT. Slupik et al. [51] suggested that several hours of tape placement were necessary to obtain a stimulating effect of the KT due to the time necessary for cutaneous mechanoreceptors to improve their neuronal excitability and thus muscle function [52]. It is possible that a longer period of application might be necessary to detect changes. However, we observed no effect on pain intensity at 24, 48 and 72 h of tape application.

Conclusions

This is the first study to assess KT efficacy on subjects who underwent surgery for shoulder rotator cuff tears. We observed some beneficial effects on muscular activity, particularly a decrease in upper trapezius activity, which is often over-activated, during maximal isometric contraction. The other results are in accordance with literature. We do not have clinical evidence to recommend the use of KT either to increase mobility or muscle strength or to diminish pain during activity. Future studies with a larger sample size are needed to confirm our results, especially those evaluating the effect of KT on muscular recruitment.

Abbreviations
DASH: Disabilities of the arm shoulder and hand; EMG: Electromyogram; KT: Kinesiotape; MVIC: Maximal voluntary isometric contraction; NT: No tape; ROM: Range of motion; RVC: Reference voluntary contraction; ST: Sham tape; VAS: Visual analogue scale for pain intensity; VAS$_{max}$: Maximal pain intensity; VAS$_{MVIC}$: Pain intensity after isometric force assessment; VAS$_{ROM}$: Pain intensity at end point of range of motion; VAS$_{waking\ up}$: Pain intensity at waking up

Acknowledgements
The authors thank the physiotherapists who participated in the creation of the study protocol and/or applied the tape: Grégoire Fanti, Valentin Sarrasin, Florent Burtin, Bianca Wynants, Valérie Klingele, Christian Favre, as well as Thomas Nesa who contributed to electromyographic data collection. The authors thank the surgeons who performed surgery on our subjects: Beat Moor, Alexandre Diederichs, Francesco Marbach and Nicolas Riand.

Funding
There was no external funding or sponsoring in this study. The material costs were funded through the physiotherapy department of the Clinique romande de réadaptation.

Authors' contributions

FR and MK conceived and designed the work; FR acquired the data; PV and BL analysed the data; RF, BL and MK interpreted the data; FR and MK drafted the article, PV and BL reviewed critically the article for important intellectual content; and all authors read and approved the final version to be published.

Competing interests

The authors declare that they have no competing interests.

Author details

[1]Department of Physiotherapy, Clinique romande de réadaptation Suva, Sion, Switzerland. [2]Institute for Research in Rehabilitation, Clinique romande de réadaptation Suva, Sion, Switzerland. [3]Department of Musculoskeletal Rehabilitation, Clinique romande de réadaptation Suva, Sion, Switzerland.

References

1. Pichonnaz C, Milliet J, Farron A, Luthi F. Update on the postsurgical shoulder rotator cuff rehabilitation. Rev Med Suisse. 2016;12:1278–83.
2. Kase K, Wallis J, Kase T. Clinical therapeutic applications of the Kinesio taping method. Tokio: Kinesio Taping Association International 3rd ed. 2013.
3. Kinesio HK: The original from Dr. Kenzo Kaze since 1979. Accessed 26 May 2017 [http://www.kinesiotaping.com/about/].
4. Morichon A, Pallot A. Taping: trial by evidence? Review of systematic reviews. Kinesither Rev. 2014;14(147):34–66.
5. Lim EC, Tay MG. Kinesio taping in musculoskeletal pain and disability that lasts for more than 4 weeks: is it time to peel off the tape and throw it out with the sweat? A systematic review with meta-analysis focused on pain and also methods of tape application. Br J Sports Med. 2015;49(24):1558–66.
6. Parreira Pdo C, Costa Lda C, Hespanhol LC Jr, Lopes AD, Costa LO. Current evidence does not support the use of Kinesio taping in clinical practice: a systematic review. J Physiother. 2014;60(1):31–9.
7. Montalvo AM, Cara EL, Myer GD. Effect of kinesiology taping on pain in individuals with musculoskeletal injuries: systematic review and meta-analysis. Phys Sportsmed. 2014;42(2):48–57.
8. Morris D, Jones D, Ryan H, Ryan CG. The clinical effects of Kinesio(R) Tex taping: a systematic review. Physiother Theory Pract. 2013;29(4):259–70.
9. Kalron A, Bar-Sela S. A systematic review of the effectiveness of Kinesio taping--fact or fashion? Eur J Phys Rehabil Med. 2013;49(5):699–709.
10. Montalvo AM, Buckley WE, Wayne S, Giampietro LV. An evidence-based practice approach to the efficacy of Kinesio taping for improving pain and quadriceps performance in physically-active patellofemoral pain syndrome patients. J Nov Physiother. 2013;3(3):151.
11. Mostafavifar M, Wertz J, Borchers J. A systematic review of the effectiveness of kinesio taping for musculoskeletal injury. Phys Sportsmed. 2012;40(4):33–40.
12. Bassett KT, Lingman SA, Ellis RF. The use and treatment efficacy of kinaesthetic taping for musculoskeletal conditions: a systematic review. N Z J Physiother. 2010;38(2):56–62.
13. Hsu YH, Chen WY, Lin HC, Wang WT, Shih YF. The effects of taping on scapular kinematics and muscle performance in baseball players with shoulder impingement syndrome. J Electromyogr Kinesiol. 2009;19(6):1092–9.
14. Kaya DO, Baltaci G, Toprak U, Atay AO. The clinical and sonographic effects of kinesiotaping and exercise in comparison with manual therapy and exercise for patients with subacromial impingement syndrome: a preliminary trial. J Manip Physiol Ther. 2014;37(6):422–32.
15. Kaya E, Zinnuroglu M, Tugcu I. Kinesio taping compared to physical therapy modalities for the treatment of shoulder impingement syndrome. Clin Rheumatol. 2011;30(2):201–7.
16. Thelen MD, Dauber JA, Stoneman PD. The clinical efficacy of kinesio tape for shoulder pain: a randomized, double-blinded, clinical trial. J Orthop Sports Phys Ther. 2008;38(7):389–95.
17. Shakeri H, Keshavarz R, Arab AM, Ebrahimi I. Clinical effectiveness of kinesiological taping on pain and pain-free shoulder range of motion in patients with shoulder impingement syndrome: a randomized, double blinded, placebo-controlled trial. Int J Sports Phys Ther. 2013; 8(6):800–10.
18. Simsek HH, Balki S, Keklik SS, Ozturk H, Elden H. Does Kinesio taping in addition to exercise therapy improve the outcomes in subacromial impingement syndrome? A randomized, double-blind, controlled clinical trial. Acta Orthop Traumatol Turc. 2013;47(2):104–10.
19. Sahin Onat S, Bicer S, Sahin Z, Kucukali Turkyilmaz A, Kara M, Ozbudak Demir S. Effectiveness of Kinesiotaping and subacromial corticosteroid injection in shoulder impingement syndrome. Am J Phys Med Rehabil. 2016;95(8):553–60.
20. Kocyigit F, Acar M, Turkmen MB, Kose T, Guldane N, Kuyucu E. Kinesio taping or just taping in shoulder subacromial impingement syndrome? A randomized, double-blind, placebo-controlled trial. Physiother Theory Pract. 2016;32(7):501–8.
21. Goksu H, Tuncay F, Borman P. The comparative efficacy of kinesio taping and local injection therapy in patients with subacromial impingement syndrome. Acta Orthop Traumatol Turc. 2016;50(5):483–8.
22. Keenan KA, Akins JS, Varnell M, Abt J, Lovalekar M, Lephart S, Sell TC. Kinesiology taping does not alter shoulder strength, shoulder proprioception, or scapular kinematics in healthy, physically active subjects and subjects with subacromial impingement syndrome. Phys Ther Sport. 2017;24:60–6.
23. Fayad F, Lefevre-Colau MM, Gautheron V, Mace Y, Fermanian J, Mayoux-Benhamou A, Roren A, Rannou F, Roby-Brami A, Revel M, et al. Reliability, validity and responsiveness of the French version of the questionnaire quick disability of the arm, shoulder and hand in shoulder disorders. Man Ther. 2009;14(2):206–12.
24. Gummesson C, Ward MM, Atroshi I. The shortened disabilities of the arm, shoulder and hand questionnaire (QuickDASH): validity and reliability based on responses within the full-length DASH. BMC Musculoskelet Disord. 2006;7:44.
25. Burrus C, Deriaz O, Luthi F, Konzelmann M. Role of pain in measuring shoulder strength abduction and flexion with the constant-Murley score. Ann Phys Rehabil Med. 2017;60(4):258–62.
26. Hermens HJ, Freriks B, Disselhorst-Klug C, Rau G. Development of recommendations for SEMG sensors and sensor placement procedures. J Electromyogr Kinesiol. 2000;10(5):361–74.
27. Criswell E. Cram's introduction to surface electromyography. 2nd ed. Sudbury, Massachussets: Jones and Bartlett Publishers; 2011.
28. Bao S, Mathiassen SE, Winkel J. Normalizing upper trapezius EMG amplitude: comparison of different procedures. J Electromyogr Kinesiol. 1995;5(4):251–7.
29. Knutson LM, Soderberg GL, Ballantyne BT, Clarke WR. A study of various normalization procedures for within day electromyographic data. J Electromyogr Kinesiol. 1994;4(1):47–59.
30. Brox JI, Roe C, Saugen E, Vollestad NK. Isometric abduction muscle activation in patients with rotator tendinosis of the shoulder. Arch Phys Med Rehabil. 1997;78(11):1260–7.
31. Muir SW, Corea CL, Beaupre L. Evaluating change in clinical status: reliability and measures of agreement for the assessment of glenohumeral range of motion. N Am J Sports Phys Ther. 2010;5(3):98–110.
32. Hirschmann MT, Wind B, Amsler F, Gross T. Reliability of shoulder abduction strength measure for the constant-Murley score. Clin Orthop Relat Res. 2010;468(6):1565–71.
33. Leggin BG, Neuman RM, Iannotti JP, Williams GR, Thompson EC. Intrarater and interrater reliability of three isometric dynamometers in assessing shoulder strength. J Shoulder Elb Surg. 1996;5(1):18–24.
34. Clark P, Lavielle P, Martinez H. Learning from pain scales: patient perspective. J Rheumatol. 2003;30(7):1584–8.
35. Farrar JT, Young JP Jr, LaMoreaux L, Werth JL, Poole RM. Clinical importance of changes in chronic pain intensity measured on an 11-point numerical pain rating scale. Pain. 2001;94(2):149–58.
36. Crossley KM, Bennell KL, Cowan SM, Green S. Analysis of outcome measures for persons with patellofemoral pain: which are reliable and valid? Arch Phys Med Rehabil. 2004;85(5):815–22.
37. van der Meijden OA, Westgard P, Chandler Z, Gaskill TR, Kokmeyer D, Millett PJ. Rehabilitation after arthroscopic rotator cuff repair: current concepts review and evidence-based guidelines. Int J Sports Phys Ther. 2012;7(2):197–218.
38. Kronberg M, Nemeth G, Brostrom LA. Muscle activity and coordination in the normal shoulder. An electromyographic study. Clin Orthop Relat Res. 1990;257:76–85.
39. Lin JJ, Hsieh SC, Cheng WC, Chen WC, Lai Y. Adaptive patterns of movement during arm elevation test in patients with shoulder impingement syndrome. J Orthop Res. 2011;29(5):653–7.

40. Lin JJ, Lim HK, Soto-quijano DA, Hanten WP, Olson SL, Roddey TS, Sherwood AM. Altered patterns of muscle activation during performance of four functional tasks in patients with shoulder disorders: interpretation from voluntary response index. J Electromyogr Kinesiol. 2006;16(5):458–68.

41. Cools AM, Declercq GA, Cambier DC, Mahieu NN, Witvrouw EE. Trapezius activity and intramuscular balance during isokinetic exercise in overhead athletes with impingement symptoms. Scand J Med Sci Sports. 2007;17(1):25–33.

42. Lin JJ, Hung CJ, Yang PL. The effects of scapular taping on electromyographic muscle activity and proprioception feedback in healthy shoulders. J Orthop Res. 2011;29(1):53–7.

43. Benedetti F, Mayberg HS, Wager TD, Stohler CS, Zubieta JK. Neurobiological mechanisms of the placebo effect. J Neurosci. 2005;25(45):10390–402.

44. Aytar A, Ozunlu N, Surenkok O, Baltacı G, Oztop P, Karatas M. Initial effects of kinesio® taping in patients with patellofemoral pain syndrome: a randomized, double-blind study. Isokinet Exerc Sci. 2011;19(2):135–42.

45. Osorio JA, Vairo GL, Rozea GD, Bosha PJ, Millard RL, Aukerman DF, Sebastianelli WJ. The effects of two therapeutic patellofemoral taping techniques on strength, endurance, and pain responses. Phys Ther Sport. 2013;14(4):199–206.

46. Lee CR, Lee DY, Jeong HS, Lee MH. The effects of Kinesio taping on VMO and VL EMG activities during stair ascent and descent by persons with patellofemoral pain: a preliminary study. J Phys Ther Sci. 2012;24:153–6.

47. Oliveira AK, Borges DT, Lins CA, Cavalcanti RL, Macedo LB, Brasileiro JS. Immediate effects of Kinesio taping((R)) on neuromuscular performance of quadriceps and balance in individuals submitted to anterior cruciate ligament reconstruction: a randomized clinical trial. J Sci Med Sport. 2016;19(1):2–6.

48. Csapo R, Alegre LM. Effects of Kinesio((R)) taping on skeletal muscle strength-a meta-analysis of current evidence. J Sci Med Sport. 2015;18(4):450–6.

49. Zhang AL, Montgomery SR, Ngo SS, Hame SL, Wang JC, Gamradt SC. Analysis of rotator cuff repair trends in a large private insurance population. Arthroscopy. 2013;29(4):623–9.

50. Van Linthoudt D, Deforge J, Malterre L, Huber H. Rotator cuff repair. Long-term results. Joint Bone Spine. 2003;70(4):271–5.

51. Slupik A, Dwornik M, Bialoszewski D, Zych E. Effect of Kinesio taping on bioelectrical activity of vastus medialis muscle. Preliminary report. Ortop Traumatol Rehabil. 2007;9(6):644–51.

52. Kim H, Lee B. The effects of kinesio tape on isokinetic muscular function of horse racing jockeys. J Phys Ther Sci. 2013;25(10):1273–7.

The predictive value of preoperative neutrophil-lymphocyte ratio (NLR) on the recurrence of the local pigmented villonodular synovitis of the knee joint

Guanglei Zhao[†], Jin Wang[†], Jun Xia[*], Yibing Wei, Siqun Wang, Gangyong Huang, Feiyan Chen, Jie Chen, Jingsheng Shi and Yuanqing Yang

Abstract

Background: To explore and evaluate the predictive value of preoperative Neutrophil-lymphocyte ratio (NLR) on the recurrence of pigmented villonodular synovitis (PVNS) of the knee joint treated by arthroscopic surgery combining local radiotherapy.

Methods: Sixty pathological-proven PVNS cases of the knee joint in our department from April 2006 to March 2017 were included. All of them are treated by arthroscopic synovectomy combined with adjuvant radiotherapy. The pre-operative hematological indexes such as c-reactive protein (CRP), erythrocyte sedimentation rate (ESR), NLR, Platelet-lymphocyte ratio (PLR) and Lymphocyte-monocyte ratio (LMR) were collected retrospectively and their relationship with postoperative recurrence was analyzed by using univariate and multivariate analysis, the receiver operating characteristic curves (ROC curve), the Kappa correspondence test and the Mc Nemar Chi-square test.

Results: All 60 patients were followed up for a median of 52.8 months (7–138 months) and the recurrence rate is about 23.3% (14/60). There is a significant difference in NLR between the recurrent and non-recurrent group ($P = 0.002$). It had a certain correlation with postoperative recurrence (correlation coefficient $r = 0.438$, $P = 0.001$). The optimal thresholds in ROC curve were 2.42 (sensitivity 71.4%, specificity 78.3% respectively). which had predictive ability for recurrence after arthroscopic treatment.

Conclusion: The preoperative NLR is an easy and cost-effective predictor for relapse in PVNS of the knee joint after the arthroscopic surgery combined with local radiotherapy, which is of profound significance to guide clinical work.

Keywords: Pigmented villonodular synovitis, Recurrence, NLR

Background

Pigmented villonodular synovitis (PVNS) is a rare and benign disease of the synovial membrane characterized by abnormal synovium proliferation and hemosiderin deposition. According to previously reported statistics, the incidence rate is about 1.8/100000. It mostly affects the knee joint [1, 2], but can occurs in any synovial joint including the hip, ankle and elbow joint [3, 4]. The PVNS can be classified into the localized and diffuse forms (LPVNS and DPVNS) [5]. The etiology of the PVNS is still unknown yet while it was regarded as an inflammatory disorder in the past decades. Some risk factors have been recognized such as the trauma, chronic inflammation, and abnormal lipid metabolism [6]. Furthermore, PVNS would invade the adjacent bone and soft tissue leading to the bone errosion and the deformity of the involved joint [7, 8]. The high recurrence rate and metastasis risk of PVNS had also been reported

---

* Correspondence: hudbt17089@gmail.com
[†]Guanglei Zhao and Jin Wang contributed equally to this work.
Division of orthopaedic surgery, Huashan Hospital, Fudan University, Shanghai 200040, China

[9], hence, up to now, PVNS has been considered to be a neoplastic-like disorder of the synovium, with synovitis as a secondary reaction in PVNS [10].

Many researchers has found that some hematological parameters like CRP [11], platelet volume [12], NLR [13] and PLR [14] are closely related with the outcomes of many diseases such as inflammatory disease, autoimmune disease and neoplastic disease [15]. Notably, NLR, PLR or LMR are new, simple and cost-effective predictors for prognosis. A meta-analysis conducted by Zhang J [16] found that the elevated NLR has a close relationship with the poorer overall survival of colorectal cancer (HR = 1.92 95%CI = 1.57–2.34; $P < 0.00001$). Kaida T et al. [17] also reported that PLR is an independent predictive factor of recurrence beyond the Milan criteria after liver resection for patients with hepatocellular carcinoma (odds ratio, 2.55; 95% confidence interval, 1.17–5.49; $P = 0.018$). However, there have been no reports regarding the relationship between NLR, PLR or LMR and the relapse of PVNS of knee joint, in addition, no quantitative parameters now can predict the recurrence of the PVNS of knee joint effectively.

In this study, we retrospectively reviewed the clinical characteristics, blood indexes, and recurrence of sixty cases diagnosed with LPVNS of knee joint in our department. The purpose of the present study is to explore the relationship between the NLR, PLR or LMR and the recurrence of the PVNS of knee joint. We hypothesized that some of these parameters could be used as new predictors for the recurrence of LPVNS of knee joint which were treated by arthroscopic surgery and adjuvant radiotherapy.

Methods
Patients
Huashan Hospital follow-up system (HSFS) is a database established on the inpatient and outpatient database. The HSFS comprises medical complete records of inpatient and outpatient. Sixty patients histopathological diagnosed with knee PVNS (29 men and 31 women) are included in this study at orthopedic department of Huashan Hospital from April 2006 to March 2017. The study was approved by the Ethical Committee in Huashan Hospital. Baseline data including age, sex, height, weight, body mass index, X rays, Magnetic Resonance images (MRI), and results of laboratory tests including neutrophil, lymphocyte, monocyte, platelet counts, erythrocyte sedimentation rate (ESR), C-reactive protein(CRP) were collected from HSFS in the study. Chronic synovitis, such as rheumatoid synovitis and synovial chondromatosis were excluded. All enrolled participants had no history of trauma and surgery when initially visited our department. Repeated swelling, pain and limited joint function were the main clinical manifestation and the time between symptom onset and hospital admission ranged from 2 months to 8 years.

Peroperative examinations
All patients received routine blood test and imaging examination including X rays and magnetic resonance image scan (MRI) before the surgery. In addition, the function of the involved knee joint before the surgery was assessed using Knee Society Score (KSS) and the Lyshoml Knee Score system.

Surgical procedures
All patients underwent comprehensive arthroscopic synovectomy in supine position under general anesthesia by an experienced surgeon. The pneumatic tourniquet (55-65 KPa) was used to stop the bleeding. Briefly, the standard anterolateral and anteromedial approaches were adopted and two 1 cm incisions was made on both sides of the patellar ligament in the front of the involved knee joint. Under the arthroscopic camera, the whole knee joint cavity was examined systematically according to the following order, suprapatellar bursa, patellofemoral joint, medial and lateral recess of the knee joint, tibiofemoral joint, meniscus and the anterior cruciate ligament. The abnormal synovial was removed as much as possible by using radiofrequency vaporization and shaving instruments. For PVNS lesions in the posterior joint, which was difficult to access from the anterior portals, the patients were placed prone. Posterolateral and posteromedial portals were used, and the PVNS lesions were removed as described before. Pathological examination of the abnormal synovium was performed routinely for each case. At the end of the procedure, surgeon would examine entire knee carefully again (Fig. 1). Finally, the wound was closed in layers.

Postoperative management
On the first day after surgery, Wound compression and ice compress were used as usual and patients were encouraged to start range of motion (ROM) exercise after removing the thick dressing on the next day. Furthermore, the patients were permitted to conduct full weight-bearing as long as they can tolerate the pain and the non-steroid anti-inflammatory drugs or analgesics and decongestants are provided to relieve the pain. All patients discharged with a significant improvement in range of motion of the affected knee joint (0–90 degrees). Importantly, in order to reduce the local recurrence rate, patients were all advised to the Cancer Hospital of Fudan University for adjuvant radiotherapy 4–6 weeks after the surgery (average total dose is 2000 cGy to 3000 cGy, 10–15 times).

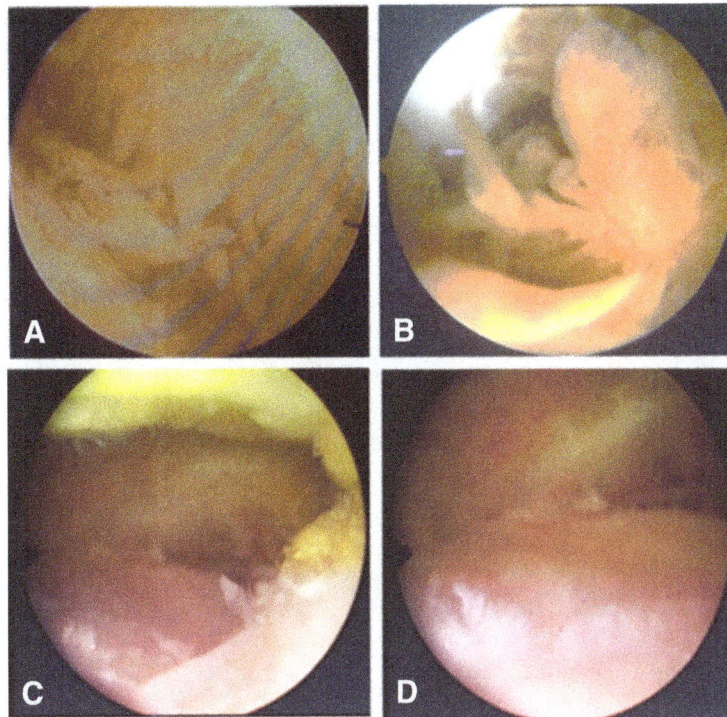

Fig. 1 Macroscopic examination of the synovium before and after the arthroscopic synovectomy. (**a-b**) hypertrophied synovium with villous transformation and haemosiderin deposition before the surgery, (**c-d**) images of the knee joint after the synovectomy

Follow up

All 60 patients were followed through outpatient visit or telephone. The postoperative recurrence is defined as reoccurred joint swelling and pain 6 months after the treatment with typical appearance of PVNS on MRI images [18]. All patients were divided into the recurrent and non-recurrent group according to the outcome of the follow-up. The symptoms, Lysholm score and American KSS score were recorded before surgery and at final follow up evaluation or at the time of recurrence.

Data analysis

The normal distribution of the data was assessed using the Kolmogorov–Smirnov test, the normally distributed data are presented as the means ± standard deviation (X ± SD) and M (P25, P75) for non-normally distributed variables. Clinical characteristics were compared between the recurrent group and non-recurrent group using Pearson's X^2 test for categorical variables and independent t-test for continuous variables. Spearman correlation was applied to assess correlations between relpase and the preoperative NLR. Receiver operating characteristic (ROC) analysis was used for evaluation of predictive markers in the recurrence of the knee PVNS. The optimal cutoff values of several markers including NLR, PLR, LMR that the best distinguished recurrent group from the non-recurrent group was

determined with the maximum value of Youden's index, which was calculated by sensitivity + 1-specificity [19]. The overall diagnostic accuracy and predictive ability were estimated based on the area under the curve (AUC) which is reported with its standard error. A multivariable analysis was performed with significant markers from ROC curves to determine which of them are independently associated with the relapse of knee PVNS. McNemar test and Kappa consistency test were also conducted to evaluate the effectiveness of the predictors. All Statistical analysis were performed with the SPSS software for windows (version 20.0; SPSS, Chicago, IL). $P < 0.05$ was considered statistically significant.

Results

Sixty patients pathological diagnosed with PVNS were included (26 right knee, 34 left knee). The median age was 32 (range 14–75) years. On the MRI, the low signal intensity was presented on both T1 and T2 weighted images before the operation [18, 20]. The median duration of follow up was 52.8 (7–138) months and no complication of skin or wound infection was observed. Fourteen patients recurred and the median relapse time was 33.75 (20–51) months. Among the recurrent group, 3 patients underwent total knee arthroplasty and others received a second arthroscopy surgery.

Table 1 Clinical characteristics of all patients (* means statistical difference $P < 0.05$)

	Total	Recurrent	Non-recurrent	P value
Patients (n)	60	14	46	–
Age (years)	32.00 (26.25–47.00)	35.50 (28.75–50.00)	32.00 (26.00–48.25)	0.45
Gender (F/M)	31/29	6/8	25/21	0.45
Body mass index (kg/m^2)	22.81 ± 1.81	23.31 ± 1.12	22.65 ± 1.95	0.12
Knee(L/R)	34/26	5/9	29/17	0.07
WBC (10^9/L)	6.57 (5.54–8.21)	7.01 (5.57–8.38)	6.57 (5.35–8.28)	0.51
ESR (mm/h)	14.00 (11.25–19.00)	16.50 (10.00–27.00)	13.50 (11.75–17.25)	0.208
CRP (mg/L)	13.30 (6.34–21.25)	17.31 (10.45–27.55)	12.51 (6.17–15.86)	0.04*
Neutrophils (10^9/L)	3.59 (2.92–4.53)	4.07 (3.22–5.36)	3.26 (2.52–4.51)	0.134
Platelets (10^9/L)	242.00 (189.75–281.25)	260.50 (235.00–282.25)	233.50 (180.75–278.50)	0.21
Lymphocytes (10^9/L)	1.87 (1.50–2.19)	1.83 (1.30–2.23)	1.87 (1.57–2.11)	0.69
Monocytes (10^9/L)	0.38 (0.32–0.46)	0.35 (0.32–0.46)	0.38 (0.32–0.46)	0.49
PLR	125.29 (105.04–152.58)	127.96 (104.05–233.92)	124.07 (105.71–148.65)	0.23
NLR	1.89 (1.40–2.50)	2.63 (2.05–2.84)	1.77 (1.36–2.25)	0.002*
LMR	4.76 (4.02–5.87)	4.75 (3.78–5.80)	4.76 (4.03–5.94)	0.68

Table 1 shows the clinical characteristics of the recurrent and non-recurrent group. The recurrent group showed higher NLR and CRP than non-recurrent group ($P_{NLR} = 0.002$, $P_{CRP} = 0.04$). There were no significant difference in other characteristics including PLR and LMR between the two groups ($P_{PLR} = 0.23$, $P_{LMR} = 0.68$).

The univariate and multivariate analysis were also performed with significant markers from ROC curves to determine which of them are independently associated with the diagnosis for relapse. The results indicates that NLR was significantly associated for prediction of relapse (odds ratio = 7.999, $P = 0.017$) (Table 2).

The optimal cutoff value that best distinguished recurrent from non-recurrent was determined at the maximum value, which was calculated by sensitivity + 1-specificity in the ROC curves. The ROC analysis of ESR, CRP, NLR, PLR and LMR showed the area under the curve (AUC) were 0.578 (95% CI = 0.443–0.704), 0.679 (95% CI = 0.545–0.793), 0.775 (95% CI = 0.649–

0.873), 0.607 (95% CI = 0.473–0.731) and 0.537 (95% CI = 0.404–0.667) respectively (Fig. 2). Among the variables, the AUC of the NLR is the largest (AUC = 0.775, 95% CI = 0.649–0.873) and the optimal cut-off value is 2.42 for distinguishing the relapse which means when the NLR value is above 2.42 before treatment, the patient is more likely to have a relapse after the surgery. The Kappa test results (Kappa = 0.432, $P = 0.001$) and McNemar Chi-square test ($P = 0.180$) indicated that the NLR is valuable index for predicting the relapse.

The lyshoml and KSS score both improved in the two groups after the surgery though there is no significant difference before surgery and at the time of relapse in the recurrent group. Tables 3 and 4 shows that recurrent patients had poorer joint function than non-recurrent patients before the treatment did. In recurrent group, the knee functional score was higher at the time of relapse than that before operation while no significant difference was obtained. However, in non-recurrent group,

Table 2 Multiple logistic regression analysis of factors associated with relapse of PVNS of the knee joint. OR: odds ratio, 95% CI: 95% confidence intervals

	Univariate analysis			Multivariate analysis		
	OR	95% CI	p-value	OR	95% CI	p-value
Gender	1.587	0.475–5.307	0.453	1.217	0.176–8.411	0.842
Age	1.017	0.975–1.060	0.442	0.982	0.918–1.051	0.596
Body mass index	1.249	0.866–1.802	0.233	1.065	0.652–1.741	0.800
ESR	1.063	0.983–1.148	0.126	1.084	0.968–1.214	0.162
CRP	1.074	1.004–1.149	0.038*	1.113	1.004–1.235	0.043*
Neutrophils	1.467	0.884–2.434	0.138	1.063	0.478–2.363	0.823
NLR	6.595	1.877–23.170	0.003*	7.999	1.451–44.103	0.017*

*P values represent statistically significant differences

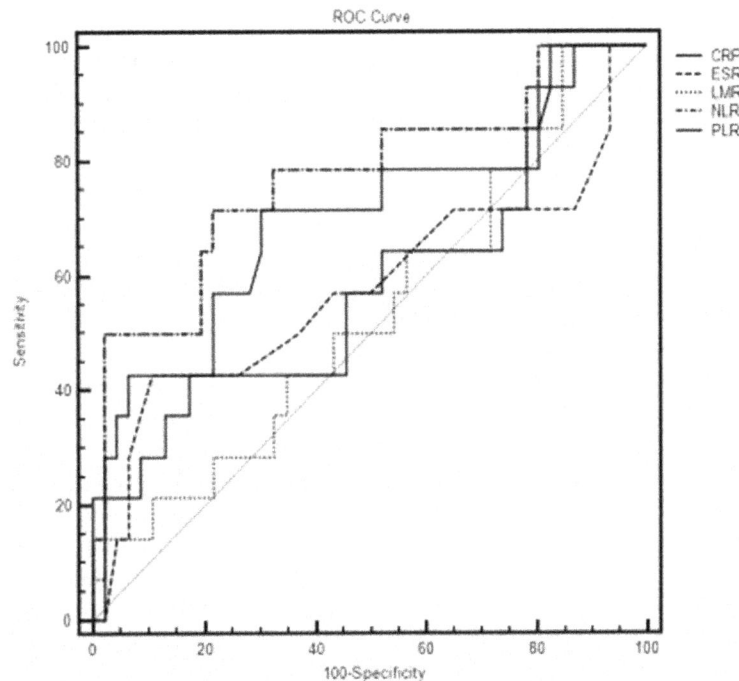

Fig. 2 Receiver operating characteristic (ROC) curves for the neutrophil-to-lymphocyte ratio (NLR), Platelet-lymphocyte ratio (PLR), Lymphocyte-monocyte ratio (LMR) erythrocyte sedimentation rate (ESR), and C-reactive protein (CRP)

most patients were satisfied with the greatly improved knee joint function and the difference in Lyshoml score and KSS score were statistically significant ($P < 0.001$) before surgery and at final follow up.

Discussion

This is the first study to explore the relationship between preoperative hematological parameters and the recurrence of the PVNS of the knee joint. Our results indicate that the preoperative NLR is a useful predictive biomarker for the recurrence of PVNS. In our research, the NLR is significantly higher in the recurrence group ($P = 0.002$), besides, the NLR shows good correlation with the relapse and has a high sensitivity and specificity to predict the postoperative relapse with a cutoff value of 2.42.

The PVNS is a locally aggressive, neoplastic-like disorder of synovial tissue that it would cause functional deterioration of the involved joint. The recurrence rate of the PVNS is as high as 10–50% for the residual diseased synovium after the simple synovectomy [21]. Isart

A et al. [22] also reported a high recurrence of PVNS (61.5%, 8/13) after arthroscopic synovectomy. Moreover, it is almost impossible to resect the pathological synovium completely by open access or arthroscopic therapy [23]. So the high recurrence rate is still an intractable clinical issue despite many reports have claimed that adjuvant local radiotherapy after the synovectomy may be a salvage option [24]. What's more, the non-specific symptoms of PVNS at its early stage often contribute to a delay in establishing a diagnosis, and the joint arthroplasty is the curative surgery in the terminal stage cases with severe bone erosion. So the early diagnosis of relapse is necessary in PVNS after the first treatment for its high recurrence rate. However, there has been no effective quantitatively marker for the relapse. The pathological examination is the gold standard and the MRI is the mostly used radiological tool for monitoring the relapse of PVNS. However, the MRI is qualitative and expensive and not available in some remote districts, additionally, the pathological examination always needs a second invasive procedure. Hence, finding an easy,

Table 3 The knee joint function in recurrent group

	Preoperative	Relapse / final follow up	P value
KSS clinical score	59.13 ± 7.59 (48–73)	64.88 ± 9.03 (50–77)	0.218
KSS function score	54.38 ± 18.20 (15–72)	60.38 ± 19.32 (20–78)	0.559
Lyshoml score	57.38 ± 12.91 (40–72)	62.38 ± 13.25 (43–76)	0.486

Table 4 The knee joint function in non-recurrent
group (*means statistical difference $P < 0.05$)

	Preoperative	Final follow up	P value
KSS clinical score	68.12 ± 3.96	87.44 ± 5.20	< 0.001*
KSS function score	70.28 ± 4.88	88.92 ± 6.95	< 0.001*
Lyshoml score	66.96 ± 8.70	84.32 ± 9.72	< 0.001*

non-invasive and cost-effective biomarker for relapse is a great challenge for surgeons.

The NLR can be obtained simply from neutrophil and lymphocyte counts. In addition, the NLR is cheaper relatively and it is obtainable in most medical institution for the blood routine examination is one of the routine preoperative test. Sever studies have demonstrated that the NLR、LMR and PLR are significantly associated with the outcome of many diseases. For example, Kucuk A et al. [25] reported that the NLR is obviously higher in Ankylosing spondylitis (AS) patients compared to controls. (NLR = 2.47 ± 1.33, 1.72 ± 0.47, respectively, $P < 0.0001$). Additionally, there is a significant difference between the severe AS disease activity and the mild AS disease activity (NLR = 2.72 ± 1.41, 2.20 ± 1.19, $P = 0.001$). The results of the ROC analysis (cutoff value = 1.91, sensitivity 69%, specificity 54%) also proved that NLR is a simple and inexpensive marker to indicate disease activity in patients with AS in daily clinical practice. Lin JP et al. [26] found preoperative LMR is an independent prognostic factor for GC which can improve the predictability of individual survival and recurrence of gastric cancer. Moreover, the predictive value of the NLR, LMR or PLR have been found in more and more diseases including the diabetes, hypertension, pancreatic cancer and hepatocellular carcinoma [27–29].

To our knowledge, there have been no report about the NLR, LMR or PLR in predicting the recurrence of the knee PVNS. In our study, 60 patients diagnosed with LPVNS were enrolled. With respect to the gender ratio, our result (1.07, 31/29) was similar to those reported in Portugal (1.15) [30]. The BMI has no significant difference between two groups All participants received an arthroscopic synovectomy for the diagnosis of the LPVNS, and Xie et al. [15] found that no significant recurrence difference was identified between PVNS patients that were treated with open versus arthroscopic surgery ($p = 0.78$). In addition, the knee arthroscopic surgery, a minimally invasive surgery, is beneficial for fast recovery and shorter the hospitalization time. What's more, the local adjuvant radiotherapy was applied to decrease the local relapse as much as possible. In a multicenter retrospective study, the recurrence rate in patients with knee PVNS is 24% (42/175) [2]. In our study, the recurrence rate is about 23.3% (14/60) which is consistent with the literatures. Among all hematologic indexes, Only CRP and NLR are significantly higher in

recurrent patients ($P_{CRP} = 0.04$, $P_{NLR} = 0.002$). Other parameters like WBC, Neutrophils count and ESR are higher in recurrent group compared to controls, but don't reach a statistical difference ($P_{WBC} = 0.51$, $P_{ESR} = 0.208$) which may implied that the PVNS is not a simple inflammatory disease. The results of ROC analysis and the multivariate analysis (Odds ratio = 7.99, 95% CI = 1.451–44.103, $P = 0.017$) indicated that the NLR may be a valuable marker for predicting relapse of knee PVNS after the treatment.

Limitations
There were also some limitations in our study. Firstly, the number of the participants is relatively small for the low incidence of the PVNS, so the larger clinical researches with longer-term follow up are needed. VSecondly, all the patients enrolled in our study received the arthroscopic synovectomy and radiotherapy. Therefore, the effect of the surgical methods on the relapse is unknown. Thirdly, the mean duration of symptoms before the treatment is not included in our study for its inaccuracy.

Conclusion
Our report suggests that the preoperative NLR is a valuable marker to predict the relapse of Knee PVNS treated by arthroscopic synovectomy combining radiotherapy. Our study indicated that these patients (preoperative NLR > 2.42) should be closely followed after the operation for the higher possibility of relapse. We hope this study could provide the orthopedic clinicians with a new method for predicting the postoperative recurrence of patients with PVNS.

Abbreviations
AUC: Area under the curve; CRP: C-reactive protein; ESR: Erythrocyte sedimentation rate; HSFS: Huashan Hospital follow-up system; KSS: Knee Society Score; LMR: Lymphocyte-monocyte ratio; MRI: Magnetic Resonance images; NLR: Neutrophil-lymphocyte ratio; PLR: Platelet-lymphocyte ratio; PVNS: Pigmented villonodular synovitis; ROC: Receiver operating characteristic; ROM: Range of motion

Authors' contributions
GLZ and JW were involved in all the work of the article. JX were involved in the data collection and analysis. YBW, SQW, GYH, FYC, JC, JSS and YQY were involved in data collection. All authors have read and approved the manuscript, and ensure that this is the case.

Competing interests
The authors declare that they have no competing interests.

References

1. Myers BW, Masi AT. Pigmented villonodular synovitis and tenosynovitis: a clinical epidemiologic study of 166 cases and literature review. Medicine (Baltimore). 1980;59:223–38.

2. Xie GP, Jiang N, Liang CX, et al. Pigmented villonodular synovitis: a retrospective multicenter study of 237 cases. PLoS One. 2015;10:e0121451.

3. Wong JJ, Phal PM, Wiesenfeld D. Pigmented villonodular synovitis of the temporomandibular joint: a radiologic diagnosis and case report. J Oral Maxillofac Surg. 2012;70:126–34.

4. Lu H, Chen Q, Shen H. Pigmented villonodular synovitis of the elbow with rdial, median and ulnar nerve compression. Int J Clin Exp Pathol. 2015;8:14045–9.

5. Abdul-Karim FW, el-Naggar AK, Joyce MJ, Makley JT, Carter JR. Diffuse and localized tenosynovial giant cell tumor and pigmented villonodular synovitis: a clinicopathologic and flow cytometric DNA analysis. Hum Pathol. 1992;23:729–35.

6. Ottaviani S, Ayral X, Dougados M, Gossec L. Pigmented villonodular synovitis: a retrospective single-center study of 122 cases and review of the literature. Semin Arthritis Rheum. 2011;40:539–46.

7. Baba S, Motomura G, Fukushi J, et al. Osteonecrosis of the femoral head associated with pigmented villonodular synovitis. Rheumatol Int. 2017;37:841–5.

8. Descamps F, Yasik E, Hardy D, Lafontaine M, Delince P. Pigmented villonodular synovitis of the hip. A case report and review of the literature. Clin Rheumatol. 1991;10:184–90.

9. Yoon HJ, Cho YA, Lee JI, Hong SP, Hong SD. Malignant pigmented villonodular synovitis of the temporomandibular joint with lung metastasis: a case report and review of the literature. Oral Surg Oral Med Oral Pathol Oral Radiol Endod. 2011;111:e30–6.

10. Yudoh K, Matsuno H, Nezuka T, Kimura T. Different mechanisms of synovial hyperplasia in rheumatoid arthritis and pigmented villonodular synovitis: the role of telomerase activity in synovial proliferation. Arthritis Rheum. 1999;42:669–77.

11. Ide S, Toiyama Y, Okugawa Y, et al. Clinical significance of C-reactive protein-to-albumin ratio with rectal Cancer patient undergoing Chemoradiotherapy followed by surgery. Anticancer Res. 2017;37:5797–804.

12. Wang X, Cui MM, Xu Y, et al. Decreased mean platelet volume predicts poor prognosis in invasive bladder cancer. Oncotarget. 2017;8:68115–22.

13. Liao LJ, Hsu WL, Wang CT, et al. Prognostic impact of pre-treatment neutrophil-to-lymphocyte ratio (NLR) in nasopharyngeal carcinoma: a retrospective study of 180 Taiwanese patients. Clin Otolaryngology. 2018;43(2):463–469.

14. Cetinkaya M, Buldu I, Kurt O, Inan R. Platelet-to-lymphocyte ratio: a new factor for predicting systemic inflammatory response syndrome after percutaneous Nephrolithotomy. Urol J. 2017;14:4089–93.

15. Yang Z, Zhang Z, Lin F, et al. Comparisons of neutrophil-, monocyte-, eosinophil-, and basophil- lymphocyte ratios among various systemic autoimmune rheumatic diseases. APMIS. 2017;125:863–71.

16. Zhang J, Zhang HY, Li J, Shao XY, Zhang CX. The elevated NLR, PLR and PLT may predict the prognosis of patients with colorectal cancer: a systematic review and meta-analysis. Oncotarget. 2017;8:68837–46.

17. Kaida T, Nitta H, Kitano Y, et al. Preoperative platelet-to-lymphocyte ratio can predict recurrence beyond the Milan criteria after hepatectomy for patients with hepatocellular carcinoma. Hepatol Res. 2017;47:991–9.

18. Cheng XG, You YH, Liu W, Zhao T, Qu H. MRI features of pigmented villonodular synovitis (PVNS). Clin Rheumatol. 2004;23:31–4.

19. Bewick V, Cheek L, Ball J. Statistics review 13: receiver operating characteristic curves. Crit Care. 2004;8:508–12.

20. Mandelbaum BR, Grant TT, Hartzman S, et al. The use of MRI to assist in diagnosis of pigmented villonodular synovitis of the knee joint. Clin Orthop Relat Res. 1988(231):135–139.

21. Murphey MD, Rhee JH, Lewis RB, Fanburg-Smith JC, Flemming DJ, Walker EA. Pigmented villonodular synovitis: radiologic-pathologic correlation. Radiographics. 2008;28:1493–518.

22. Isart A, Gelber PE, Besalduch M, et al. High recurrence and good functional results after arthroscopic resection of pigmented villonodular synovitis. Revista espanola de cirugia ortopedica y traumatologia. 2015;59:400–5.

23. Shabat S, Kollender Y, Merimsky O, et al. The use of surgery and yttrium 90 in the management of extensive and diffuse pigmented villonodular synovitis of large joints. Rheumatology (Oxford). 2002;41:1113–8.

24. Horoschak M, Tran PT, Bachireddy P, et al. External beam radiation therapy enhances local control in pigmented villonodular synovitis. Int J Radiat Oncol Biol Phys. 2009;75:183–7.

25. Kucuk A, Uslu AU, Ugan Y, et al. Neutrophil-to-lymphocyte ratio is involved in the severity of ankylosing spondylitis. Bratislavske lekarske listy. 2015;116:722–5.

26. Lin JP, Lin JX, Cao LL, et al. Preoperative lymphocyte-to-monocyte ratio as a strong predictor of survival and recurrence for gastric cancer after radical-intent surgery. Oncotarget. 2017;8:79234–47.

27. Hong YF, Chen ZH, Wei L, et al. Identification of the prognostic value of lymphocyte-to-monocyte ratio in patients with HBV-associated advanced hepatocellular carcinoma. Oncol Lett. 2017;14:2089–96.

28. Xue P, Hang J, Huang W, et al. Validation of lymphocyte-to-monocyte ratio as a prognostic factor in advanced pancreatic Cancer: an east Asian cohort study of 2 countries. Pancreas. 2017;46(8):1011–1017.

29. Guo X, Zhang S, Zhang Q, et al. Neutrophil:lymphocyte ratio is positively related to type 2 diabetes in a large-scale adult population: a Tianjin chronic low-grade systemic inflammation and health cohort study. Eur J Endocrinol. 2015;173:217–25.

30. Coutinho M, Laranjo A, Casanova J. Pigmented Villonodular synovitis: a diagnostic challenge. Review of 28 cases. Acta reumatologica portuguesa. 2012;37:335–41.

13

Bone morphogenetic proteins – 7 and – 2 in the treatment of delayed osseous union secondary to bacterial osteitis in a rat model

Lars Helbig[1†], Georg W. Omlor[1*†] (iD), Adriana Ivanova[1], Thorsten Guehring[2], Robert Sonntag[3], J. Philippe Kretzer[3], Susann Minkwitz[4], Britt Wildemann[4,5] and Gerhard Schmidmaier[1]

Abstract

Background: Bone infections due to trauma and subsequent delayed or impaired fracture healing represent a great challenge in orthopedics and trauma surgery. The prevalence of such bacterial infection-related types of delayed non-union is high in complex fractures, particularly in open fractures with additional extensive soft-tissue damage. The aim of this study was to establish a rat model of delayed osseous union secondary to bacterial osteitis and investigate the impact of rhBMP-7 and rhBMP-2 on fracture healing in the situation of an ongoing infection.

Methods: After randomization to four groups 72 Sprague-Dawley rats underwent a transverse fracture of the midshaft tibia stabilized by intramedullary titanium K-wires. Three groups received an intramedullary inoculation with *Staphylococcus aureus* (10^3 colony-forming units) before stabilization and the group without bacteria inoculation served as healing control. After 5 weeks, a second surgery was performed with irrigation of the medullary canal and local rhBMP-7 and rhBMP-2 treatment whereas control group and infected control group received sterile saline. After further 5 weeks rats were sacrificed and underwent biomechanical testing to assess the mechanical stability of the fractured bone. Additional micro-CT analysis, histological, and histomorphometric analysis were done to evaluate bone consolidation or delayed union, respectively, and to quantify callus formation and the mineralized area of the callus.

Results: Biomechanical testing showed a significantly higher fracture torque in the non-infected control group and the infected rhBMP-7- and rhBMP-2 group compared with the infected control group ($p < 0.001$). RhBMP-7 and rhBMP-2 groups did not show statistically significant differences ($p = 0.57$). Histological findings supported improved bone-healing after rhBMP treatment but quantitative micro-CT and histomorphometric results still showed significantly more hypertrophic callus tissue in all three infected groups compared to the non-infected group. Results from a semiquantitative bone-healing-score revealed best bone-healing in the non-infected control group. The expected chronic infection was confirmed in all infected groups.

Conclusions: In delayed bone healing secondary to infection rhBMP treatment promotes bone healing with no significant differences in the healing efficacy of rhBMP-2 and rhBMP-7 being noted. Further new therapeutic bone substitutes should be analyzed with the present rat model for delayed osseous union secondary to bacterial osteitis.

Keywords: Animal model, Rat, Delayed osseous union, Osteitis, Biomechanical testing, Micro-CT, Bone morphogenetic protein 7, Bone morphogenetic protein 2

* Correspondence: Georg.omlor@med.uni-heidelberg.de
†Lars Helbig and Georg W. Omlor contributed equally to this work.
[1]Clinic for Orthopedics and Trauma Surgery, Center for Orthopedics, Trauma Surgery and Spinal Cord Injury, Heidelberg University Hospital, Schlierbacher Landstrasse 200a, 69118 Heidelberg, Germany
Full list of author information is available at the end of the article

Background

Bacterial bone infections due to trauma with subsequent delayed or impaired fracture healing are highly feared complications in orthopedics and traumatology and represent a great challenge. Open fractures in particular exhibit an incidence of osteitis as high as 55% [1]. Bacteria colonizing implants can interfere with physiological bone formation and remodeling mechanisms and lead to a higher risk of impaired fracture healing [1, 2]. In most cases, *Staphylococcus aureus* (*S. aureus*) is responsible for infection. The bacterium can infiltrate osteoblasts, builds biofilms and mutates into its small colony variants form, all leading to a high antibiotic resistance [1, 3, 4]. Therefore currently available therapeutic options must involve not only antibiotic treatment but also repeated surgical debridement, potentially exacerbating extensive bone defects [4]. Furthermore, prolonged treatment of delayed fracture healing may have a profound effect on both the medical and emotional condition of the patient as well as his financial and professional security [5].

Bone morphogenetic proteins (BMPs), already established as a useful addition to classic therapy in cases of non-union and delayed fracture union, have not been sufficiently investigated in infected fractures of the long bones [6]. Only rhBMP-2 was evaluated on surgical infections in a rabbit posterolateral lumbar fusion model showing an insignificant trend toward improved fusion rate and less mortality [7]. BMP-application is officially not indicated in the situation of an infected non-union of the long bones, because scientific data in the literature is insufficient. Currently, BMPs can only be used off-label in the situation of an infection.

BMPs are naturally responsible for the induction of osteogenic differentiation of mesenchymal stem cells and for angiogenesis and show limited expression during delayed fracture healing [8–10]. Recombinant(rh)BMP-2 and rhBMP-7 have been proven to promote fracture healing both in delayed fracture healing and non-union animal models [11–14]. RhBMP-2 has shown high potential in the treatment of open fractures in clinical trials, leading to faster union establishment, lower infection rate and lower number of surgeries needed [15–17]. Similarly, rhBMP-7 could enhance the efficacy and the treatment success of non-union in the combined therapy with autologous cancellous bone [18].

The outcome of BMP-enhanced treatment of delayed fracture healing in the situation of an ongoing low-grade bone infection has not yet been sufficiently explored.

Therefore, the goal of this study was to investigate the impact of rhBMP-7 and rhBMP-2 on fracture healing in an animal model of delayed osseous union secondary to chronic bacterial osteitis [19]. The hypothesis was that rhBMP-7 and rhBMP-2 may improve bone healing in the situation of an infection without significant differences between both factors. Primary objective was the fracture torque in biomechanical evaluations, secondary objectives were radiological and histological outcome.

Methods

Preparation of bacterial inoculum

Bone infection in this study was induced by the bacterium *Staphylococcus aureus subsp. aureus* Rosenbach (ATCC® 49,230™) – a strain isolated from a patient with chronic osteomyelitis and effectively used in the induction of bone infections before [20]. The needed amount of 10^3 colony-forming units (CFU) had already been determined in a previous study [19]. Bacterial cultivation was performed according to the official product instruction, using Trypticase Soy Broth (TSB) for liquid cultures and blood agar plates for plating (Becton, Dickinson and Company, New Jersey, USA). All cultures were handled under sterile conditions and incubated under permanent oxygen supply at a temperature of 37 °C. Bacterial CFU counts on blood agar plates and spectrophotometric measurements of liquid cultures were performed to establish a calibration formula. An overnight culture of *S-. aureus* in TSB, containing 10^3 CFU in 10 μl was used for each surgery.

Animals and surgical procedure

All experiments were approved by the Animal Experimentation Ethics Committee of Karlsruhe (35–9185.81/ G-171/11). 72 four-months old female Sprague Dawley rats (Charles River Laboratories, Germany) with an average weight of 296 g were divided into four study groups with 18 rats per group. Two of the groups were used as controls with induction of a bone infection (+S. aureus) or without infection (control). The animals in the two other groups were used as study groups for the treatment with rhBMP-7 (rhBMP-7 + S. aureus) or rhBMP-2 (rhBMP-2 + S. aureus).

Surgery preparation and follow-up

Prior to surgery, general anesthesia was performed by a weight-adapted subcutaneous injection of medetomidine (Dorbene Vet 1 mg/ml), midazolam (Dormicum 15 mg/3 ml) and fentanyl (Fentanyl – Janssen 0.05 mg/ml) after sedation with isoflurane in a sedation box. Additional preparation for surgery included shaving and disinfecting the right hind leg of the rat and covering the animal body with sterile sheets. Body temperature and anesthesia depth were tested periodically during surgery. After completion of the surgical procedure an anesthesia antidote mixture of atipamezole (Antisedan 5 mg/ml), flumazenil (Flumazenil Kabi 0.1 mg/ml) and naloxone (Naloxon Incresa 0,4 mg/ml) was injected. Clinical condition and body weight were controlled and a three-day post-operative analgesic medication with buprenorphine (Temgesic) was applied.

Fracture and infection model

During the first surgery all right tibiae were fractured and a bacterial infection was induced in the infection groups. A 5 mm incision through the skin and fasciae medial to the ligamentum patellae was followed by drilling a 1 mm hole through the cortical tibial bone at the proximal metaphysis to access the medullar cavity. Afterwards intramedullary reaming without irrigation was performed using a 0.8 mm k-wire up to the distal part of the medullar cavity. Tibia and fibula were then fractured using an established fracture device [12, 19]. The right hind leg was placed on a metal plate and a weight of 600 g was fixated 15 cm above the leg with a removable pin. Removal of the pin resulted in a sudden free fall of the weight and a consequent transverse fracture of tibia and fibula (AO 42-A3) with a momentum of 1.03 kg m/s. The bacterial inoculum of 10^3 CFU / 10 µl S. aureus was injected with a microliter syringe into the medullar cavity of all tibiae in the infection groups. All animals of the control group received the same procedure using a sham liquid of 10 µl sterile Tryptic Soy Broth (TSB). A closed reduction of the fracture was performed with 0.8 mm k-wire ostheosynthesis. The fascia and skin were sutured in a single-knot technique.

Growth factor application

All animals received second surgery five weeks after the first surgery. The skin incision was placed over the scar of the previous suturing. The k-wire was carefully removed and the medullar cavity was irrigated with sterile saline. All animals of the control and infected control group received an intramedullary injection of a control fluid of 30 µl sterile saline at the fracture site. The other infected animals received an intramedullary injection of 30 µg rhBMP-7 (1 µg/µl in sterile saline, Olympus, USA) or 25 µg rhBMP-2 (1 µg/µl in sterile saline, Medtronic, USA) respectively. A new k-wire was applied for osteosynthesis and the skin and fascia were sutured in a single-knot technique.

Body weight and body temperature

Rectal body temperature was measured and body weight was determined with a precision scale on post-operative days 0, 7, 14, 35, 42 and 70. Further indications for local or systemic infections were evaluated.

Sacrifice

The animals were sacrificed with CO_2 in a sedation box. The right tibiae of the hind legs were dissected under sterile conditions. The entire soft tissue was removed from bones.

Biomechanical testing

At the 10 weeks endpoint the intramedullary implants were carefully removed (Control group: 9 samples; infected control group: 9; rhBMP-7 group: 8; rhBMP-2 group: 7). Both tibiae were dissected free from soft tissue for biomechanical torsional testing. After dissection of the bones, the proximal and distal ends were placed into two embedding molds (Technovit 4071, Heraeus Kulzer GmbH, Germany) while using a fixture device to avoid any preloading of the bones prior to testing. The lower embedding mold was connected to a pivoted axis while rotation of the upper mold was restrained (Fig. 1). A linear, constant rotation (10°/min) was applied by the biomechanical testing device while the resultant torque was recorded (8661–4500-V0200, Burster, Germany) until bony fracture occurred. For biomechanical testing a comparison with the contralateral tibiae of each animal was done.

Micro-CT

The fractured tibiae of all animals were scanned with the SkyScan 1076 in-vivo micro-computertomograph (Brucker micro-CT, Belgium) at the endpoint (10 weeks after fracture). The tibiae were scanned with an isotropic pixel size of 18 µm and energy settings of 100 kV (voltage), 400 ms (exposure time) and 100 µA (current) through a 1.0-mm aluminium filter. Image reconstruction, including ring artifact reduction (20/20), beam hardening correction (30%) and smoothing (1/10) was performed using the SkyScan NRecon software (v. 1.6.9.8, Brucker microCT, Belgium).

Qualitative evaluation of the datasets was performed by simultaneously viewing multiple orthogonal slices in SkyScan DataViewer (v. 1.4, Brucker microCT, Belgium). Additionally, new bone formation at the fracture site, bridging of the fracture and bone remodeling were analyzed semi-quantitatively adopted from the scoring system of Lane and Sandhu and given points from 0 (absent), 1 (25%), 2 (50%), 3 (75%) to 4 (100%) [21]. Hence, the highest possible score was 12 points. The scoring system was used as "bone-healing-score". The modified score of An and Friedman was used to determine the grade of osteitis at the endpoint [22, 23]. The score of An and Friedman is a radiographic scoring system for assessing the development and progression of osteomyelitis in a rabbit model. This score was used in the study as "bone-infection-score". Seven characteristic parameters were analyzed: periosteal reaction (1), osteolysis (2), soft tissue swelling (3), deformity (4), general impression (5), sequester formation (6) and spontaneous fracture (7). For evaluation of the parameter 1 to 5, the

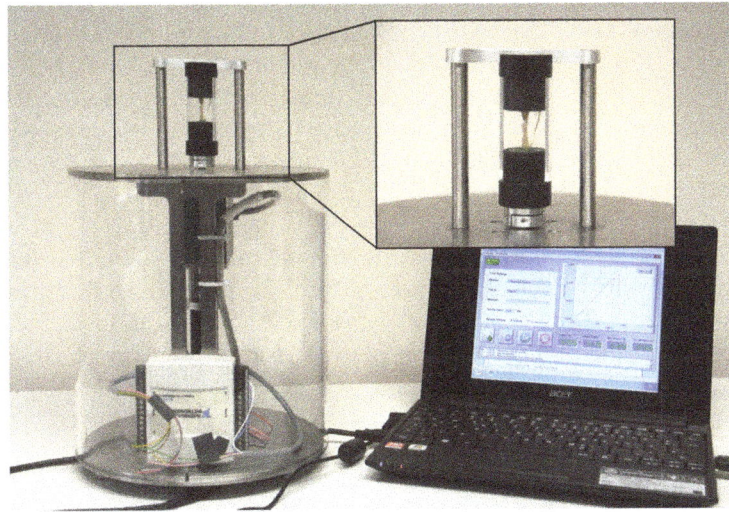

Fig. 1 Biomechanical torsional testing machine with bone segment fixed in vertical direction by two embedding molds (detail view). A linear, constant rotation speed of 10°/min was applied to measure the resultant torque needed to induce re-fracture

tibia was divided into three regions of interest (ROI) – proximal epiphysis, diaphysis and distal epiphysis, and a score from 0 (absent), 1 (mild), 2 (moderate) to 3 (severe) was given to each ROI. For parameters 6 and 7 the whole tibia was graded with a score of either 0 (absent) or 1 (present). Therefore, the highest possible score was 47.

Bone morphometry of the 3D-dataset was performed using the software CTAn (v. 1.13.2.1., Brucker microCT, Belgium). The volume of interest (VOI) for each tibia was defined as the bone area in between 3.5 mm proximal and distal to the fracture line (400 slices) [24, 25]. The following parameters were used for bone morphometry of the VOI for each animal at the endpoint after 10 weeks: tissue volume (TV), bone volume (BV) and bone volume fraction (BV/TV).

Histology

The tibiae from each group were randomly harvested for histological evaluation at the endpoint after 10 weeks as previously described (Control group: 9 samples; infected control group: 7; rhBMP-7 group: 6; rhBMP-2 group: 7) [26]. Surrounding muscles and intramedullary implant were carefully removed. After fixation for 2 days in 10% normal buffered formaldehyde, dehydration was done in ascending concentrations of ethanol and followed by undecalcified embedding in methylmethacrylate (Technovit 9100, Heraeus Kulzer GmbH, Germany). Longitudinal sections in a sagittal plane were cut at 6 μm with a Leica SM 2500 s microtome (Bensheim, Germany) with a 40° stainless-steel knife. Different stains were used, including von Kossa/Safranin-O, Masson Goldner and Gram stain for microscopic visualization of mineralized bone, cartilage and *S. aureus* in the tissue and bone, respectively. Evaluation was performed with a Leica DM-RB

microscope (Bensheim, Germany). Qualitative changes were first evaluated in representative slides depicting the fracture gap area. Further histological parameters were measured with an image analysis system (Zeiss KS 400, Germany) at a magnification of × 1.6 to calculate structural indices as described previously [26]. The region of interest was defined at 3.5 mm proximally and distally to the center of the fracture gap. The total diameter of the callus was included in the ROI. For quantitative histomorphometric analysis, the area of the total callus (Total callus area; [mm^2]), the area of the periosteal callus (periosteal callus area; [mm^2]), and the mineralized periosteal bone area of the periosteal total callus area (periosteal bone area/periosteal total area; [%]) were measured and compared between the four groups.

Statistics

Primary outcome measure was fracture torque in biomechanical analysis. Secondary outcome measures were the results from the bone-healing-score and the bone-infection-score, and the results from quantitative micro CT and histomorphometry. The sample size planning showed an effect size f of 0.82 and an actual power of 0.878 with a sample size of 6 animals per group. A final sample size of 9 animals per group was chosen to compensate drop-outs. The post hoc power analysis provided an effect size f of 0.71 and an actual power of 0.918 for the biomechanical evaluations as the primary end point. For descriptive statistics, mean and standard deviation (SD) were calculated for continuous, median, and interquartile ranges for ordinal variables. Group comparisons were performed using one-way analysis of variance (ANOVA) for independent samples. All tests were two-sided and a p-value ≤0.05 was considered significant. Statistical analysis was performed with SPSS software (v. 22.0, IBM Corporation, USA).

Results

Body weight and body temperature
No significant differences of body weight and body temperature were detected between the four groups. Body weight moderately decreased in the four groups during the first two weeks after surgery, but the animals continuously gained weight afterwards reaching normal weight again at the endpoint. Body temperature remained stable in all groups during the 10 weeks follow-up.

Drop-outs
Three animals died at the first and second operation, respectively, due to complications with general anesthesia. Two animals were sacrificed because of a postoperative infected hematoma. Further 5 specimens had to be excluded due to technical problems during the preparation of the tibiae.

Biomechanical testing
The K-wires could be removed easily in all cases, with no differences detected between the groups. At the contralateral non-fractured side, all groups did not show statistically significant differences ($p = 0.9$). Average fracture torques (Nm) was 0.213 +/− 0.022 Nm in the control group, 0.227 +/− 0.087 Nm in the infected control group, 0.227 +/− 0.074 Nm in the rhBMP-7 group and 0.206 +/− 0.035 Nm in the rhBMP-2 group at the non-fractured side. At the fractured side, Fracture torques (Nm) in the rhBMP-2, rhBMP-7, and control group were significantly higher than in the infected control group ($p < 0.001$) (Fig. 2). The differences between the rhBMP-7 group and rhBMP-2 group were not

statistically significant ($p = 0.6$) (Fig. 2). The fractured tibiae of the control group showed an average fracture torque of 0.212 +/− 0.012 Nm, the rhBMP-7 group an average fracture torque of 0.209 +/− 0.026 Nm and the rhBMP-2 group a fracture torque of 0.203 +/− 0.018 Nm compared to 0.147 +/− 0.019 Nm in the infected control group (Fig. 2).

Micro-CT results
Micro-CT pictures of the non-infected control group showed increased consolidation with complete bridging of the fracture gap compared with both rhBMP-groups and the infected control group at the endpoint (Fig. 3). Compared to the non-infected control group, all infected groups (infected control group (*S. aureus*), rhBMP-7 group (rhBMP-7 + *S. aureus*), rhBMP-2 group (rhBMP-2 + *S. aureus*)) showed increased hypertrophic callus formation. Most callus was visible in the infected control group. Callus formation showed no differences between the rhBMP-7 and the rhBMP-2 group (Fig. 3).

The non-infected control group presented a significantly higher bone-healing-score representative for best bone healing and bridging ($p < 0.001$) and a significantly lower bone-infection-score compared to all other three groups ($p < 0.001$). The scores of both rhBMP-groups (rhBMP-7 + *S. aureus*, rhBMP-2 + *S. aureus*) did not reach the level of the control group, but they showed better results than the infected control group (*S. aureus*) with fewer signs of osteitis, more bone formation and enhanced bone remodeling (Fig. 4a and b).

Quantitative callus evaluation revealed that bone volume (BV) and tissue volume (TV) of the non-infected control group were significantly lower than of the infected groups (infected control group, rhBMP-7 group, rhBMP-2 group) (Fig. 5a and b). Additionally, the rhBMP-2 group and the rhBMP-7 group showed a

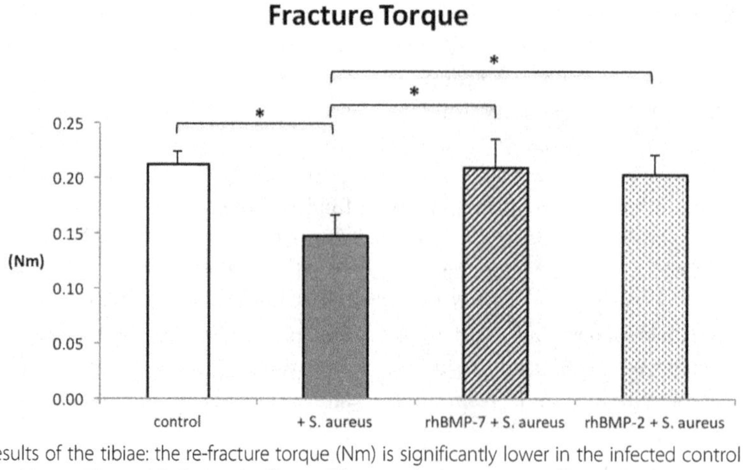

Fig. 2 Mechanical testing results of the tibiae: the re-fracture torque (Nm) is significantly lower in the infected control group than in the other three groups at the endpoint. Lines with asterisk depict significant differences between groups (* $p < 0.001$)

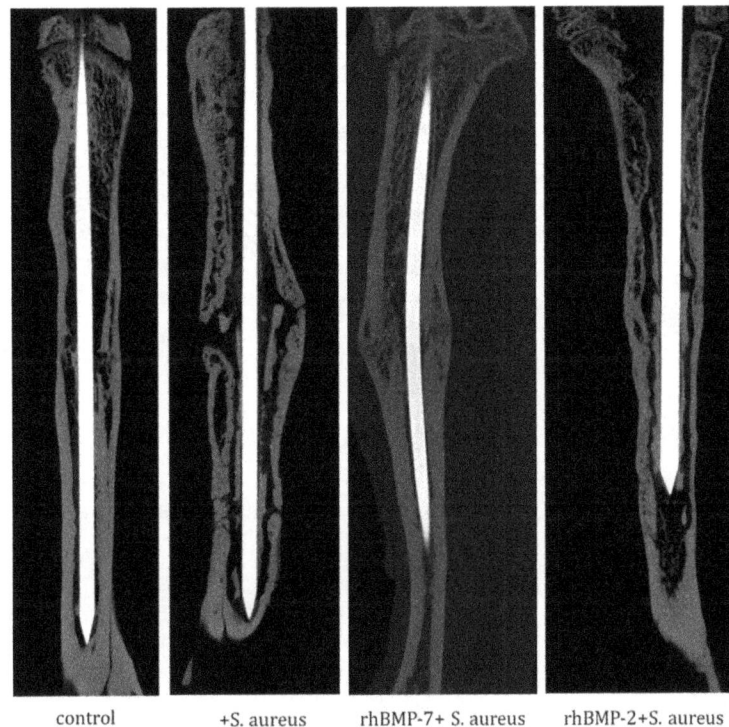

|control|+S. aureus|rhBMP-7+ S. aureus|rhBMP-2+S. aureus|

Fig. 3 Micro computed tomography (micro-CT) of the right tibiae of Sprague-Dawley rats at the endpoint. Fracture, bacterial infection or sham infection, and intramedullary stabilization with titanium Kirschner wires was performed 10 weeks before; application of rhBMP-7, rhBMP-2 or sterile saline was done 5 weeks before analysis. Improved consolidation of the fracture gap is recognizable in the control group compared to the three infected groups. Considerable differences in callus formation between both rhBMP groups were not detected

significantly lower bone volume fraction compared to the control group. There were no statistically significant differences between the infected control group and both rhBMP-groups (Fig. 5c).

Histology

Qualitative evaluation of histological slides showed good callus formation and progressed bone remodeling with few connective tissue in the non-infected control group. In the infected control group, more fibroblasts and cartilage were observed in the fracture region (Figs. 6 and 7: II). Both rhBMP groups showed partially remodeled fractures at the endpoint with only moderately remaining cartilage or fibrous tissue (Figs. 6 and 7: III and IV). Gram stain showed *S. aureus* in the orginal cortex and cancellous bone in all specimens of the three infected groups (Fig. 8). The bacteria were encapsulated in the cortex fragments. *S. aureus* was not found in the newly formed woven bone in all three infected groups. There were no significant differences between the three infected groups. Additionally, the three infected groups showed a second cortex in the histology. Significant differences between these groups were not detectable.

Histomorphometric analyses of the periosteal callus area showed significant differences in the infected control group ($p = 0.009$) and the rhBMP-2 group ($p = 0.037$) compared to non-infected controls (Fig. 9a). Analysis of callus composition still revealed significantly less mineralized bone tissue in the periosteal callus in the rhBMP-2 ($p = 0.005$) and rhBMP-7 group ($p = 0.05$) compared to non-infected controls (Fig. 9b). Infected controls and both rhBMP groups did not show significant differences ($p = 0.8$ (rhBMP-7) and $p = 0.3$ (rhBMP-2)).

Discussion

In this study, we have evaluated the effect of recombinant human bone morphogenetic proteins – 7 and – 2 for the treatment of delayed osseous union secondary to bacterial osteitis in our animal model using micro-CT examinations, qualitative histology, histomorphometric evaluations, and biomechanical investigations. To our knowledge this is the first study, which compared recombinant human bone morphogenetic proteins – 7 and – 2 in an in vivo animal model of delayed osseous union in the situation of an ongoing bacterial bone infection.

We have chosen rhBMP-7 and -2 in our study setting, because these growth factors have been established clinically in the treatment of non-union [15, 27–29]. Giannoudis et al. [29] could show a synergistic effect of

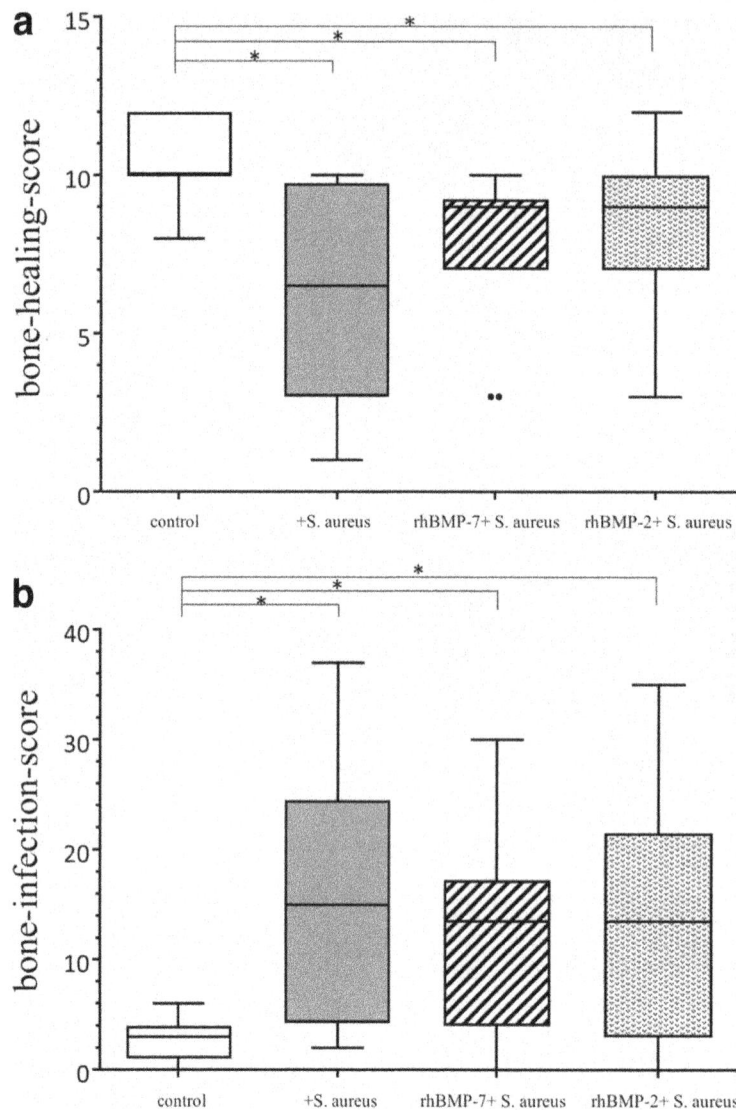

Fig. 4 Outcome of (**a**) the bone-healing-score adapted from Lane & Sandhu with a maximal score of 12 points and (**b**) the bone-infection-score adapted from An & Friedman with seven characteristic parameters for a maximal score of 47 points. Both scores are significantly different between the control group and the three infected groups. Lines with asterisk depict significant differences between groups (* $p < 0.05$)

autograft and bone morphogenetic protein – 7 in the therapy of atrophic humeral, femoral and tibial non-union with a healing rate of 100% in 45 patients. Govender et al. [15] investigated rhBMP-2 in the treatment of open tibial fractures and showed better fracture- and wound-healing and reduced infection rate. Similar effects have been described by others [30, 31]. Significant differences in the effectiveness of both factors or synergistic effects have not been described.

According to micro-CT-scans and histology, treatment with rhBMPs was unable to achieve a complete union in the situation of infection during the follow-up period, but we could find positive effects on bone healing in biomechanical evaluations as well as in the semi-quantitative bone-healing-score and in callus histology. Biomechanical

investigations and scoring of the micro-CT images revealed significantly more stability and healing in the infected rhBMP groups equal to non-infected controls if compared to the infected control group. Thus, the findings indicate that rhBMP treatment is possibly able to improve bone healing in the setting of infection, although it has no direct effect on the infection with *S. aureus* [32]. In this regard, our investigations supported the results in the literature [33, 34]. All infected groups, no matter if rhBMP therapy was added or not showed significantly increased mineralized callus (BV) and soft-tissue callus (TV), but a significantly decreased bone volume fraction (BV/TV) in quantitative micro-CT evaluation as well as larger periosteal callus areas and smaller mineralized periosteal bone areas of the periosteal total callus area in histology. This

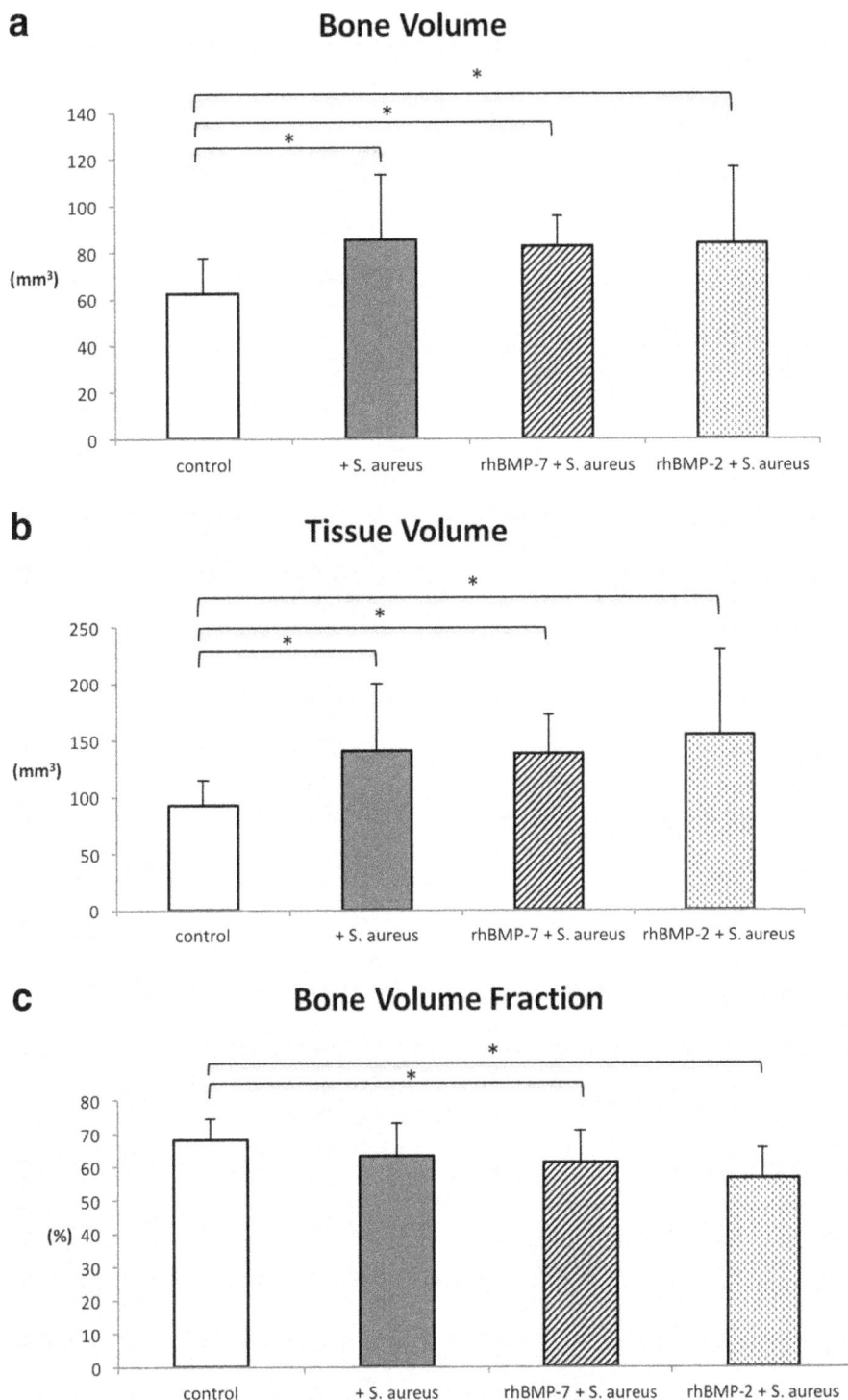

Fig. 5 Quantitative micro-CT evaluation of bone volume (mm^3) (**a**), tissue volume (mm^3) (**b**) and bone volume fraction (%) (**c**) of the four groups at the endpoint. Lines with asterisk depict significant differences between groups (* $p < 0.05$)

may be interpreted as a hypertrophic callus, explaining less stability compared with the non-infected control group. In agreement with other studies, Schmidmaier et al. [28] and Bode et al. [35] postulated that an infection or an instable fixation are the cause of a hypertrophic

non-union formation. They recommend repeated debridements in case of infected, especially open fractures, with stable osteosynthesis depending on the type of the fracture to prevent non-union. In the present study, histology further showed some qualitative differences of the callus. In

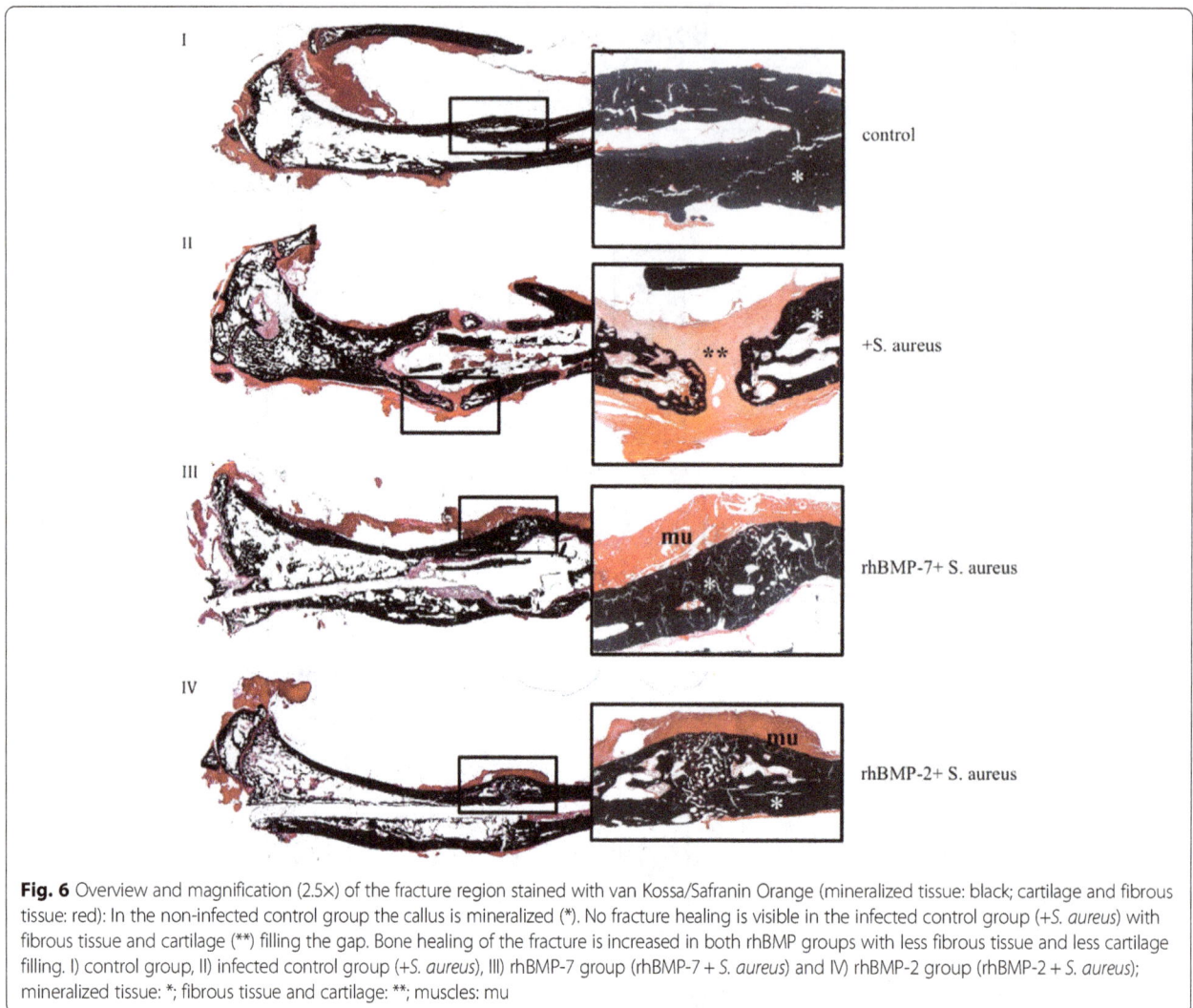

Fig. 6 Overview and magnification (2.5×) of the fracture region stained with van Kossa/Safranin Orange (mineralized tissue: black; cartilage and fibrous tissue: red): In the non-infected control group the callus is mineralized (*). No fracture healing is visible in the infected control group (+*S. aureus*) with fibrous tissue and cartilage (**) filling the gap. Bone healing of the fracture is increased in both rhBMP groups with less fibrous tissue and less cartilage filling. I) control group, II) infected control group (+*S. aureus*), III) rhBMP-7 group (rhBMP-7 + *S. aureus*) and IV) rhBMP-2 group (rhBMP-2 + *S. aureus*); mineralized tissue: *; fibrous tissue and cartilage: **; muscles: mu

rhBMP specimens, we saw increased signs of fracture remodeling with only moderately remaining cartilage and fibrous tissue. These changes seemed less pronounced in infected controls without rhBMP treatment. In contrast to the study of Chen et al. [33, 34], which used a rat femur model with a segmental chronically infected bone defect, we were not able to achieve significantly more newly mineralized callus compared to infected controls in our animal model. A possible reason for this better mineralization might be the additional antibiotic treatment in the study of Chen et al.

As a limitation of our study, we did not analyze longer follow-up times, so further effects might have been detectable after the analyzed duration of 5 weeks after rhBMP treatment. Furthermore, we were not able to specifically identify or quantify the underlying mechanisms for the increased stability, possibly due to technical limitations as the bone specimen had to be collected, removed from soft tissue, further prepared and fixed before cutting into 6 μm sections for

histological slides. Hence, semi-quantitative histological assessment of the callus architecture was not possible. Nevertheless, signs of partial fracture remodeling were mainly found in rhBMP specimen contrary to more fibroblasts and remaining cartilage in infected controls.

Clinical studies such as the BESTT study (BMP-2 Evaluation in Surgery and Tibial Trauma) have presented both an accelerated healing process and a lower infection rate after treatment with rhBMP-2 [15]. Similarly successful results were obtained by a combined two-step non-union therapy with rhBMP-7 after osteomyelitis [36]. However, it should be taken into consideration that clinical routine therapy of bone infections also involves debridement of necrotic bone, soft tissue management and antibiotic therapy [4, 37]. These procedures lead to reduction of bacterial load and open the way for osteoprogenitor cells from the periosteum, blood vessels and soft tissue into the defect [38, 39]. Similar procedure was used in the rhBMP-2 and rhBMP-7 studies in a rat model of Chen et al. [33]. In the experimental setting of

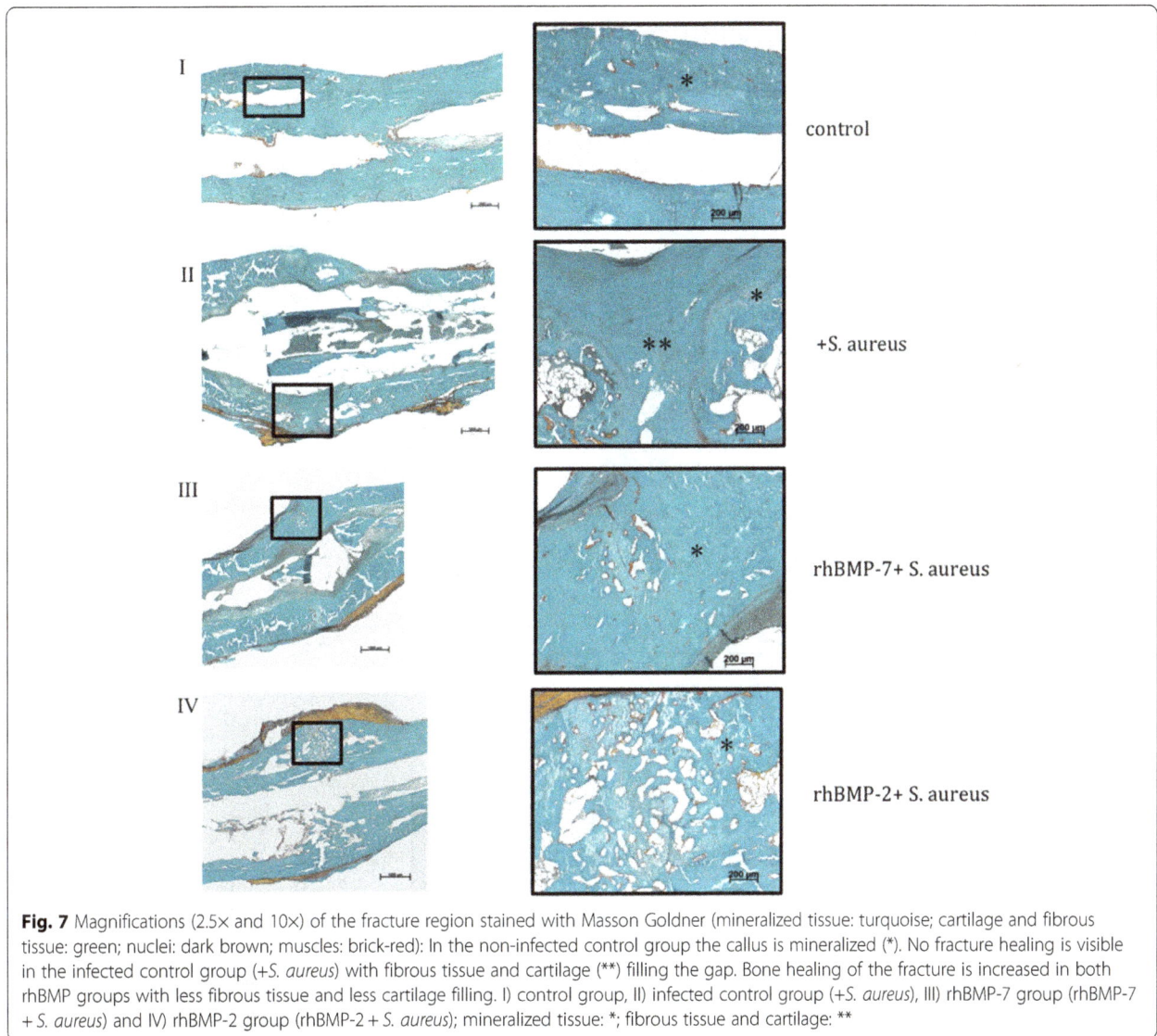

Fig. 7 Magnifications (2.5× and 10×) of the fracture region stained with Masson Goldner (mineralized tissue: turquoise; cartilage and fibrous tissue: green; nuclei: dark brown; muscles: brick-red): In the non-infected control group the callus is mineralized (*). No fracture healing is visible in the infected control group (+*S. aureus*) with fibrous tissue and cartilage (**) filling the gap. Bone healing of the fracture is increased in both rhBMP groups with less fibrous tissue and less cartilage filling. I) control group, II) infected control group (+*S. aureus*), III) rhBMP-7 group (rhBMP-7 + *S. aureus*) and IV) rhBMP-2 group (rhBMP-2 + *S. aureus*); mineralized tissue: *; fibrous tissue and cartilage: **

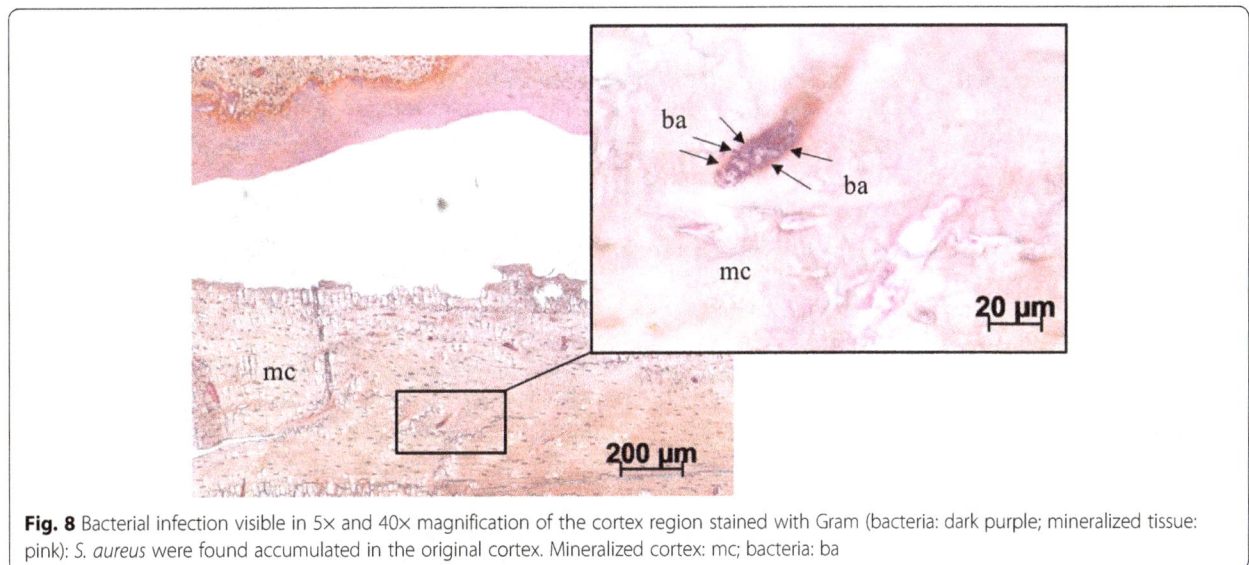

Fig. 8 Bacterial infection visible in 5× and 40× magnification of the cortex region stained with Gram (bacteria: dark purple; mineralized tissue: pink): *S. aureus* were found accumulated in the original cortex. Mineralized cortex: mc; bacteria: ba

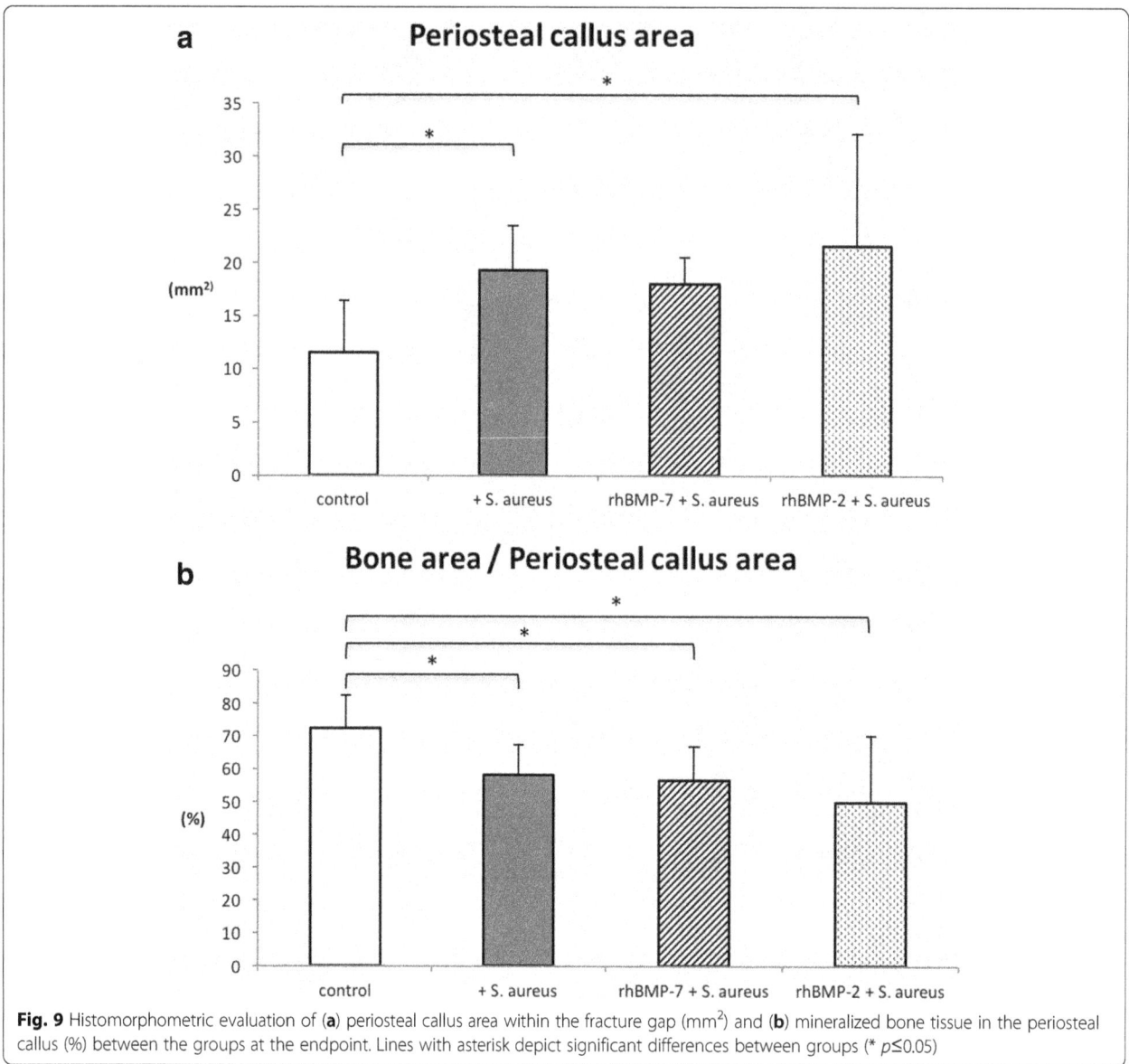

Fig. 9 Histomorphometric evaluation of (**a**) periosteal callus area within the fracture gap (mm^2) and (**b**) mineralized bone tissue in the periosteal callus (%) between the groups at the endpoint. Lines with asterisk depict significant differences between groups (* $p \leq 0.05$)

our study only intramedullary irrigation with sterile saline, rhBMPs application and k-wire replacement were performed, which will have maintained a high bacterial burden in the bone. Most clinical cases of unsuccessful non-union treatment reveal subclinical infection [36]. This clinical experience, together with the findings of the current animal study suggest that an ongoing bone infection will hamper bone healing with potentially reduced effectiveness of the rhBMPs. Further in-vivo studies might help to get further information on this topic. RhBMP application in an animal model together with differently concentrated bacterial suspensions and without could be analyzed, to determine potential bacterial-dose-dependent effects. Also adverse effects have been described in the literature for rhBMP therapy [40–43] but were not found in the present animal study

at least in the short term, as we did not find rhBMP associated side-effects or complications such as heterotopic ossifications or induction of neoplasms [42, 43].

Future studies should investigate later time-points of bone healing in order to compare the biomechanical, histological and radiological results with the present study. Other growth factor application systems as well as other antibacterial or bone stimulating substances and osteosynthesis techniques [44] could also be analyzed with the present animal model considering their effectiveness in case of infection. The long-term goal would be to establish a material or a combination of materials and techniques that have osteoinductive and osteoconductive but also antimicrobial effects to provide bone healing within a short operation and healing period.

Conclusions

We could establish a rat model of delayed osseous union secondary to experimental fracture and bone infection with biomechanical, histological, and micro-CT evaluation after treatment with rhBMP-2 and rhBMP-7 compared to infected and non-infected controls. The induced bone infection caused quantitatively more callus tissue in all infected groups. In the infected control group callus was biomechanically less stable and showed less bridging. RhBMP treatment increased biomechanical stability of the callus without significant differences between rhBMP-2 and rhBMP-7. Our results demonstrate that rhBMP treatment can improve bone-healing in the situation of a chronic bone infection supporting clinical use in complicated infected non-unions.

Abbreviations

BV: bone volume; CFU: Colony-Forming Unit; CT: Computer Tomography; rhBMP: Recombinant human Bone Morphogenetic Protein; ROI: Region of interest; S. aureus: Staphylococcus aureus; TSB: Tryptic Soy Broth; TV: Tissue volume; VOI: Volume of interest

Acknowledgements

The present study was financially supported by the Center for Orthopedics, Trauma Surgery and Spinal Cord Injury, Heidelberg University Hospital. The authors thank our institutional statistician Simone Gantz for statistical analyses.

Funding

Financial support was provided by non-profit organizations exclusively (Center for Orthopedics, Trauma Surgery and Spinal Cord Injury, Heidelberg University Hospital).

Authors` contributions

LH and GO participated in the study design, animal surgeries, analysis of the findings, and drafting of the final manuscript. LH and GO contributed equally to this work. AI participated in the animal surgeries, analysis of the findings and helped draft the final manuscript. TG participated in the study design, analysis of the findings and helped draft the final manuscript. JPK and RS participated in the biomechanical testing and analysis of the findings. SM and BW participated in the histological evaluations, analysis of the findings and helped draft the final manuscript. GS participated in the study design, analysis of the findings and helped draft the final manuscript. All authors have read and approved the final manuscript.

Competing interests

All authors declare that they have no competing interests. One author (BW) is a member of the editorial board of this journal.

Author details

[1]Clinic for Orthopedics and Trauma Surgery, Center for Orthopedics, Trauma Surgery and Spinal Cord Injury, Heidelberg University Hospital, Schlierbacher Landstrasse 200a, 69118 Heidelberg, Germany. [2]Clinic for Trauma and Orthopaedic Surgery, BG Trauma Center Ludwigshafen at Heidelberg University Hospital, Ludwig-Guttmann-Strasse 13, 67071 Ludwigshafen on the Rhine, Germany. [3]Laboratory of Biomechanics and Implant Research, Clinic for Orthopedics and Trauma Surgery, Heidelberg University Hospital, Schlierbacher Landstrasse 200a, 69118 Heidelberg, Germany. [4]Berlin-Brandenburg Center for Regenerative Therapies, Charité—Universitätsmedizin Berlin, 13353 Berlin, Germany. [5]Experimental Trauma Surgery, Universitätsklinikum Jena, 07747 Jena, Germany.

References

1. Josse J, Velard F, Gangloff SC. Staphylococcus aureus vs Osteoblast: Relationship and Consequences in Osteomyelitis. Front Cell Infect Microbiol. 2015;5:85.
2. Papakostidis C, Kanakaris NK, Pretel J, Faour O, Morell DJ, Giannoudis PV. Prevalence of complications of open tibial shaft fractures stratified as per the Gustilo-Anderson classification. Injury. 2011;42:1408–15.
3. Wright JA, Nair SP. Interaction of staphylococci with bone. Int J Med Microbiol. 2010;300:193–204.
4. Walter G, Kemmerer M, Kappler C, Hoffmann R. Treatment algorithms for chronic osteomyelitis. Dtsch Arztebl International. 2012;109:257–64.
5. Hak DJ, Fitzpatrick D, Bishop JA, Marsh JL, Tilp S, Schnettler R, Simpson H, Alt V. Delayed union and nonunions: epidemiology, clinical issues, and financial aspects. Injury. 2014;45(Suppl 2):S3–7.
6. Nair MB, Kretlow JD, Mikos AG, Kasper FK. Infection and tissue engineering in segmental bone defects--a mini review. Curr Opin Biotechnol. 2011;22: 721–5.
7. Miller CP, Simpson AK, Whang PG, Erickson BP, Waked WR, Lawrence JP, Grauer JN. Effects of recombinant human bone morphogenetic protein 2 on surgical infections in a rabbit posterolateral lumbar fusion model. Am J Orthop (Belle Mead NJ). 2009;38:578–84.
8. Giannoudis PV, Einhorn TA, Marsh D. Fracture healing: the diamond concept. Injury. 2007;38(Suppl 4):S3–6.
9. Schwabe P, Simon P, Kronbach Z, Schmidmaier G, Wildemann B. A pilot study investigating the histology and growth factor content of human non-union tissue. Int Orthop. 2014;38:2623–9.
10. Garcia P, Pieruschka A, Klein M, Tami A, Histing T, Holstein JH, Scheuer C, Pohlemann T, Menger MD. Temporal and spatial vascularization patterns of unions and nonunions: role of vascular endothelial growth factor and bone morphogenetic proteins. J Bone Joint Surg Am. 2012;94:49–58.
11. Cook SD, Wolfe MW, Salkeld SL, Rueger DC. Effect of recombinant human osteogenic protein-1 on healing of segmental defects in non-human primates. J Bone Joint Surg Am. 1995;77:734–50.
12. Schmidmaier G, Wildemann B, Cromme F, Kandziora F, Haas NP, Raschke M. Bone morphogenetic protein-2 coating of titanium implants increases biomechanical strength and accelerates bone remodeling in fracture treatment: a biomechanical and histological study in rats. Bone. 2002;30: 816–22.
13. Wildemann B, Lange K, Strobel C, Fassbender M, Willie B, Schmidmaier G. Local BMP-2 application can rescue the delayed osteotomy healing in a rat model. Injury. 2011;42:746–52.
14. Vogelin E, Jones NF, Huang JI, Brekke JH, Lieberman JR. Healing of a critical-sized defect in the rat femur with use of a vascularized periosteal flap, a biodegradable matrix, and bone morphogenetic protein. J Bone Joint Surg Am. 2005;87:1323–31.
15. Govender S, Csimma C, Genant HK, Valentin-Opran A, Amit Y, Arbel R, Aro H, Atar D, Bishay M, Borner MG, et al. Recombinant human bone morphogenetic protein-2 for treatment of open tibial fractures: a prospective, controlled, randomized study of four hundred and fifty patients. J Bone Joint Surg Am. 2002;84-A:2123–34.
16. Jones AL, Bucholz RW, Bosse MJ, Mirza SK, Lyon TR, Webb LX, Pollak AN, Golden JD, Valentin-Opran A. Recombinant human BMP-2 and allograft compared with autogenous bone graft for reconstruction of diaphyseal tibial fractures with cortical defects. A randomized, controlled trial. J Bone Joint Surg Am. 2006;88:1431–41.
17. Swiontkowski MF, Aro HT, Donell S, Esterhai JL, Goulet J, Jones A, Kregor PJ, Nordsletten L, Paiement G, Patel A. Recombinant human bone morphogenetic protein-2 in open tibial fractures. A subgroup analysis of data combined from two prospective randomized studies. J Bone Joint Surg Am. 2006;88:1258–65.
18. Moghaddam-Alvandi A, Zimmermann G, Buchler A, Elleser C, Biglari B, Grutzner PA, Wolfl CG. Results of nonunion treatment with bone morphogenetic protein 7 (BMP-7). Unfallchirurg. 2012;115:518–26.
19. Helbig L, Guehring T, Rosenberger S, Ivanova A, Kaeppler K, Fischer CA, Moghaddam A, Schmidmaier G. A new animal model for delayed osseous union secondary to osteitis. BMC Musculoskelet Disord. 2015;16:362.
20. Lucke M, Schmidmaier G, Sadoni S, Wildemann B, Schiller R, Stemberger A, Haas NP, Raschke M. A new model of implant-related osteomyelitis in rats. J Biomed Mater Res B Appl Biomater. 2003;67:593–602.

21. Lane JM, Sandhu HS. Current approaches to experimental bone grafting. Orthop Clin North Am. 1987;18:213–25.

22. An YH, Friedman RJ. Animal models of orthopedic implant infection. J Invest Surg. 1998;11:139–46.

23. Lucke M, Wildemann B, Sadoni S, Surke C, Schiller R, Stemberger A, Raschke M, Haas NP, Schmidmaier G. Systemic versus local application of gentamicin in prophylaxis of implant-related osteomyelitis in a rat model. Bone. 2005; 36:770–8.

24. Bosemark P, Isaksson H, McDonald MM, Little DG. Augmentation of autologous bone graft by a combination of bone morphogenic protein and bisphosphonate increased both callus volume and strength. Acta Orthop. 2013;84:106–11.

25. Otsu N. A threshold selection method from gray-level histograms. IEEE Trans Syst Man Cybern. 1979;9:62–6.

26. Fassbender M, Minkwitz S, Thiele M, Wildemann B. Efficacy of two different demineralised bone matrix grafts to promote bone healing in a critical-size-defect: a radiological, histological and histomorphometric study in rat femurs. Int Orthop. 2014;38:1963–9.

27. Garrison KR, Shemilt I, Donell S, Ryder JJ, Mugford M, Harvey I, Song F, Alt V. Bone morphogenetic protein (BMP) for fracture healing in adults. Cochrane Database Syst Rev. 2010:CD006950.

28. Schmidmaier G, Moghaddam A. Long bone nonunion. Z Orthop Unfall. 2015;153:659–76.

29. Giannoudis PV, Kanakaris NK, Dimitriou R, Gill I, Kolimarala V, Montgomery RJ. The synergistic effect of autograft and BMP-7 in the treatment of atrophic nonunions. Clin Orthop Relat Res. 2009;467:3239–48.

30. Guelcher SA, Brown KV, Li B, Guda T, Lee BH, Wenke JC. Dual-purpose bone grafts improve healing and reduce infection. J Orthop Trauma. 2011;25:477–82.

31. Brown KV, Li B, Guda T, Perrien DS, Guelcher SA, Wenke JC. Improving bone formation in a rat femur segmental defect by controlling bone morphogenetic protein-2 release. Tissue Eng Part A. 2011;17:1735–46.

32. Dusane DH, Kyrouac D, Petersen I, Bushrow L, Calhoun JH, Granger JF, Phieffer LS, Stoodley P. Targeting intracellular Staphylococcus aureus to lower recurrence of orthopaedic infection. J Orthop Res. 2018;36:1086-1092.

33. Chen X, Schmidt AH, Tsukayama DT, Bourgeault CA, Lew WD. Recombinant human osteogenic protein-1 induces bone formation in a chronically infected, internally stabilized segmental defect in the rat femur. J Bone Joint Surg Am. 2006;88:1510–23.

34. Chen X, Schmidt AH, Mahjouri S, Polly DW Jr, Lew WD. Union of a chronically infected internally stabilized segmental defect in the rat femur after debridement and application of rhBMP-2 and systemic antibiotic. J Orthop Trauma. 2007;21:693–700.

35. Bode G, Strohm PC, Sudkamp NP, Hammer TO. Tibial shaft fractures - management and treatment options. A review of the current literature. Acta Chir Orthop Traumatol Cechoslov. 2012;79:499–505.

36. Moghaddam A, Zietzschmann S, Bruckner T, Schmidmaier G. Treatment of atrophic tibia non-unions according to 'diamond concept': results of one- and two-step treatment. Injury. 2015;46(Suppl 4):S39–50.

37. Chadayammuri V, Hake M, Mauffrey C. Innovative strategies for the management of long bone infection: a review of the Masquelet technique. Patient safety in surgery. 2015;9:32.

38. Gerstenfeld LC, Cullinane DM, Barnes GL, Graves DT, Einhorn TA. Fracture healing as a post-natal developmental process: molecular, spatial, and temporal aspects of its regulation. J Cell Biochem. 2003;88:873–84.

39. Marsell R, Einhorn TA. The biology of fracture healing. Injury. 2011;42:551–5.

40. Brannan PS, Gaston RG, Loeffler BJ, Lewis DR. Complications with the use of BMP-2 in scaphoid nonunion surgery. J Hand Surg Am. 2016;41:602–8.

41. Tannoury CA, An HS. Complications with the use of bone morphogenetic protein 2 (BMP-2) in spine surgery. Spine J. 2014;14:552–9.

42. Shi L, Sun W, Gao F, Cheng L, Li Z. Heterotopic ossification related to the use of recombinant human BMP-2 in osteonecrosis of femoral head. Medicine (Baltimore). 2017;96:e7413.

43. Hughes AP, Taher F, Farshad M, Aichmair A. Multiple myeloma exacerbation following utilization of bone morphogenetic protein-2 in lateral lumbar interbody fusion: a case report and review of the literature. Spine J. 2014;14: e13–9.

44. Nguyen AH, Kim S, Maloney WJ, Wenke JC, Yang Y. Effect of coadministration of vancomycin and BMP-2 on cocultured Staphylococcus aureus and W-20-17 mouse bone marrow stromal cells in vitro. Antimicrob Agents Chemother. 2012;56:3776–84.

14

Lower serum clusterin levels in patients with erosive hand osteoarthritis are associated with more pain

Tereza Kropáčková[1,2], Olga Šléglová[1,2], Olga Růžičková[1,2], Jiří Vencovský[1,2], Karel Pavelka[1,2] and Ladislav Šenolt[1,2*]

Abstract

Background: The aims of this study were to analyse the serum concentrations of clusterin (CLU) in patients with hand osteoarthritis (OA) and in healthy controls, to compare CLU levels between patients with erosive and non-erosive disease, and to examine the association of CLU levels with clinical and laboratory parameters.

Methods: A total of 135 patients with hand OA (81 with erosive and 54 with non-erosive disease) and 53 healthy individuals were included in this study. All patients underwent clinical and hand joint ultrasound examination. The Australian/Canadian (AUSCAN) hand osteoarthritis index, algofunctional index and a visual analogue scale (VAS) for the measurement of pain were assessed. Serum levels of CLU were measured by an enzyme-linked immunosorbent assay (ELISA).

Results: Serum levels of CLU were significantly lower in patients with hand OA than in control subjects ($p < 0.0001$). In addition, patients with erosive hand OA had significantly lower CLU levels than those with non-erosive disease ($p = 0.044$). Negative correlations between CLU levels and pain as assessed by the AUSCAN score and the VAS were found in patients with erosive hand OA ($r = -0.275$; $p = 0.013$ and $r = -0.220$; $p = 0.049$, respectively).

Conclusion: The present study demonstrates that lower concentrations of CLU are found in hand OA patients than in healthy individuals, especially in those with erosive disease, and that CLU concentrations have a negative association with hand pain.

Keywords: Hand osteoarthritis, Erosive osteoarthritis, Clusterin

Background

Osteoarthritis (OA) of the hands is a degenerative joint disease primarily affecting the interphalangeal and thumb base joints. Hand OA is common among the elderly, especially in women. It may cause pain and disability, and it negatively affects the patients' quality of life [1, 2]. The erosive form of hand OA is defined radiographically by its subchondral erosion, cortical destruction and subsequent reparative changes, which may include bony ankylosis. Erosive OA typically has an abrupt onset and is accompanied by local inflammation and worse symptoms than non-erosive disease [3].

Clusterin (CLU), also known as apolipoprotein J, is a protein that is involved in a number of biological processes, including inflammation and apoptosis. CLU exists in several distinct isoforms that differ in their structure, function and localization. The predominant isoform, secretory clusterin (sCLU), is a heterodimeric glycoprotein that acts as a molecular chaperone [4] and exhibits anti-apoptotic and pro-survival activities [5]. Nuclear clusterin (nCLU) arises via an alternative splicing of the *CLU* gene leading to exclusion of exon II [6] and acts as a pro-apoptotic molecule [7]. Cellular forms of CLU are relatively rare, and their function is still poorly understood, but it does not appear that they affect the apoptotic pathway [8].

Clusterin is produced in many tissues, including articular cartilage and the synovium. Higher expression of CLU mRNA has been reported in early OA than in normal cartilage [9]. In advanced OA cartilage, CLU mRNA

* Correspondence: senolt@revma.cz
[1]Institute of Rheumatology, Prague, Czech Republic
[2]Department of Rheumatology, 1st Faculty of Medicine, Charles University, Prague, Czech Republic

expression was reduced in comparison with that found in early OA. Based on these results, the authors proposed a potential role of CLU in the maintenance of articular cartilage. The upregulated expression of CLU in early OA might reflect an effort of chondrocytes to protect and repair the cartilage tissue while the downregulated CLU mRNA expression and consequently the loss of this protection in the advanced OA cartilage accompanies the final degenerative stage of the disease [9]. Fandridis et al. detected increased expression of sCLU mRNA in advanced OA compared with the expression of that in healthy cartilage. Moreover, they found higher serum sCLU levels in patients with advanced OA than in healthy individuals. Therefore, CLU could be suggested as a biomarker reflecting cartilage tissue changes [10].

CLU mRNA expression in synovial tissue is decreased in rheumatoid arthritis (RA) compared with its expression in OA or healthy tissue, but the protein levels in synovial fluid are equally present in RA and OA [11]. In cultured fibroblast-like synoviocytes (FLS), CLU inhibits nuclear factor (NF)-κB activation and modulates the expression of genes in the response to tumor necrosis factor (TNF)-α stimulation [11, 12]. Recently, sCLU has been shown to inhibit osteoclast proliferation and differentiation, and its protective role against bone erosions has been suggested [13].

The aims of this study were therefore to compare the serum levels of CLU between patients with hand OA and healthy subjects and between OA patients with erosive and non-erosive disease and to investigate the association of CLU levels with measures of disease severity.

Methods
Patients
A total of 135 patients with hand OA (81 with the erosive and 54 with the non-erosive form) and 53 healthy individuals were included in this study. The demographic and clinical characteristics of the subjects are summarized in Table 1. The exclusion criteria for all subjects were the presence of systemic inflammatory disease or cancer; the healthy controls showed no clinical signs of hand OA. All patients fulfilled the American College of Rheumatology (ACR) classification criteria for hand OA [14]; patients with erosive disease had at least one interphalangeal joint with radiographic signs of erosions. Ultrasound of all joints of both hands for the detection of osteophytes and the assessment of power Doppler (PD) and gray scale (GS) synovitis was performed by two ultrasonographers using Esaote Mylab 60 equipment (Esaote S.p.A., Genova, Italy) using a linear transducer with a 18 MHz frequency. Synovitis in the GS and PD were scored semiquantitatively (0–3) as described

Table 1 Characteristics of patients with hand OA and control subjects

	OA patients (n = 135)	Erosive (n = 81)	Non-erosive (n = 54)	Controls (n = 53)
Age, years	66.3 ± 8.3	67.6 ± 8.6*	64.3 ± 7.3	64.6 ± 7.6
Sex, female/male	120/15	74/7	46/8	48/5
CRP, mg/l	3.2 ± 3.9	3.4 ± 4.1	2.9 ± 3.7	3.3 ± 5.1
BMI, kg/m²	27.2 ± 4.2	27.5 ± 4.5	26.8 ± 3.7	NA
Disease duration, years	4.4 ± 5.2	4.4 ± 5.1	4.5 ± 5.5	NA
AUSCAN	22.5 ± 10.5	23.9 ± 11.1*	20.3 ± 9.1	NA
AUSCAN - pain	8.4 ± 4.2	9.0 ± 4.4*	7.5 ± 3.8	NA
AUSCAN - stiffness	1.9 ± 0.9	2.0 ± 0.9	1.9 ± 0.9	NA
AUSCAN - function	12.0 ± 6.4	12.8 ± 6.8	10.9 ± 5.6	NA
Algofunctional index	18.6 ± 5.9	19.5 ± 6.4	17.2 ± 4.8	NA
VAS - pain, mm	44.2 ± 22.7	46.7 ± 24.0	40.3 ± 20.3	NA
US osteophytes, n	12.8 ± 5.1	14.0 ± 4.6**	11.0 ± 5.4	NA
GS synovitis (total)	7.5 ± 8.7	9.3 ± 9.2***	4.8 ± 7.2	NA
GS synovitis (joint count)	5.5 ± 6.4	6.5 ± 6.6***	3.9 ± 5.8	NA
PD synovitis (total)	2.0 ± 2.7	2.5 ± 3.1*	1.3 ± 1.9	NA
PD synovitis (joint count)	1.7 ± 2.1	2.1 ± 2.3**	1.1 ± 1.6	NA
Knee OA, n (%)	59 (44)	35 (43)	24 (44)	NA
Hip OA, n (%)	40 (30)	27 (33)	13 (24)	NA
Knee and hip OA, n (%)	28 (21)	18 (22)	10 (19)	NA

The data are presented as the mean ± the standard deviation. * $p < 0.05$, ** $p < 0.01$, *** $p < 0.001$ compared with non-erosive. (*AUSCAN* Australian/Canadian, *BMI* body mass index, *CRP* C-reactive protein, *GS* gray scale, *OA* osteoarthritis, *PD* power Doppler, *US* ultrasound, *VAS* visual analogue scale)

earlier [15]. The ultrasonographers were unaware of patient's clinical examination and laboratory findings. Inter- and intra-observer reliability has recently been published with moderate to very good results [15]. The clinical examinations were performed by qualified rheumatologists. Pain, stiffness and function were assessed by Australian/Canadian (AUSCAN) hand osteoarthritis index [16]. Hand disability was further determined using an algofunctional index [17]. A visual analogue scale (VAS) was used for the assessment of pain. Radiographs of the knees and hips were evaluated for the presence of OA using the Kellgren-Lawrence system in all patients [18]. Written informed consent from each subject was obtained prior to enrolment, and the study was approved by the local ethics committee.

Laboratory measurements
Peripheral blood samples were obtained from all individuals and immediately centrifuged. The serum samples were stored at − 80 °C until their analysis. C-reactive protein (CRP) levels were measured turbidimetrically using the Beckman Coulter AU system (Beckman Coulter, Brea, CA, USA). The serum CLU concentrations were analysed by an enzyme-linked immunosorbent assay (ELISA) in compliance with the manufacturer's instructions (BioVendor, Brno, Czech Republic). The samples from the patients and the healthy individuals were analysed together in each ELISA plate. As claimed by the manufacturer, the antibodies used in this ELISA are specific for human CLU, the assay detection limit is 5 ng/ml and the detection range is

5–160 ng/ml. The manufacturer's stated intra-assay and inter-assay coefficients of the variations are 6.2 and 7.8%, respectively. The final absorbance was detected using a Sunrise ELISA reader (Tecan, Salzburg, Austria), with 450 nm as the primary wavelength.

Statistical analysis
The data are presented as the mean and standard deviation (SD) unless stated otherwise. Data were analysed using a GraphPad Prism 6 (GraphPad Software, San Diego, CA, USA). The normal distribution was assessed by the D'Agostino and Pearson omnibus normality test. For the comparison between groups, the unpaired t-test or Mann-Whitney test were used. Pearson's and Spearman's correlation coefficients were calculated to assess the relationship between the CLU levels and other parameters. P-values less than 0.05 were considered statistically significant.

Results
The patients and the control group did not differ in age, gender or CRP levels. However, the patients with erosive OA were older than those with non-erosive disease ($p = 0.023$). The CRP levels were comparable between both of the groups with hand OA. The AUSCAN total score and its subscale for pain were significantly higher in patients with erosive than in those with non-erosive OA ($p = 0.048$ and $p = 0.032$, respectively). Patients with erosive OA had more osteophytes ($p = 0.003$) and higher GS and PD synovitis total scores ($p < 0.001$ and $p = 0.014$, respectively) as well as higher number of affected

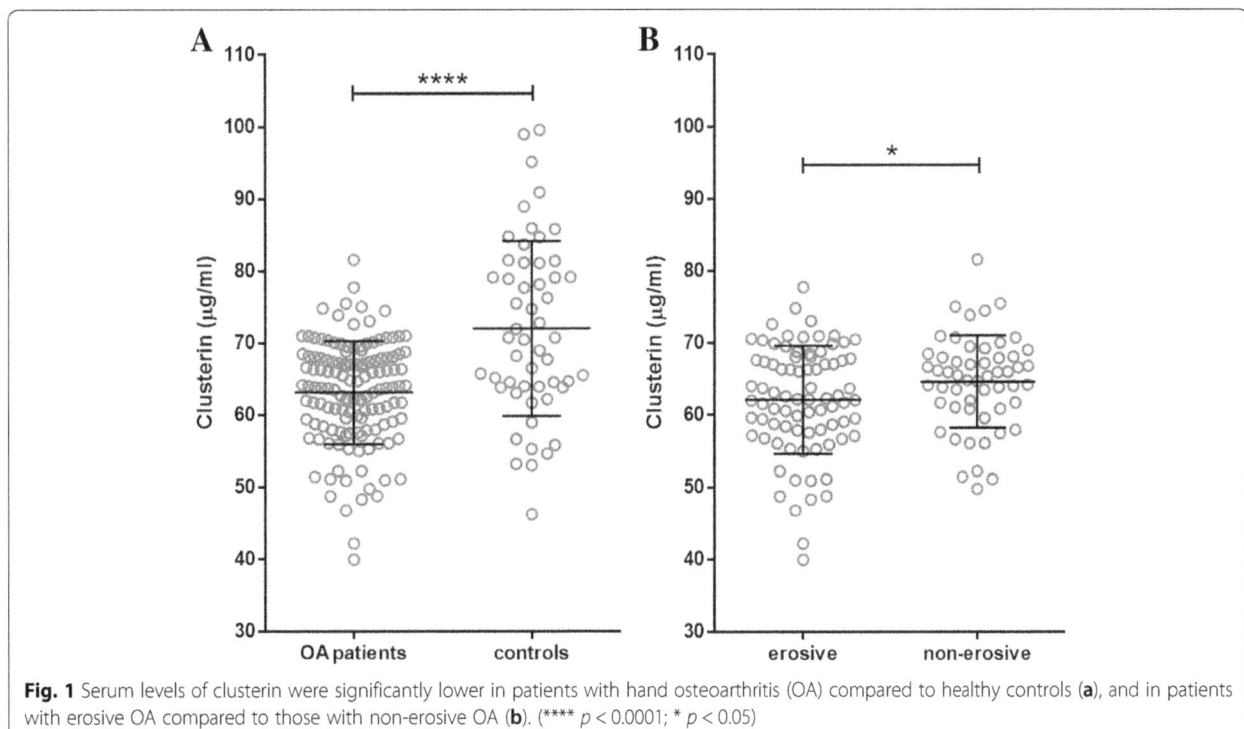

Fig. 1 Serum levels of clusterin were significantly lower in patients with hand osteoarthritis (OA) compared to healthy controls (**a**), and in patients with erosive OA compared to those with non-erosive OA (**b**). (**** $p < 0.0001$; * $p < 0.05$)

joints ($p < 0.001$ and $p = 0.009$, respectively) compared to those with non-erosive disease (Table 1).

Clusterin levels are lower in patients with hand OA

The serum concentrations of CLU were significantly lower in the patients with hand OA than in the healthy subjects (63.12 ± 7.17 vs 72.02 ± 12.19 µg/ml; $p < 0.0001$) (Fig. 1a). After dividing the patients into disease subsets, the difference remained statistically significant for both erosive ($p < 0.0001$) and non-erosive ($p < 0.0001$) OA. Moreover, the patients with erosive disease had significantly lower CLU levels than those with non-erosive OA (62.11 ± 7.51 vs 64.64 ± 6.42 µg/ml; $p = 0.044$) (Fig. 1b). The CLU levels in hand OA patients were not affected by the concurrent presence of knee and/or hip OA (63.35 vs 62.95 µg/ml for knee OA, 62.98 vs 63.18 µg/ml for hip OA, 63.47 vs 63.03 µg/ml for knee and hip OA; $p > 0.05$ for all comparisons).

Clusterin levels are inversely associated with pain in patients with erosive hand OA

Associations of CLU levels with clinical and laboratory parameters are shown in Table 2. There were no significant correlations between the CLU levels and the algofunctional index and total AUSCAN score in any of the patients with hand OA; however, among those with erosive disease, the CLU levels were negatively correlated with pain as assessed by the AUSCAN and the VAS ($r = -0.275$; $p = 0.013$ and $r = -0.220$; $p = 0.049$, respectively) (Fig. 2). The CLU concentrations were not associated with age, sex or body mass index. There were also no significant correlations between the CLU levels and disease duration, CRP levels, ultrasound-determined synovitis and osteophytes.

Discussion

In this study, we found lower levels of CLU in patients with hand OA than in healthy subjects and an inverse association between CLU levels and pain in patients with erosive disease.

Erosive hand OA is a more severe form of hand OA than non-erosive OA, both clinically and radiographically, and is accompanied by worse pain and disability [19, 20]. In our study, we found significantly higher scores on the AUSCAN and its pain subscale in patients with erosive than in patients with non-erosive OA. Inflammatory signs were also reported to be more frequent in erosive than in non-erosive disease [21, 22]. In addition, Punzi et al. [23] found higher CRP levels in erosive OA patients than in those with non-erosive hand OA and suggested CRP as a potential marker of disease activity. However, no differences in the CRP levels between erosive and non-erosive OA were found in other studies [24, 25]. A number of other biomarkers have been studied in hand OA, including markers of inflammation [26]. Recently,

Table 2 Correlations between serum CLU levels, clinical and laboratory parameters

	OA patients	Erosive	Non-erosive
AUSCAN	r = -0.087	r = -0.151	r = 0.100
	p = 0.318	p = 0.179	p = 0.470
AUSCAN - pain	r = -0.166	r = -0.275	r = 0.071
	p = 0.054	p = 0.013	p = 0.610
AUSCAN - stiffness	r = -0.107	r = -0.124	r = -0.097
	p = 0.218	p = 0.271	p = 0.487
AUSCAN - function	r = -0.009	r = -0.066	r = 0.144
	p = 0.914	p = 0.558	p = 0.299
Algofunctional index	r = -0.139	r = -0.151	r = -0.075
	p = 0.107	p = 0.179	p = 0.590
VAS – pain , mm	r = -0.084	r = -0.220	r = 0.201
	p = 0.331	p = 0.049	p = 0.145
CRP, mg/l	r = 0.037	r = -0.004	r = 0.117
	p = 0.674	p = 0.969	p = 0.401
Disease duration, years	r = -0.032	r = -0.024	r = -0.011
	p = 0.713	p = 0.832	p = 0.938
US osteophytes, n	r = 0.156	r = 0.189	r = 0.214
	p = 0.072	p = 0.091	p = 0.120
GS synovitis (total)	r = 0.007	r = 0.042	r = 0.130
	p = 0.937	p = 0.711	p = 0.349
GS synovitis (joint count)	r = 0.001	r = 0.023	r = 0.133
	p = 0.990	p = 0.840	p = 0.339
PD synovitis (total)	r = 0.083	r = 0.111	r = 0.217
	p = 0.341	p = 0.324	p = 0.114
PD synovitis (joint count)	r = 0.079	r = 0.097	r = 0.236
	p = 0.362	p = 0.389	p = 0.085

AUSCAN Australian/Canadian, *CRP* C-reactive protein, *GS* gray scale, *OA* osteoarthritis, *PD* power Doppler, *US* ultrasound, *VAS* visual analogue scale

Fioravanti et al. [27] reported significantly higher levels of serum myeloperoxidase (MPO) in patients with hand OA than in healthy controls. Moreover, patients with erosive OA showed significantly elevated MPO levels than those with non-erosive OA, which confirmed the results of a previous study [28] and further supported the involvement of inflammation in the pathogenesis of hand OA, especially in the erosive disease. In the present study, we observed higher ultrasound-determined synovitis total scores as well as the number of affected joints in patients with erosive OA compared to those with non-erosive disease. However, no significant differences in the CRP levels between the two subgroups of patients were found.

In this study, we found lower serum levels of CLU in the patients with hand OA than in the healthy controls. Several other studies have investigated CLU in OA [9–11]; however, this is the first study to explore the CLU levels in patients with hand OA. The expression of CLU mRNA

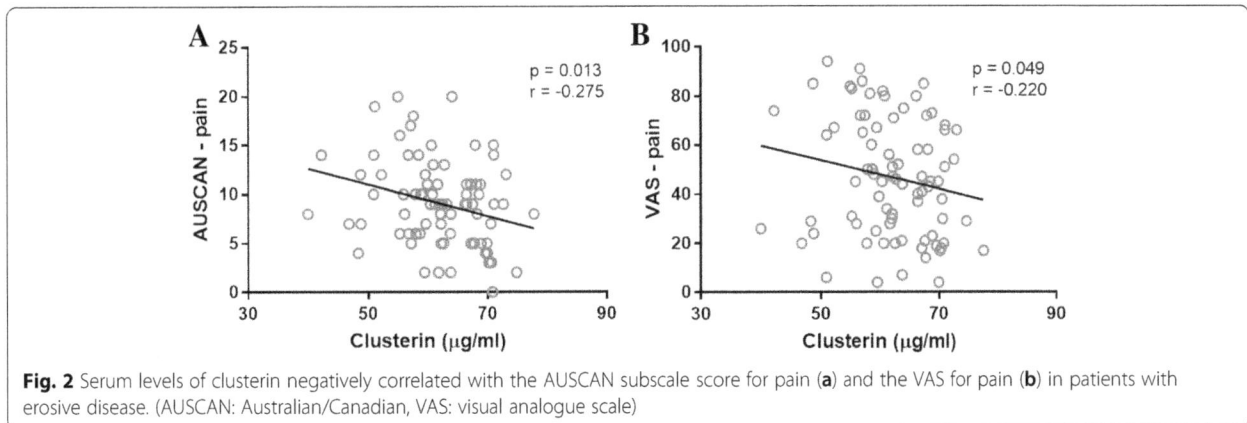

Fig. 2 Serum levels of clusterin negatively correlated with the AUSCAN subscale score for pain (**a**) and the VAS for pain (**b**) in patients with erosive disease. (AUSCAN: Australian/Canadian, VAS: visual analogue scale)

has been reported to be higher in OA than in healthy cartilage [9, 10]. Fandridis et al. [10] also reported higher serum levels of CLU in patients with knee and hip OA than in healthy controls. The reason for these apparently contradictory results may be caused by the different locations of the affected joints. Nevertheless, we did not find any differences in the CLU levels between the hand OA patients with and without knee and/or hip OA. It is also important to note that, in our study, the samples obtained from the patients and the healthy subjects were analysed at the same time, whereas Fandridis et al. used the data from the healthy controls from their previous study and analysed only the patient group [10].

A previous study has shown that CLU mRNA expression in synovial tissue is lower in patients with RA than in patients with OA and healthy individuals [11]. We found significantly lower serum levels of CLU in patients with erosive OA compared with patients with non-erosive hand OA. Bone erosions are present in RA as well as in erosive OA, although their locations differ. The lower expression of CLU in these diseases may be explained by the potentially protective role of CLU against the development of bone erosions [13]. A recent study also suggests a protective function of CLU in inflammation and autoimmune diseases [29], which is in agreement with the study of Newkirk et al. [30] that reported lower serum concentrations of CLU in systemic lupus erythematosus and found negative correlations among CLU levels, disease activity and disease symptoms. In our study, we reported a negative correlation between the CLU levels and hand pain in patients with erosive OA. No such association was found in patients with non-erosive disease. Therefore, we can speculate that CLU may play a role in the pathology of erosive hand OA.

This study has several limitations. First, its design was cross-sectional. Therefore, a long-term prospective study is needed to further investigate the role of CLU in hand OA. Second, CLU levels might be affected due to the effects of other involved joints or diseases. However, we did not observe a difference in the CLU levels between the hand OA patients with and without radiographic hip and/or knee joint involvement.

Conclusions

In conclusion, we demonstrate here for the first time that lower serum levels of CLU are found in patients with hand OA, especially in those with erosive disease, and that a negative association exists between CLU concentrations and hand pain. These data suggest a possible involvement of CLU in the pathophysiology of erosive hand OA and further support its role in the development of bone erosions.

Abbreviations
ACR: American College of Rheumatology; AUSCAN: Australian/Canadian; BMI: Body mass index; CLU: Clusterin; CRP: C-reactive protein; ELISA: Enzyme-linked immunosorbent assay; FLS: Fibroblast-like synoviocytes; GS: Gray scale; nCLU: Nuclear clusterin; NF: Nuclear factor; OA: Osteoarthritis; PD: Power Doppler; RA: Rheumatoid arthritis; sCLU: Secretory clusterin; TNF: Tumor necrosis factor; US: Ultrasound; VAS: Visual analogue scale

Acknowledgements
The authors thank Zdena Leopoldová for technical and administrative assistance.

Funding
This study was supported by the Ministry of Health, Czech Republic, research project AZV no. 18-01-00542.

Authors' contributions
TK performed the laboratory and statistical analysis, and drafted the manuscript. OŠ, OR, KP and LŠ made clinical assessments and contributed to data acquisition and interpretation. JV and KP revised the manuscript critically for important intellectual content. LŠ made substantial contributions to study concept and design, and revised the final draft of the manuscript. All authors read and approved the final version of the manuscript.

Competing interests
All authors declare no competing interests.

References
1. Dahaghin S, Bierma-Zeinstra SMA, Ginai AZ, Pols HAP, Hazes JMW, Koes BW. Prevalence and pattern of radiographic hand osteoarthritis and association with pain and disability (the Rotterdam study). Ann Rheum Dis. 2005;64:682–7.
2. Zhang Y, Niu J, Kelly-Hayes M, Chaisson CE, Aliabadi P, Felson DT. Prevalence of symptomatic hand osteoarthritis and its impact on functional status among the elderly: the Framingham study. Am J Epidemiol. 2002;156:1021–7.

3.   Zhang W, Doherty M, Leeb BF, Alekseeva L, Arden NK, Bijlsma JW, et al. EULAR evidence-based recommendations for the diagnosis of hand osteoarthritis: report of a task force of ESCISIT. Ann Rheum Dis. 2009;68:8–17.

4.   Poon S, Easterbrook-Smith SB, Rybchyn MS, Carver JA, Wilson MR. Clusterin is an ATP-independent chaperone with very broad substrate specificity that stabilizes stressed proteins in a folding-competent state. Biochemistry. 2000;39:15953–60.

5.   Trougakos IP, Lourda M, Antonelou MH, Kletsas D, Gorgoulis VG, Papassideri IS, et al. Intracellular clusterin inhibits mitochondrial apoptosis by suppressing p53-activating stress signals and stabilizing the cytosolic Ku70-Bax protein complex. Clin Cancer Res. 2009;15:48–59.

6.   Leskov KS, Klokov DY, Li J, Kinsella TJ, Boothman DA. Synthesis and functional analyses of nuclear clusterin, a cell death protein. J Biol Chem. 2003;278:11590–600.

7.   Kim N, Yoo JC, Han JY, Hwang EM, Kim YS, Jeong EY, et al. Human nuclear clusterin mediates apoptosis by interacting with Bcl-XL through C-terminal coiled coil domain. J Cell Physiol. 2012;227:1157–67.

8.   Prochnow H, Gollan R, Rohne P, Hassemer M, Koch-Brandt C, Baiersdörfer M. Non-secreted clusterin isoforms are translated in rare amounts from distinct human mRNA variants and do not affect Bax-mediated apoptosis or the NF-κB signaling pathway. PLoS One. 2013;8:e75303.

9.   Connor JR, Kumar S, Sathe G, Mooney J, O'Brien SP, Mui P, et al. Clusterin expression in adult human normal and osteoarthritic articular cartilage. Osteoarthr Cartil. 2001;9:727–37.

10. Fandridis E, Apergis G, Korres DS, Nikolopoulos K, Zoubos AB, Papassideri I, et al. Increased expression levels of apolipoprotein J/clusterin during primary osteoarthritis. In Vivo (Brooklyn). 2011;25:745–9.

11. Devauchelle V, Essabbani A, De Pinieux G, Germain S, Tourneur L, Mistou S, et al. Characterization and functional consequences of underexpression of clusterin in rheumatoid arthritis. J Immunol. 2006;177:6471–9.

12. Falgarone G, Essabbani A, Dumont F, Cagnard N, Mistou S, Chiocchia G. Implication of clusterin in TNF-α response of rheumatoid synovitis: lesson from in vitro knock-down of clusterin in human synovial fibroblast cells. Physiol Genomics. 2012;44:229–35.

13. Choi B, Kang S-S, Kang S-W, Min B-H, Lee E-J, Song D-H, et al. Secretory clusterin inhibits osteoclastogenesis by attenuating M-CSF-dependent osteoclast precursor cell proliferation. Biochem Biophys Res Commun. 2014;450:105–9.

14. Altman R, Alarcón G, Appelrouth D, Bloch D, Borenstein D, Brandt K, et al. The American College of Rheumatology criteria for the classification and reporting of osteoarthritis of the hand. Arthritis Rheum. 1990;33:1601–10.

15. Hurnakova J, Zavada J, Hanova P, Hulejova H, Klein M, Mann H, et al. Serum calprotectin (S100A8/9): an independent predictor of ultrasound synovitis in patients with rheumatoid arthritis. Arthritis Res Ther. 2015;17:252.

16. Bellamy N, Campbell J, Haraoui B, Gerecz-Simon E, Buchbinder R, Hobby K, et al. Clinimetric properties of the AUSCAN osteoarthritis hand index: an evaluation of reliability, validity and responsiveness. Osteoarthr Cartil. 2002;10:863–9.

17. Dreiser RL, Maheu E, Guillou GB, Caspard H, Grouin JM. Validation of an algofunctional index for osteoarthritis of the hand. Rev Rhum Engl Ed. 1995;62:43S–53S.

18. Kellgren JH, Lawrence JS. Radiological assessment of osteo-arthrosis. Ann Rheum Dis. 1957;16:494–502.

19. Addimanda O, Mancarella L, Dolzani P, Punzi L, Fioravanti A, Pignotti E, et al. Clinical and radiographic distribution of structural damage in erosive and nonerosive hand osteoarthritis. Arthritis Care Res. 2012;64:1046–53.

20. Bijsterbosch J, Watt I, Meulenbelt I, Rosendaal FR, Huizinga TWJ, Kloppenburg M. Clinical burden of erosive hand osteoarthritis and its relationship to nodes. Ann Rheum Dis. 2010;69:1784–8.

21. Kortekaas MC, Kwok W-Y, Reijnierse M, Huizinga TWJ, Kloppenburg M. In erosive hand osteoarthritis more inflammatory signs on ultrasound are found than in the rest of hand osteoarthritis. Ann Rheum Dis. 2013;72:930–4.

22. Haugen IK, Mathiessen A, Slatkowsky-Christensen B, Magnusson K, Bøyesen P, Sesseng S, et al. Synovitis and radiographic progression in non-erosive and erosive hand osteoarthritis: is erosive hand osteoarthritis a separate inflammatory phenotype? Osteoarthr Cartil. 2016;24:647–54.

23. Punzi L, Ramonda R, Oliviero F, Sfriso P, Mussap M, Plebani M, et al. Value of C reactive protein in the assessment of erosive osteoarthritis of the hand. Ann Rheum Dis. 2005;64:955–7.

24. Filková M, Senolt L, Braun M, Hulejová H, Pavelková A, Sléglová O, et al. Serum hyaluronic acid as a potential marker with a predictive value for further radiographic progression of hand osteoarthritis. Osteoarthr Cartil. 2009;17:1615–9.

25. Dolzani P, Assirelli E, Pulsatelli L, Addimanda O, Mancarella L, Peri G, et al. Systemic inflammation and antibodies to citrullinated peptides in hand osteoarthritis. Clin Exp Rheumatol. 29:1006–9.

26. Lennerová T, Pavelka K, Šenolt L. Biomarkers of hand osteoarthritis. Rheumatol Int. 2018;38:725–35.

27. Fioravanti A, Tenti S, Pulsatelli L, Addimanda O. Could myeloperoxidase represent a useful biomarker for erosive osteoarthritis of the hand? Scand J Rheumatol. 2018;1-3. doi: https://doi.org/10.1080/03009742.2017.1386796. [Epub ahead of print]

28. Punzi L, Ramonda R, Deberg M, Frallonardo P, Campana C, Musacchio E, et al. Coll2-1, Coll2-1NO2 and myeloperoxidase serum levels in erosive and non-erosive osteoarthritis of the hands. Osteoarthr Cartil. 2012;20:557–61.

29. Cunin P, Beauvillain C, Miot C, Augusto J-F, Preisser L, Blanchard S, et al. Clusterin facilitates apoptotic cell clearance and prevents apoptotic cell-induced autoimmune responses. Cell Death Dis. 2016;7:e2215.

30. Newkirk MM, Apostolakos P, Neville C, Fortin PR. Systemic lupus erythematosus, a disease associated with low levels of clusterin/apoJ, an antiinflammatory protein. J Rheumatol. 1999;26:597–603.

15

The multidisciplinary treatment of osteosarcoma of the proximal tibia: a retrospective study

Junqi Huang[1], Wenzhi Bi[2*], Gang Han[2], Jinpeng Jia[2], Meng Xu[2] and Wei Wang[2]

Abstract

Background: Survival and reconstruction constitute important challenges in multimodal treatment of osteosarcoma of the proximal tibia. The purpose of this study was to assess the efficacy and prognosis of neoadjuvant chemotherapy and custom-designed endoprosthetic arthroplasty.

Methods: A total of 69 patients with osteosarcoma of the proximal tibia were evaluated, including 43 males and 26 females, treated with multidisciplinary limb-salvage remedy from October 2003 to December 2013. They were at least 12 years old (mean, 20 years; range, 12–57 years). The gap between tumor and main artery/nerve was showed in MRI. Mean follow up was 69.5 months (range, 9–144 months). Kaplan-Meier survival curves were generated to assess prognosis and relapse rate. The initial symptoms and disease duration for each patient were recorded. Correlation analyses were performed for the association of various parameters with prognosis. Functional outcomes were evaluated using the Musculoskeletal Tumor Society (MSTS) guidelines after 6 months postoperatively, to analyze the relation between bone excision size and function recovery.

Results: The resection lengths measured intraoperatively ranged from 80 to 230 mm, and contained 3 cm of normal bone around the tumor. A total of 3 courses of preoperative chemotherapy were administered to all cases. At final follow-up, 1 case showed recurrence. Meanwhile, 8 patients (11.6%) died from lung metastasis. Post-operative infection occurred in 3 patients; 1 case was maintained with revision surgery. Two cases underwent amputation. The mean MSTS system score was 21.6.

Conclusions: The multidisciplinary treatment result in an overall positive outcome, with improved function.

Keywords: Osteosarcoma, Tibia, Arthroplasty, Reconstruction, Survival

Background

Osteosarcoma is a malignant tumor originated from a mesenchymal stem cell precursor that produces immature woven bone (osteoid) after becoming malignant [1]. It is the most common solid bone cancer, occurring in 2–3 per 106,000 individuals [2]. Previously, this disease was only treated by amputation; however, effective neoadjuvant/preoperative and postoperative adjuvant chemotherapy regimens allow safe limb-sparing resections, improving survival rates [3, 4]. Indeed, with the recent availability of multimodal treatment combining imaging, chemotherapy, and surgical techniques, 70–85% of malignant tumors are efficiently treated with limb salvage [5, 6], and long-term survival for patients with localized osteosarcoma now reaches approximately 60% [7, 8]. Limb-sparing surgery yields good oncological and functional outcomes, as well as satisfactory psychological results [9]. Despite multiple reports regarding the operative techniques, such as allografts and arthrodesis, the choice for reconstructing bone and soft-tissue defects after resection remains a serious challenge [10]. Meanwhile, complications after allografts reconstruction limited its application [11]. The arthrodesis had poor joint activity.

Prosthetic implantation has been proposed to result in physical improvement, but most individuals develop dismal femur lesions [11, 12]. According to any reports, overall survival is reduced due to recurrence [13, 14].

* Correspondence: 13011277676@163.com
[2]Department of Orthopaedics, PLA General Hospital, Beijing 100853, China
Full list of author information is available at the end of the article

The proximal tibia is second only to distal femur in osteosarcoma frequency [5], with about 75% of all patients suffering from osteosarcoma around knee [15]. Unlike other sites, resection of osteosarcoma of the proximal tibia meeting the wide incision principle causes the loss of bone and patellar tendon; indeed, tibial growth plate will not return to normal after implantation of a distal femoral prosthesis [16, 17]. This likely increases the likelihood of relapse. In addition, periprosthetic-related accidents after surgery are numerous, including infections, aseptic loosening, wear of joint components, dislocations, prosthesis breakage, and fatigue; fractures are also common in the long run [18]. Interestingly, medial gastrocnemius rotational flap was shown to decrease soft tissue defects and the risk of infection [19]. We hypothesized that neoadjuvant chemotherapy combined custom designed prosthesis for osteosarcoma treatment would result in improved function and prolonged survival. Therefore, this study aimed to retrospectively assess the efficacy of neoadjuvant chemotherapy and custom-designed endoprosthetic arthroplasty for the treatment of osteosarcoma of the proximal tibia.

Methods
Study design
This retrospective cohort study assessed patients with osteosarcoma of the proximal tibia treated in our institution, between October 2003 and December 2013. It was approved by Ethics Committee of our hospital; informed consent was obtained from all patients.

Patients
A total of sixty-nine patients who underwent neoadjuvant chemotherapy and hinge prosthesis, extensor function reconstruction of the proximal tibia after wide resection for osteosarcoma were assessed. There were forty-three males (62.3%) and twenty-six females (37.7%), averaging 20 years old (range, 12–57). The patients, diagnosed with stage IIB(Ennecking system, no metastasis) osteosarcoma by biopsy and imaging, were included if meeting the following eligibility criteria: complete neoadjuvant chemotherapy, no invasion of tibial artery and vein on imaging (MRI), no invasion of tibial (peroneal) nerve on imaging (MRI), no preoperative metastasis. Exclusion criteria included skin ulceration, tumor surrounding popliteal artery, metastasis showed on imaging. Data (e.g. Initial symptoms before treatment and their durations) were collected from medical records.

X-ray and MRI were taken before neoadjuvant chemotherapy and surgery. When imaging examination and laboratory examination were finished, biopsy was conducted in our institution. The pathologic report was confirmed by chief pathologist.

Chemotherapy
Neoadjuvant chemotherapy was administered after positive pathology. Every cycle consisted of ifosfamide (2 g/m^2/day on days 1 to 5) and doxorubicin (40 mg/m^2/day on day 5). Based on physical condition and efficiency of multi-agents, additional drug was methotrexate 8 g/m^2/day on day 3 (children) or cisplatin 120 mg/m^2/day on day 6 (adults). Three and six courses, respectively, were administered preoperatively and postoperatively as standard therapy. Blood, liver function, renal function, and electrolyte assessment was performed during chemotherapy. About 1 month was allowed after every cycle. Complete standard therapy was executed unless patients showed intolerance.

Surgery
All patients receiving 3 courses of chemotherapy were submitted to plain radiography, magnetic resonance imaging (MRI) and chest CT before surgery [20]. These tests determined the resection realm and prosthesis size. A rotary hinge endoprostheses was applied. An anteromedial incision started proximally at the distal third of the femur and extended below the lesion. The biopsy site was excised with a 3 cm margin. The medial sural artery supplying the medial gastrocnemius was preserved. The patellar ligament was detached 3 cm proximal to its insertion, and the knee capsule was incised 3 cm from tibial insertion. A specimen was collected 3 cm outside the normal tissue, based on T1 imaging data. The length of resection tumor was measured intraoperatively. It determined to choose the same standard prosthesis. An artificial joint was implanted using the cemented technique for component insertion. The extensor mechanism was advanced, and the remaining patellar tendon attached to the prosthesis where had immobilized groove. An allograft like LARS ligament was used to prolong tendon when residual patellar tendon had not sufficient to insert in prosthetic fixed groove. In case the muscle and deep fascia did not inadequately cover the prosthesis after wide resection, a medial gastrocnemius rotation flap would repair the passive spacer. Antibiotic was infused for a week after surgery.

Postoperative care, indicators and follow up
The affected extremity flexion was kept slightly moist, with a drain left until the fluid is minimal. Antibiotics were routinely administered 1 week postoperatively. Knee extension was kept for 3 weeks to allow healing of knee extensor reconstruction. Active and active-assisted exercises were then encouraged, with the purpose to recover the range of motion and strength. Regarding the time of arthroplasty, the Musculoskeletal Tumor Society (MSTS) 93 scoring system was applied to comparably assess the muscle function 6 months postoperatively through outpatient review. Follow up was performed in outpatient service and by telephone. The **indices assessed** were pain,

range of motion, emotional acceptance, supports (brace, cane, and crutches), walking ability and gait. Lung CT and X-ray of the affected limb were reviewed in outpatient service every 6 months, to detect local control and distant metastasis.

Statistics

Data were presented as mean ± standard deviation (SD) or percentage, as appropriate. Correlation analyses were performed to determine the associations of various parameters with prognosis (survival, recurrence and metastasis). Kaplan-Meier survival curves were generated to assess overall 3- and 5-year patient survival rates. The correlation between prosthesis length and rehabilitation function was also evaluated. Function scores were based on MSTS indication, with 30 as maximum score and normal function. Any complication was considered to be related to prosthesis performance.

Results

Baseline patient data

All the patients underwent en block resection confirmed by pathology postoperatively and custom-designed prostheses arthroplasty for reconstruction. The clinical information was uncovered in Table 1. Precisely, the patients included 62.3 and 37.7% male and female individuals, respectively. Initial symptoms were pain and swelling in 19 patients (27.5%), pain in 41 (59.4%), and swelling in 9 (13.1%). The symptoms had lasted for 5 ± 10 (ranging from 1 to 20) months. Metal on polyethylene locking mechanism was used in prostheses.

Limb function

Limb function was evaluated in all patients by the MSTS 93 system 6 months postoperatively [21]. A mean score of 21.6 was obtained, with values between 19 and 28. The range of knee motion was from 60°to 110°. 17 patients (24.6%) exercised to improve limb function 12 months

Table 1 Baseline characteristics of patients

Parameter	Value
Gender	
Male	43(62.3%)
Female	26(37.7%)
Initial symptom	
Pain+swelling	19(27.5%)
Pain	41(59.4%)
Swelling	9(13.1%)
Average symptom duration	5 ± 10 months
Average follow-up	69.5 ± 4.3 months
Prosthetic complication	3(infection) 2(ligament Breakage)

postoperatively. The mean MSTS score was 22.3. The range of knee motion between 60°and 120°. Meanwhile, bone resection size was 13 cm (ranging 10 to 16 cm). Limb function was not associated with bone loss or exercise ($p > 0.05$ in correlation analyses). Figure 1 was the postoperative view of the prosthesis.

Prognosis and survival

Every patient was reexamined per 6 months. The examination contained limb X-ray, lung CT. Mean of follow up time was 75.9 months, with 95% confidence intervals between 67.4 and 84.4 months. At the last follow-up, 54 patients (78.3%) were continuously event-free, and 3 (6.5%) had evidence of infection; meanwhile, 8 patients (11.6%) had died of disease-related complications. The 3- and 5-year overall survival rates were 91.3% and 87%, respectively, as obtained by Kaplan-Meier analysis (Fig. 2). One case of local recurrence was observed after 5 months postoperatively; amputation was conducted and adjuvant chemotherapy added for two courses, and lung metastasis finally caused death 18 months after confirmed diagnosis. Correlation analyses indicated no significant associations of pain accompanying swelling or symptom duration before treatment with prognosis (both $p > 0.05$).

Complications

Among the 3 cases with infection, 2 selected limb amputation for lack of money. The prosthesis was removed and bone cement containing vancomycin was implanted in 1 patient. Vancomycin and ceftriaxone were used when infection was confirmed. Revision surgery was conducted and drug withdrawal when infection indexes, such as C-reactive protein (CRP) and erythrocyte sedimentation rate (ESR) returned to normal. No infection was further verified by joint fluid culture. To date, no prosthesis-related disease has been recorded. Breakage of the wire fixing the patellar ligament occurred in 2 cases; this was removed and a second surgery was performed.

Discussion

This study aimed to evaluate the efficacy of neoadjuvant chemotherapy and custom-designed endoprosthetic arthroplasty for treating osteosarcoma of the proximal tibia, and showed that the multidisciplinary treatment result in improved prognosis and survival.

It is critical to identify effective approaches for lesion treatment. With the introduction of chemotherapy, 5 year survival has dramatically improved in the last decades [22, 23], allowing limb salvage [22, 24]. However, the best association for neoadjuvant drug had not yet been confirmed. In the current study, we combined triplet regimen for increase of drug tolerance. The 5-year overall survival was 87%.

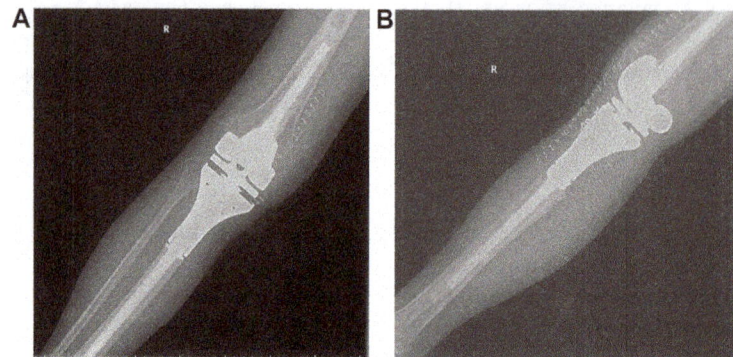

Fig. 1 The graph shows front (**a**) and side (**b**) appearance of prosthesis postoperatively

Prosthetic arthroplasty does not increase death and recurrence [25], providing an improved limb function [26]. According to the special anatomy of the proximal tibia, knee extensor mechanism reconstruction after resection is of utmost importance. Previous reports examined the artificial ligaments, osteotomized fibula, and autologous fasciae for reconstruction [27–29]. However, complications associated with proximal tibia prosthesis are common: it results in poor patellar tendon reattachment, infection, poor skin covering, mechanical wearing and loosening, and damage to neurovascular structures [10, 20, 30]. Based on en block resection, we preserved the normal patellar ligament for reattachment to the prosthesis by a wire. To minimize the incidence of loosening, synovitis, and trauma, allografts were selected in the combination method [31]. This reinforced the patellar tendon, and no case of poor reattachment was found in this retrospective study. When the preserved tendon was

inadequate because of wide excision or excessive soft tissue removed from the anteromedial tibia, a medial gastrocnemius flap was employed to keep stretches stable and supply a comprehensive surrounding [32, 33], which shortened infection and promoted healing as observed during follow up.

Variable rates of infection in tumor endoprostheses have been reported [34, 35]. Operative time, blood loss and wound complications are risk factors for infection [36]. Despite conformation to asepsis, infection was found in 3 patients, as described above, probably due to immune suppression by chemotherapy and soft-tissue defects. The prosthesis was removed after infection was diagnosed, and antibiotic cement was placed as proposed previously [37]. Revision was not carried out until normal levels of blood infection markers were obtained. Of note, debridement and retention for management of early and late acute infections have significant success rates [36], likely providing

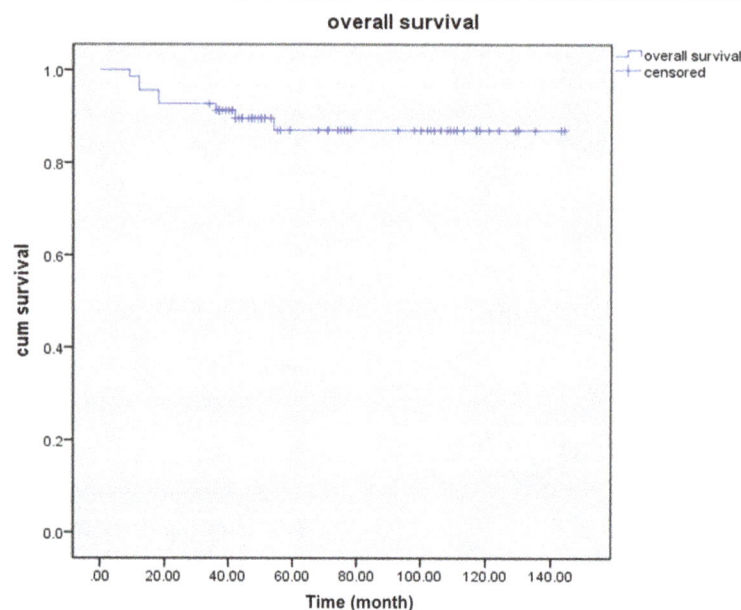

Fig. 2 Overall survival was assessed by the by Kaplan-Meier method. The 3- and 5-year overall survival rates were 91.3% and 87%, respectively

an approach to resist microbial infection. Meanwhile, we found that infection incidence was plummeting among patients with medial gastrocnemius flap transposition.

No patient had aseptic loosening, whose incidence for proximal tibia reduced compared with that obtained for dismal femur. Indeed, mechanics indicated that the more pressure dismal femur prosthesis bears, the higher risk. Meanwhile, extensor mechanism in this study was stabilized with bone-muscle flap. The prosthesis matching the medullary space and enhanced cement promise low risk of loosening. Furthermore, other complications, such as injury of artery and nerve, were not found in this study; the reason might be that preoperative MRI clearly revealed anatomy around the knee. Breakage of prosthesis handle is mostly found among children [21], and fine handle to match the diameter of medullary increases the risk of breaking. In this study, mean patient age was 20 years. Preserving enough bone cortex and using thick handle overcame these shortcomings.

Independent exercising and rehabilitation were begun at postoperative week 3 in this study, with the purpose of ensuring ligament healing. For unifying function comparison at different intervention times, we selected 6 months post-surgery as MSTS assessment point. An average functional score of 21 was obtained, and normal flexion and extension were achieved by the majority of patients. Routine walking was achieved after muscle exercise. Bone loss affected muscle function slightly. The prosthesis had the ability to rebuild the defect, but MSTS values were lower than those of distal femur [38, 39]; this may be due to the involvement of patellar ligament reconstruction. Both local control and tissue reserve were crucial in method design.

This study has several limitations. First, this was a single study, with inherent selection bias. In addition to its small sample size, the patients were assessed retrospectively. Therefore, these findings should be confirmed in larger sample, multicenter, prospective studies.

Conclusion

In summary, custom-designed endoprostheses, combined with neoadjuvant chemotherapy, result in an overall positive outcome, improving prognosis and survival. Therefore, the multidisciplinary treatment constituted an appropriate alternative in patients with osteosarcoma of the proximal tibia.

Acknowledgements
Not applicable.

Authors' contributions
JH as secondary surgeon made substantial contributions to conception and design, and acquisition of data. WB is treating surgeon for cases involved. He also made substantial contributions to manuscript revising. GH offered initial advice and acted as one of the reviewers. JJ made substantial contributions to study design, drafting the manuscript and revising it critically for important intellectual content. MX and WW was involved in the conception of the study improving it with important intellectual content. All authors read and approved the final manuscript.

Competing interests
The authors declare that they have no competing interests.

Author details
[1]Department of Orthopaedics, Mianyang Central Hospital, Mianyang 621000, Sichuan, China. [2]Department of Orthopaedics, PLA General Hospital, Beijing 100853, China.

References

1. Ene R, Sinescu RD, Ene P, Popescu D, Cirstoiu MM, Cirstoiu FC. Proximal tibial osteosarcoma in young patients: early diagnosis, modular reconstruction. Rom J Morphol Embryol. 2015;56(2):413–7.
2. Stiller CA, Bielack SS, Jundt G, Steliarova-Foucher E. Bone tumours in European children and adolescents, 1978-1997. Report from the automated childhood Cancer information system project. Eur J Cancer. 2006;42(13): 2124–35.
3. Sohn JH, Rha SY, Jeung HC, et al. Efficacy of pre- and postoperative chemotherapy in patients with osteosarcoma of the extremities. Cancer Res Treat. 2001;33(6):520–6.
4. Ritter J, Bielack SS. Osteosarcoma. Ann Oncol. 2010;21(Suppl 7):vii320–5.
5. Zhang Y, Yang Z, Li X, et al. Custom prosthetic reconstruction for proximal tibial osteosarcoma with proximal tibiofibular joint involved. Surg Oncol. 2008;17(2):87–95.
6. Veth R, van Hoesel R, Pruszczynski M, Hoogenhout J, Schreuder B, Wobbes T. Limb salvage in musculoskeletal oncology. Lancet Oncol. 2003;4(6):343–50.
7. Dai X, Ma W, He X, Jha RK. Review of therapeutic strategies for osteosarcoma, chondrosarcoma, and Ewing's sarcoma. Med Sci Monit. 2011; 17(8):RA177–90.
8. Ando K, Heymann MF, Stresing V, Mori K, Redini F, Heymann D. Current therapeutic strategies and novel approaches in osteosarcoma. Cancers (Basel). 2013;5(2):591–616.
9. Gebhardt MC. What's new in musculoskeletal oncology. J Bone Joint Surg Am. 2002;84-A(4):694–701.
10. Anract P, Missenard G, Jeanrot C, Dubois V, Tomeno B. Knee reconstruction with prosthesis and muscle flap after total arthrectomy. Clin Orthop Relat Res. 2001;384:208–16.
11. Biau DJ, Dumaine V, Babinet A, et al. Allograft prosthesis composites after bone tumor resection at the proximal tibia. Clin Orthop Relat Res. 2007;456:211–7.
12. Dubousset J, Missenard G, Kalifa C. Management of osteogenic sarcoma in children and adolescents. Clin Orthop Relat Res. 1991;(270):52–9.
13. Marulanda GA, Henderson ER, Johnson DA, Letson GD, Cheong D. Orthopedic surgery options for the treatment of primary osteosarcoma. Cancer Control. 2008;15(1):13–20.
14. Campanacci L, Manfrini M, Colangeli M, Ali N, Mercuri M. Long-term results in children with massive bone osteoarticular allografts of the knee for high-grade osteosarcoma. J Pediatr Orthop. 2010;30(8):919–27.
15. Hogendoorn PC, Group EEW, Athanasou N, et al. Bone sarcomas: ESMO clinical practice guidelines for diagnosis, treatment and follow-up. Ann Oncol. 2010;21(Suppl 5):v204–13.
16. Arteau A, Lewis VO, Moon BS, Satcher RL, Bird JE, Lin PP. Tibial growth disturbance following distal femoral resection and expandable Endoprosthetic reconstruction. J Bone Joint Surg Am. 2015;97(22):e72.
17. Capanna R, Scoccianti G, Campanacci DA, Beltrami G, De Biase P. Surgical technique: extraarticular knee resection with prosthesis-proximal tibia-extensor apparatus allograft for tumors invading the knee. Clin Orthop Relat Res. 2011;469(10):2905–14.
18. Niimi R, Matsumine A, Hamaguchi T, Nakamura T, Uchida A, Sudo A. Prosthetic limb salvage surgery for bone and soft tissue tumors around the knee. Oncol Rep. 2012;28(6):1984–90.

19. Wittig JC, Villalobos CE, Hayden BL, Choi I, Silverman AM, Malawer M. Osteosarcoma of the proximal tibia: limb-sparing resection and reconstruction with a modular segmental proximal tibia tumor prosthesis. Ann Surg Oncol. 2010;17(11):3021.

20. Bi W, Wang W, Han G, Jia J, Xu M. Osteosarcoma around the knee treated with neoadjuvant chemotherapy and a custom-designed prosthesis. Orthopedics. 2013;36(4):e444–50.

21. Zeegen EN, Aponte-Tinao LA, Hornicek FJ, Gebhardt MC, Mankin HJ. Survivorship analysis of 141 modular metallic endoprostheses at early followup. Clin Orthop Relat Res. 2004;420:239–50.

22. Rosen G, Marcove RC, Caparros B, Nirenberg A, Kosloff C, Huvos AG. Primary osteogenic sarcoma: the rationale for preoperative chemotherapy and delayed surgery. Cancer. 1979;43(6):2163–77.

23. Ferrari S, Palmerini E. Adjuvant and neoadjuvant combination chemotherapy for osteogenic sarcoma. Curr Opin Oncol. 2007;19(4):341–6.

24. Hong S, Shin SJ, Jung M, et al. Comparison of long-term outcome between doublet and triplet neoadjuvant chemotherapy in non-metastatic osteosarcoma of the extremity. Oncology. 2011;80(1–2):107–17.

25. Mir O, Ropert S, Goldwasser F. Neoadjuvant chemotherapy with high-dose methotrexate in osteosarcoma. Lancet Oncol. 2008;9(12):1198.

26. Grimer RJ, Carter SR, Tillman RM, et al. Endoprosthetic replacement of the proximal tibia. J Bone Joint Surg Br. 1999;81(3):488–94.

27. Jeon DG, Kawai A, Boland P, Healey JH. Algorithm for the surgical treatment of malignant lesions of the proximal tibia. Clin Orthop Relat Res. 1999;358:15–26.

28. Ogihara Y, Sudo A, Fujinami S, Sato K. Limb salvage for bone sarcoma of the proximal tibia. Int Orthop. 1991;15(4):377–9.

29. Petschnig R, Baron R, Kotz R, Ritschl P, Engel A. Muscle function after endoprosthetic replacement of the proximal tibia. Different techniques for extensor reconstruction in 17 tumor patients. Acta Orthop Scand. 1995; 66(3):266–70.

30. Bickels J, Wittig JC, Kollender Y, et al. Reconstruction of the extensor mechanism after proximal tibia endoprosthetic replacement. J Arthroplast. 2001;16(7):856–62.

31. Yoshida Y, Osaka S, Ryu J. Reconstruction of the knee extensor mechanism in patients with a malignant bone tumor of the proximal tibia. Surg Today. 2010;40(7):646–9.

32. Ayerza MA, Aponte-Tinao LA, Abalo E, Muscolo DL. Continuity and function of patellar tendon host-donor suture in tibial allograft. Clin Orthop Relat Res. 2006;450:33–8.

33. Shimose S, Sugita T, Kubo T, Matsuo T, Ochi M. Reconstructed patellar tendon length after proximal tibia prosthetic replacement. Clin Orthop Relat Res. 2005;439:176–80.

34. Jeys LM, Kulkarni A, Grimer RJ, Carter SR, Tillman RM, Abudu A. Endoprosthetic reconstruction for the treatment of musculoskeletal tumors of the appendicular skeleton and pelvis. J Bone Joint Surg Am. 2008;90(6): 1265–71.

35. Myers GJ, Abudu AT, Carter SR, Tillman RM, Grimer RJ. Endoprosthetic replacement of the distal femur for bone tumours: long-term results. J Bone Joint Surg Br. 2007;89(4):521–6.

36. Peel T, May D, Buising K, Thursky K, Slavin M, Choong P. Infective complications following tumour endoprosthesis surgery for bone and soft tissue tumours. Eur J Surg Oncol. 2014;40(9):1087–94.

37. Brock HS, Moodie PG, Hendricks KJ, McIff TE. Compression strength and porosity of single-antibiotic cement vacuum-mixed with vancomycin. J Arthroplast. 2010;25(6):990–7.

38. Yu XC, Xu M, Xu SF, Song RX. Long-term outcomes of epiphyseal preservation and reconstruction with inactivated bone for distal femoral osteosarcoma of children. Orthop Surg. 2012;4(1):21–7.

39. Aponte-Tinao L, Ayerza MA, Muscolo DL, Farfalli GL. Survival, recurrence, and function after epiphyseal preservation and allograft reconstruction in osteosarcoma of the knee. Clin Orthop Relat Res. 2015;473(5):1789–96.

16

Lumbar spine MRI versus non-lumbar imaging modalities in the diagnosis of sacral insufficiency fracture: a retrospective observational study

Yoon Yi Kim, Bo Mi Chung* ⓘ and Wan Tae Kim

Abstract

Background: Sacral insufficiency fractures (SIFs) are a common cause of lower back pain in the elderly. However, because clinical symptoms are frequently vague and nonspecific and can mimic lumbar spine pathologies, initial imaging in SIF patients is frequently targeted at the lumbar spine rather than the sacrum, resulting in delayed diagnosis. The purpose of this study is to show the proportions of modalities used in diagnosing SIF in practice and to compare the clinical and imaging features of SIF diagnosed by lumbar spine MRI (L-spine MRI) with those diagnosed by non-lumbar imaging modalities (bone scan, pelvic bone CT, pelvis MRI).

Methods: Forty-two patients with SIF were enrolled in this study. SIFs diagnosed by L-spine were assigned to group 1 and SIFs diagnosed by non-lumbar imaging modalities (bone scan, pelvic bone CT, pelvis MRI) were assigned to group 2. The clinical and imaging features of SIFs were assessed and compared between two groups.

Results: SIF were more commonly diagnosed by L-spine MRI (group 1: $n = 27$, 64.3%) than non-lumbar imaging modalities (group 2: $n = 15$, 35.7%), which was comprised of pelvic bone CT ($n = 6$, 14.3%), bone scan ($n = 5$, 11.9%), and pelvis MRI ($n = 4$, 9.5%). Lower back pain, radiating pain and comorbid other causes of pain were more frequently identified in group 1. Fracture involving bilateral sacral ala with horizontal component was the most common shape and S2 being the most commonly involved horizontal component, without significant difference between two groups.

Conclusion: SIFs are more commonly diagnosed by L-spine MRI than non-lumbar imaging modalities, because of symptoms that mimic lumbar spine pathology and variable comorbid causes of pain. To know that L-spine MRI commonly reveal SIF and to be familiar with SIF features on L-spine MRI would help increase sensitivity in detecting this commonly underrecognized entity and achieve earlier and more appropriate management.

Keywords: Sacral insufficiency fracture, Sacrum, MRI, Lumbar spine MRI

Background

Sacral insufficiency fractures (SIFs) are a common cause of lower back pain in the elderly, with a mean age between 70 and 75 years in most studies [1–3]. They were first described as a clinical entity in 1982 by Lourie, and the awareness and reports of this entity have increased with the increasing number of elderly patients [4, 5]. American College of Radiology (ACR) appropriateness criteria recommend radiography as the first imaging study when SIF is suspected. When radiography is negative, the next imaging study recommended is pelvis MRI without intravenous contrast or bone scan, with reported high sensitivities [6]. However, because clinical symptoms are frequently vague and nonspecific and can mimic lumbar spine pathologies, initial imaging in SIF patients is frequently targeted at the lumbar spine rather than the sacrum, resulting in delayed diagnosis [1, 6–8].

Although many authors suggest radiologists and clinicians to be aware of this entity in interpreting L-spine MRI in old age patients [1, 9], there has been no study that revealed the proportion of L-spine MRI among the

* Correspondence: bom1086@naver.com
Department of Radiology, Veterans Health Service Medical Center, 53, Jinhwangdo-ro 61-gil, Gangdong-gu, Seoul 05368, Republic of Korea

modalities used in diagnosing SIFs or analyzed the difference in clinical and imaging characteristics of SIFs between the L-spine MRI and the non-lumbar imaging modalities.

The purpose of this study is to show the proportions of modalities used in diagnosing SIF in practice and to compare the clinical and imaging features of SIF diagnosed by L-spine MRI with those diagnosed by non-lumbar imaging modalities (bone scan, pelvic bone CT, pelvis MRI).

Methods

Study population

This study was approved by the institutional review board, and informed consent was waived due to the retrospective nature of the study. Figure 1 is a flowchart that summarizes the inclusion process in this study. A picture archiving and communication system (PACS) search was conducted using the keywords "sacral insufficiency fracture," "insufficiency fracture," "sacral fracture," "sacral ala" in the CT, MRI, and bone scan readings at our hospital between January 2014 and August 2017 ($n = 368$). To be enrolled in this study, patients were required to have sacral fracture confirmed on CT or MRI ($n = 65$). We excluded patients with infection or tumor at the sacrum ($n = 5$), prior sacroplasty ($n = 1$), sacral fracture by high energy trauma ($n = 4$), or isolated transverse fracture of the sacrum ($n = 13$). Finally, 42 patients (15 men, 27 women; mean age, 78.83 years; age range, 59–94 years) with SIF were enrolled in this study. Among the 42 patients, 7 patients had two imaging modalities that demonstrated SIF. In 5

patients, SIFs were initially detected by bone scan and confirmed on cross-sectional imaging (4 patients with CT, 1 patient with MRI). One patient underwent L-spine MRI and subsequent pelvis MRI, the other patient initially underwent pelvic bone CT and then bone scan. The interval between two imaging modalities ranged from 1 to 37 days. SIFs initially detected and diagnosed by L-spine were assigned to group 1 ($n = 27$). SIFs initially detected by non-lumbar imaging modalities (bone scan, pelvic bone CT, pelvis MRI) were assigned to group 2 ($n = 15$).

All patients were confirmed as having SIF based on CT or MRI findings. A retrospective review of these patients was conducted by two musculoskeletal radiologists with 2 and 13 years of experience in musculoskeletal image interpretation. An SIF was diagnosed on CT when sagittally oriented fracture lines with or without bony callous were evident at the sacral ala [1, 9]. On MRI, SIF was confirmed by detecting bone marrow edema at the sacral ala, demonstrated as a hypointense area on T1-weighted image (T1-WI) or a hyperintense area with a hypointense fracture line on fat-suppressed T2-weighted image (T2-WI) [1, 9]. In cases initially detected by bone scan, subsequent cross-sectional imaging (either CT or MRI) to confirm the diagnosis was required for patient inclusion in this study [1, 9].

The electronic medical record was reviewed for patient age, gender, body mass index (BMI), presence or absence of osteoporosis by bone mineral density (BMD), low-energy trauma history, operation history at spine or hip, past medical history, and chief complaint. The BMD

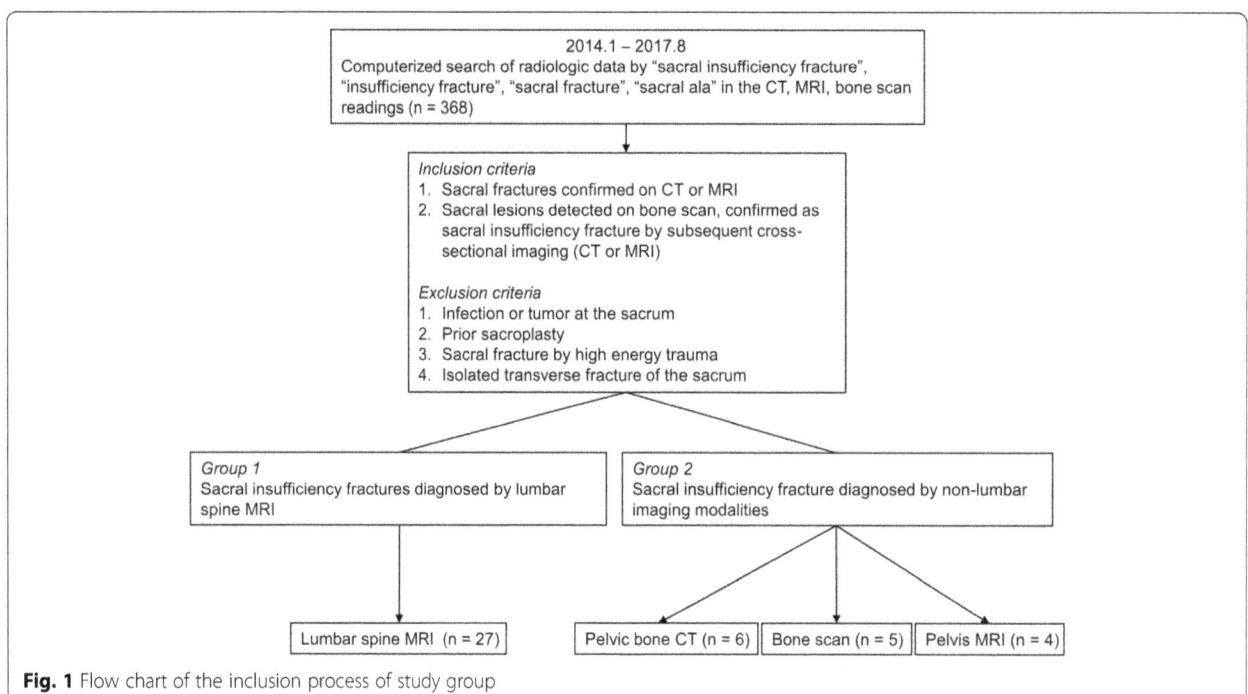

Fig. 1 Flow chart of the inclusion process of study group

and BMI were available for 23 and 33 out of a total of 42 patients, respectively. Through the review of medical records and all the imaging studies performed around the time of detection of SIF, we recorded the presence or absence of vertebral compression fractures and other causes of pain including acute vertebral compression fracture, spinal stenosis, insufficiency fracture of pelvic bone other than the sacrum, and acute hip fracture.

Image acquisition

MR images were obtained using either 1.5-T (Signa, GE) or 3-T (Magnetom Skyra, Siemens) scanners. The protocols varied somewhat depending on the machines or the clinician's request at our institution, but most patients had a combination of the following sequences: sagittal T2-WI (section thickness 4 mm; section gap 0.4–0.5 mm; matrix 448–512 × 256–448; TR 2920–3630; TE 88–114), sagittal T1-WI (section thickness 4 mm; section gap 0.4–0.5 mm; matrix 448–512 × 256–369; TR 460–652; TE 7–11), axial T2-WI (section thickness 4 mm; section gap 0.4–0.5 mm; matrix 320–448 × 202–224; TR 3590–4784; TE 95–104), and axial T1-WI (section thickness 4 mm; section gap 0.4–0.5 mm; matrix 320–448 × 202–224; TR 603–821; TE 9–14). Seventeen patients had additional sequences using fat suppression techniques including sagittal fat-suppressed T2-WI (slice thickness 4 mm; section gap 0.5 mm; matrix 352 × 224; TR 2897; TE 90) on 1.5-T and Dixon sequence water image (slice thickness 4 mm; section gap 0.4 mm; matrix 382 × 307; TR 2880–3720; TE 93) on 3-T MRI. Twenty-two patients had coronal T2-WI (section thickness 4 mm; section gap 0.4–0.5 mm; matrix 448–512 × 224–314; TR 2500–3330; TE 88–114).

The area of coverage was T10 to S3 on sagittal images, and bilateral neural foramina and bilateral sacroiliac joints were included on parasagittal images. On axial imaging, disc spaces including endplates were included for at least four levels of L2/3, L3/4, L4/5, and L5/S1. In eight patients, axial images of the sacrum to S3 level were also acquired. On coronal images, vertebral bodies and the spinal canals of lumbar spines were included, which covered variable portion of sacrum according to the degree of sacral lordosis.

CT examinations were performed using 64-channel (Sensation 64, Siemens) CT systems. The scanning parameters were tube voltage of 120 KV, quality reference tube current of 150 mA, a rotation time of 1 s, a pitch of 0.9, a collimation of 0.6 mm, and a section thickness/reconstruction interval of 2 mm. In addition to axial images, coronal and sagittal images were reformatted with section thickness/reconstruction interval of 2 mm. The field of view were variable depending on the clinician's request, but invariably included the sacrum from S1 down to below the lesser trochanters.

Image analysis

The MR images were evaluated using a PACS workstation. The evaluation of imaging features was performed by consensus of two radiologists with 2 and 13 years of experience in musculoskeletal MRI interpretation (BM C [reader 1] and WT K [reader 2], respectively). We assessed and classified the shape of all SIFs into four groups; vertical fracture at unilateral sacral ala (U), vertical fractures at bilateral sacral alae (B), vertical fracture at unilateral sacral ala with horizontal component (UH), and vertical fractures at bilateral sacral alae with horizontal component (BH). The level of horizontal component fracture was recorded. The degree of bone marrow edema around vertical fracture of sacral ala shown on T1-WI in the sagittal plane were recorded in group 1 and categorized as 'moderate' when there was diffuse bone marrow edema with barely visible normal fatty marrow (Fig. 2). The degree was recorded as 'mild' when bone marrow edema occupied between one-third and two-thirds of the diseased area (Fig. 3) and 'minimal' when only hypointense streaks or nodular lesions were seen (Fig. 4). Six months after the initial imaging analysis, reader 1 again evaluated the degree of bone marrow edema, avoiding recall bias. The reader 3 (YY K) independently rated the bone marrow edema with the same criteria. The interobserver and intraobserver agreement was evaluated.

Statistical analysis

To assess the differences in the clinical and imaging features between group 1 and 2, the Chi-square test, Fisher's exact test, Student's t test, and Mann–Whitney test were utilized for analysis. Agreement regarding the degree of bone marrow edema was statistically compared with the kappa (κ) statistics. κ values of interobserver and intraobserver agreement was assigned as follows: less than 0.20, poor; 0.21–0.40, fair; 0.41–0.60, moderate; 0.61–0.80, good; and more than 0.81, excellent [10]. A p value less than 0.05 was considered statistically significant. All analyses were performed with IBM SPSS 20 (IBM Software Inc.).

Results

Out of 42 patients, 27 SIFs were diagnosed by L-spine MRI and assigned to group 1 (64.3%). Fifteen SIFs were detected and diagnosed by non-lumbar imaging modalities and were assigned to group 2 (35.7%). Group 2 was comprised of pelvic bone CT ($n = 6$, 14.3%), bone scan ($n = 5$, 11.9%), and pelvis MRI ($n = 4$, 9.5%).

The clinical features of patients are summarized in Table 1. In terms of chief complaint, lower back pain and radiating pain were more frequently identified in group 1, whereas hip pain was more commonly associated with group 2. Other causes of pain were present in most patients ($n = 31$, 73.8%) and were significantly more

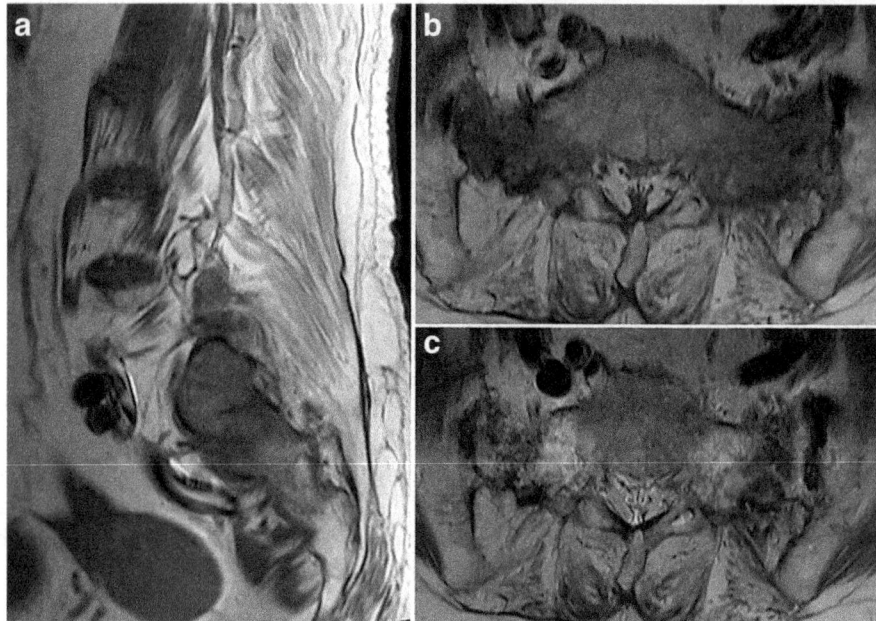

Fig. 2 A 72-year-old woman with sacral insufficiency fracture (SIF) involving the bilateral sacral alae with horizontal component. **a** Sagittal T1-weighted MR image shows diffuse signal alteration that suggests moderate bone marrow edema at the left sacral ala. **b** Axial T1-weighted MR image at the proximal S1 level shows moderate bone marrow edema at both sacral alae. **c** Axial T2-weighted MR image of the same level shows hypointense fracture lines at both sacral alae

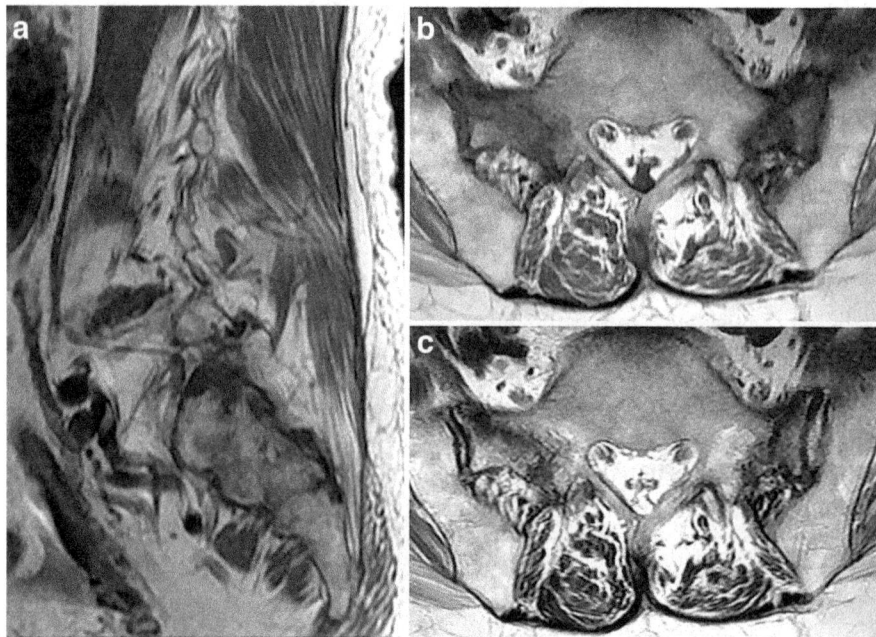

Fig. 3 A 68-year-old woman with SIF involving the bilateral sacral alae. **a** Sagittal T1-weighted MR image shows irregular signal alteration suggesting mild bone marrow edema at the left sacral alae. **b** Axial T1-weighted MR image at the proximal S1 level shows hypointense fracture lines with surrounding bone marrow edema at both sacral alae. **c** Axial T2-weighted MR image at the same level shows hypointense fracture line

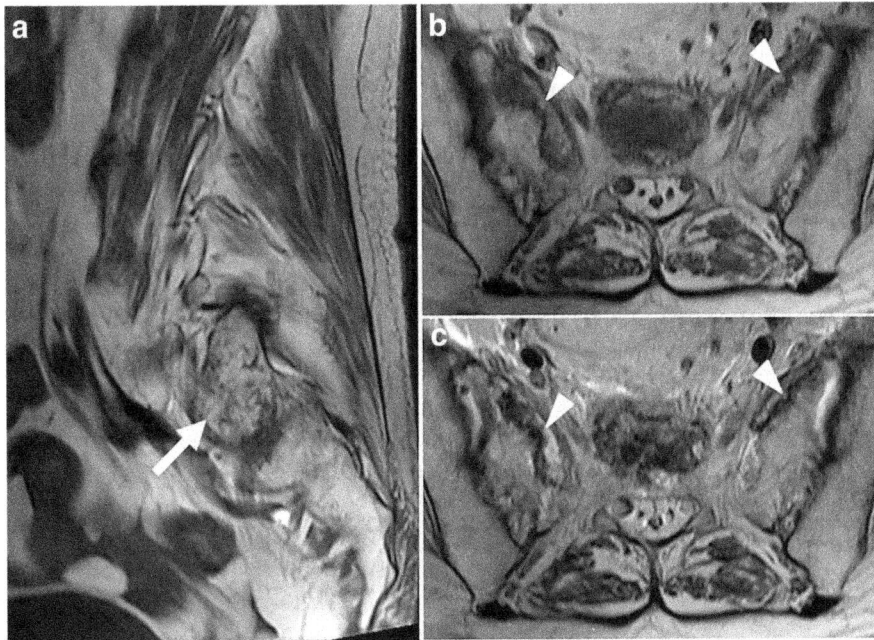

Fig. 4 An 81-year-old woman with SIF involving the bilateral sacral alae with a horizontal component (not shown). **a** Sagittal T1-weighted MR image shows hypointense streaks at the right sacral ala (arrow). **b** and **c**, Axial T1-weighted (**b**) and T2-weighted (**c**) MR images at the distal S1 level show hypointense fracture lines at both sacral alae with minimal surrounding bone marrow edema (arrowheads)

Table 1 Clinical Features of Sacral Insufficiency Fractures

	Group 1 (n = 27)	Group 2(n = 15)	Total (n = 42)	P value
Age (years)	79.5±7.8	77.7±12.1	78.8±9.3	0.599
Male:Female	12:15	3:12	15:27	0.180
Osteoporosis	8 (n = 13)	9 (n = 10)	17 (n = 23)	0.179
BMI	22.5±3.5	23.0 ±3.5	22.7±3.4	0.690
Trauma history	13	8	21	1.000
Prior surgery (hip, spine)	7	4	11	1.000
Vertebral compression fracture	18	8	26	0.511
Past medical history				
Diabetes	4	1	5	0.639
Hypertension	10	4	14	0.734
Chronic renal disease	2	1	3	1.000
Malignancy	2	6	8	0.016
Chief complaint				
Lower back pain	24	2	26	0.000
Radiating pain	10	0	10	0.007
Hip pain	2	10	12	0.000
Other cause of pain	23	8	31	0.034
Acute vertebral compression fracture	9	2	11	0.273
Spinal stenosis	17	0	17	0.000
Other PIF	3	2	5	1.000
Acute hip fracture	1	4	5	0.047

BMI body mass index, *PIF* pelvic insufficiency fracture
Values in parenthesis for osteoporosis represent the number of patients with available bone mineral density (BMD) results

common in group 1. The most common other cause of pain was spinal stenosis followed by acute vertebral compression fracture in group 1 and acute hip fracture in group 2. History of malignancy was more common in group 2. No significant difference between the two groups was noted in other clinical features.

The imaging features of SIFs are summarized in Table 2. The BH shape was the most common ($n = 28$, 66.7%), followed by UH ($n = 6$, 14.3%), B ($n = 5$, 11.9%), and U ($n = 3$, 7.1%) shapes. The most commonly involved horizontal component was S2 ($n = 14$, 41.2%). No statistically significant difference was noted between the two groups regarding fracture shape or the level of the horizontal component. On sagittal T1-WI, bone marrow edema around vertical fracture most commonly showed moderate ($n = 24$, 49%) degree, followed by mild ($n = 17$, 34.7%) or minimal (n = 6, 16.3%) degrees. The interobserver agreement between the first reading and reader 3 was good ($\kappa = 0.693$). The intraobserver agreement between the two readings by reader 1 was excellent ($\kappa = 0.831$).

Discussion

Insufficiency fractures occur when normal stresses are applied to bone with decreased density. They occur most commonly in the pelvis, including the sacrum, followed by the proximal femur and the vertebral bodies. SIFs commonly affect elderly women with osteoporosis [1, 5, 11, 12]. Antecedent trauma is not identified in two-thirds of patients and, when present, is usually minor [1, 2, 13]. Clinical features including age, gender, presence of osteoporosis, and trauma history were comparable with previous reports and showed no significant difference between the two groups.

Various modalities are in use to diagnose SIF in daily practice, and this is the first study to show the proportion of modalities and analyzed the clinical and imaging features. Although sacrum is not routinely covered completely on L-spine MRI, our study revealed that L-spine MRI was the most common modality that detected SIF ($n = 27$, 64.3%), followed by pelvic bone CT ($n = 6$, 14.3%), bone scan ($n = 5$, 11.9%), and pelvis MRI ($n = 4$, 9.5%). In 73.8% of all patients, other comorbid causes of pain were present. The advanced age of SIF patients and the risk factors represented by osteoporosis would have contributed to this result. Other cause of pain was significantly more common in group 1 and were mainly comprised of spinal stenosis and acute vertebral compression fracture. This result partly explains the frequent chief complaints of lower back pain and radiating pain in group 1. The choice of L-spine MRI seems to be effective to find both lumbar spine pathology and SIF. Acute hip fracture and hip pain complaints was more prevalent in group 2, and it explains why these SIFs were diagnosed by non-lumbar imaging studies. History of malignancy was more common in group 2, which was associated with the SIFs detected in the screening bone scan for bone metastasis in patients with malignancy history.

SIFs most commonly involve the bilateral or unilateral sacral alae, lateral to the neural foramina and medial to the sacroiliac joints. There can also be a horizontal component to the fracture through the sacral bodies [1, 14]. BH was the most common shape of SIF, and S2 was the most common horizontal level in our study, which was in accordance with the literature [14–16]. Authors expected that the fracture shape might be related with clinical presentation and the choice of modality but there was no statistically significant difference between the two groups. We excluded isolated horizontal fracture of the sacrum in this study because it is controversial whether this is really an insufficiency fracture versus a

Table 2 Imaging Features of Sacral Insufficiency Fractures

	Group 1 ($n = 27$)	Group 2($n = 15$)	Total ($n = 42$)	P value
SIF shape				0.102
U	2	1	3 (7.1%)	
B	1	4	5 (11.9%)	
UH	3	3	6 (14.3%)	
BH	21	7	28 (66.7%)	
H component level				0.158
S1	1	2	3 (8.8%)	
S1,2	2	0	2 (5.9%)	
S2	11	3	14 (41.2%)	
S2,3	3	0	3 (8.8%)	
S3	7	5	12 (35.3%)	

SIF sacral insufficiency fracture, *U* unilateral sacral ala, *B* bilateral sacral alae, *UH* unilateral sacral ala with horizontal component, *BH* bilateral sacral alae with horizontal component, *H* horizontal fracture caused by minor trauma [14, 17]. Linstrom et al. introduced isolated horizontal fracture as an atypical SIF shape in cases with unusual sacral stress patterns, such as extreme amounts of sacral lordosis. However, more commonly the horizontal component seems to develop at a later stage after loss of sacral alar support, which causes the entire weight of the upper body to be longitudinally transferred down the central portion of the sacral bodies [14, 18].

Bone scan, CT, and MRI were utilized to diagnose SIF in our study. Bone scan is one of the most sensitive examinations for the detection of SIF and regarded as gold standard for detecting insufficiency fractures for many years. Some authors have suggested that the H-shaped (Honda or butterfly) sacral pattern could be considered diagnostic in the correct clinical setting, especially if there are no other sites of abnormal uptake and no history of primary malignancy. But this characteristic pattern is seen in only 20 to 40% of patients and variations in the pattern of radiopharmaceutical activity could be seen [6, 11]. There also have been case reports of isolated metastases presenting as unilateral sacral uptake [16]. Therefore, we included only cases that were confirmed by cross-sectional imaging when bone scan suggested the possibility of SIF. CT is less sensitive for the detection of SIFs than bone scan or MRI, with a reported sensitivity between 60 and 75%, and is not typically used for first or second-line imaging tool for work up of insufficiency fractures. However, CT may offer adjunct role to confirm inconclusive or equivocal findings on bone scan or MRI [1, 6]. MRI can detect SIF very sensitively like bone scan, with higher specificity than bone scan. MRI can usually differentiate insufficiency fracture from pathologic fracture due to tumor infiltration [1]. Recent literature favors MRI for making early diagnosis of insufficiency fractures at pelvic region [1, 6, 19]. The fat suppressed images are especially sensitive for the detection of early bone marrow edema and coronal imaging of sacrum are recommended to be included in suspected cases [1, 20]. Gupta et al. reported that addition of coronal short tau inversion recovery sequence to the L-spine MRI enabled them to detect significant findings in 6.8% of patients, including SIF or sacroiliitis [21].

Although fat suppressed images can more sensitively detect bone marrow edema and coronal imaging of sacrum can better demonstrate vertically oriented fracture line, it is difficult to suspect SIF on physical examination and add these sequences before imaging, due to the ambiguity of SIF as discussed ahead [1, 20]. Therefore, we evaluated imaging features of SIF based on sagittal T1-WI, which is generally available sequence in most L-spine MRI studies. Getting used to the MRI findings with a scan range and sequences of routine L-spine

MRI would help to reduce the underrecognized SIF. The vertical sacral ala fracture most commonly showed moderate bone marrow edema (49%), followed by mild and minimal degrees. The vertical fracture of sacral ala with moderate bone marrow edema would be readily detectable. In addition, based on our result, careful detection of irregular or reticular pattern could enable the early diagnosis of the otherwise overlooked SIF.

There are several limitations in our study. First, MRI protocols were variable because of the retrospective nature of this study. Second, the distal sacrum was not entirely covered because the routine L-spine MRI covered distally to S3 body in our institution. However, the horizontal component of SIF involved S1, 2 or 3 not only in group 1 but also in group 2 which fully covered sacrum. Third, this is a single-center study. The choice of imaging modality and protocol of L-spine MRI could vary according to the clinicians and institutions. Multicenter, prospective studies are needed for further verification. Lastly, the number of SIFs diagnosed by bone scan could be underestimated because only cases confirmed on cross-sectional images were included in this study.

Conclusions

In conclusion, SIFs are more commonly diagnosed by L-spine MRI than non-lumbar imaging modalities in practice, because SIF frequently mimics lumbar spine pathology due to ambiguous symptoms and variable comorbid causes of pain. Knowing that L-spine MRI commonly reveal SIF and to be familiar with SIF features on L-spine MRI would help radiologists and clinicians to sensitively diagnose this commonly underrecognized entity and achieve earlier and more appropriate management.

Abbreviations
BMD: Bone mineral density; BMI: Body mass index; CT: Computed tomography; L-spine MRI: Lumbar spine MRI; MRI: Magnetic resonance imaging; SIF: Sacral insufficiency fracture

Funding
This study was supported by a VHS Medical Center Research Grant, Republic of Korea (grant number: VHSMC 17035).

Authors' contributions
YY K made contributions to the study design, acquisition of data, and image analysis; WT K participated in the study design, image analysis; BM C contributed to the study design, image analysis and drafting of the manuscript. All authors read and approved the final manuscript.

Competing interests
The authors declare that they have no competing interests.

References
1. Lyders EM, Whitlow CT, Baker MD, Morris PP. Imaging and treatment of sacral insufficiency fractures. AJNR Am J Neuroradiol. 2010;31(2):201–10.
2. Finiels H, Finiels PJ, Jacquot JM, Strubel D. Fractures of the sacrum caused by bone insufficiency. Meta-analysis of 508 cases. Presse Med. 1997;26(33):1568–73.

3. Frey ME, Depalma MJ, Cifu DX, Bhagia SM, Carne W, Daitch JS. Percutaneous sacroplasty for osteoporotic sacral insufficiency fractures: a prospective, multicenter, observational pilot study. Spine J. 2008;8(2):367–73.

4. Lourie H. Spontaneous osteoporotic fracture of the sacrum. An unrecognized syndrome of the elderly. JAMA. 1982;248(6):715–7.

5. Na WC, Lee SH, Jung S, Jang HW, Jo S. Pelvic insufficiency fracture in severe osteoporosis patient. Hip Pelvis. 2017;29(2):120–6.

6. Bencardino JT, Stone TJ, Roberts CC, Appel M, Baccei SJ, Cassidy RC, et al. ACR appropriateness criteria((R)) stress (fatigue/insufficiency) fracture, including sacrum, excluding other vertebrae. J Am Coll Radiol. 2017;14(5S):S293–306.

7. Tamaki Y, Nagamachi A, Inoue K, Takeuchi M, Sugiura K, Omichi Y, et al. Incidence and clinical features of sacral insufficiency fracture in the emergency department. Am J Emerg Med. 2017;35(9):1314–6.

8. Grangier C, Garcia J, Howarth NR, May M, Rossier P. Role of MRI in the diagnosis of insufficiency fractures of the sacrum and acetabular roof. Skelet Radiol. 1997;26(9):517–24.

9. Sudhir G, KL K, Acharya S, Chahal R. Sacral insufficiency fractures mimicking lumbar spine pathology. Asian Spine J. 2016;10(3):558–64.

10. Cohen J. Weighted kappa: nominal scale agreement with provision for scaled disagreement or partial credit. Psychol Bull. 1968;70(4):213–20.

11. Krestan C, Hojreh A. Imaging of insufficiency fractures. Eur J Radiol. 2009;71(3):398–405.

12. Yoder K, Bartsokas J, Averell K, McBride E, Long C, Cook C. Risk factors associated with sacral stress fractures: a systematic review. J Man Manip Ther. 2015;23(2):84–92.

13. Newhouse KE, el-Khoury GY, Buckwalter JA. Occult sacral fractures in osteopenic patients. J Bone Joint Surg Am. 1992;74(10):1472–7.

14. Linstrom NJ, Heiserman JE, Kortman KE, Crawford NR, Baek S, Anderson RL, et al. Anatomical and biomechanical analyses of the unique and consistent locations of sacral insufficiency fractures. Spine (Phila Pa 1976). 2009;34(4):309–15.

15. Weber M, Hasler P, Gerber H. Insufficiency fractures of the sacrum. Twenty cases and review of the literature. Spine (Phila Pa 1976). 1993;18(16):2507–12.

16. Fujii M, Abe K, Hayashi K, Kosuda S, Yano F, Watanabe S, et al. Honda sign and variants in patients suspected of having a sacral insufficiency fracture. Clin Nucl Med. 2005;30(3):165–9.

17. Urzua A, Marre B, Martinez C, Ballesteros V, Ilabaca F, Fleiderman J, et al. Isolated transverse sacral fractures. Spine J. 2011;11(12):1117–20.

18. Cooper KL, Beabout JW, Swee RG. Insufficiency fractures of the sacrum. Radiology. 1985;156(1):15–20.

19. Ahovuo JA, Kiuru MJ, Visuri T. Fatigue stress fractures of the sacrum: diagnosis with MR imaging. Eur Radiol. 2004;14(3):500–5.

20. Blake SP, Connors AM. Sacral insufficiency fracture. Br J Radiol. 2004;77(922):891–6.

21. Gupta R, Mittal P, Mittal A, Mittal K, Gupta S, Kaur R. Additional merit of coronal STIR imaging for MR imaging of lumbar spine. J Craniovertebr Junction Spine. 2015;6(1):12–5.

17

Infection after knee replacement: a qualitative study of impact of periprosthetic knee infection

Charlotte M Mallon[1], Rachael Gooberman-Hill[1,2] and Andrew J Moore[1]* (iD)

Abstract

Background: Approximately 340,000 knee replacements are performed each year in the USA and UK. Around 1% of patients who have had knee replacement develop deep infection around the prosthesis: periprosthetic knee infection. Treatment often requires a combination of one or more major operations and antibiotic therapy. This study aimed to understand and characterise patients' experiences of periprosthetic knee infection.

Methods: Qualitative semi-structured interviews were conducted with 16 patients (9 men, 7 women; 59–80 years, mean age 72) who experienced periprosthetic knee infection and subsequent revision treatment in six National Health Service orthopaedic departments. Interviews were audio-recorded, transcribed, anonymised and analysed thematically. The concept of biographical disruption was used to frame our analysis, and four transcripts double-coded for rigour. Patients were interviewed between two and 10 months after surgical revision.

Results: Participant experiences can be characterised according to three aspects of biographical disruption which we have used to frame our analysis: onset and the problem of recognition; emerging disability and the problem of uncertainty, and chronic illness and the mobilisation of resources. Participants' experiences of infection and treatment varied, but everyone who took part reported that infection and revision treatment had devastating effects on them. Participants described use of social and healthcare support and a need for more support. Some participants thought that the symptoms that they had first presented with had not been taken seriously enough.

Conclusions: Periprosthetic knee infection and its treatment can be life-changing for patients, and there is a need for greater support throughout treatment and lengthy recovery. Future work could look at preparedness for adverse outcomes, help-seeking in impactful situations, and information for healthcare professionals about early signs and care for periprosthetic infection.

Keywords: Periprosthetic infection, Revision, Surgical treatment, Impact, Qualitative, Biographical disruption

Background

In the USA and UK, approximately 340,000 primary knee replacements are performed each year [1, 2]. In 2015, 98,591 primary knee replacement procedures were performed in England and Wales alone [2]. Primary knee replacement is most commonly performed for osteoarthritis [3]. Although knee replacement often improves function and decreases pain, complications after knee replacement can include long-term pain [4], periprosthetic fracture [5] and prosthetic joint infection [6]. For some complications, revision surgery is required. Periprosthetic infection occurs when the tissues surrounding the prosthesis become infected, and it accounts for 25.2% of revision procedures after knee replacement [7] with reported incidence in the UK and USA ranging from 0.5 to 2% [6, 8, 9]. In 2015 in the UK, 6104 knee revision procedures were performed, of which nearly one quarter (1420 (23%)) were for infection [2].

Periprosthetic infection is commonly treated with either one-stage or two-stage revision. One-stage revision treatment consists of one major surgery, during which the prosthesis and infected tissues are removed before a new prosthesis is re-implanted [10]. Two-stage revision

* Correspondence: a.j.moore@bristol.ac.uk
[1]Bristol Medical School, University of Bristol, Bristol, UK
Full list of author information is available at the end of the article

treatment consist of two separate operations where the re-insertion of a new implant is delayed allowing for additional antibiotic therapy between surgeries, sometimes via an anti-biotic-impregnated cement spacer [10]. Two-stage surgical revision is the most common treatment for infection after joint replacement [11], however infection is costly to health services [12] – a revision for infection is more than three times that of an aseptic revision [13] – and two-stage revisions are more expensive than one-stage revisions with the patient undergoing two major surgical procedures [14, 15].

Previous research on infection after joint replacement highlights how infection and treatment can have pro-foundly negative impact on all aspects of patients' lives [16–18]. Due to the heavy physical and psychological burden of treatment that periprosthetic infection im-poses on patients and their families, there is a need for increased psychological and rehabilitative support during treatment and long-term recovery [18].

So far, research has not drawn on social science theories to extend and deepen understanding of the impact of peri-prosthetic infection on patients. In understanding the im-pact of major health and treatment events, insights from the social science of health and illness are useful, particu-larly regarding disruption to people's lives, and how people negotiate and manage major change brought about by ill-ness. Bury's work on 'biographical disruption' is widely recognised as making a major contribution to the greater understanding of experiences of health and illness events. It has been used in health research to highlight how illness disrupts people's expected life course in multiple ways, changing the structures of daily life, challenging and re-defining people's sense of identity and constructed biog-raphy [19–22]. Bury's work has been applied in diverse health contexts, including rheumatoid arthritis [19], long-term knee pain [23], osteoarthritis [24], multiple scler-osis, cerebral palsy, blindness [25]; Meniere's disease [26] and cancer [27, 28]. Bury describes three aspects of disrup-tion that take place in the experience of chronic illness: on-set and the problem of recognition; emerging disability and the problem of uncertainty, and chronic illness and the mobilisation of resources [19]. In exploring the biograph-ical impact of illness, Bury [29] conceptualises the symp-toms of chronic illness as having two distinct meanings: *meaning as consequence*: the problems experienced by people as a result of activity restriction, social disadvantage and their impact on daily life; and *meaning as significance*: the connotations that illnesses carry, in a cultural context. Critique of Bury's work often focusses on these two distinct meanings and the degrees to which each is true, with the concept of 'normal illness' [20] set against that which is disruptive. The concept of biographical disruption is "pred-icated in large part on an adult-centred model of illness de-noting the shift from a normal state of health to one of illness" [25]. Based on our previous work [18],

periprosthetic infection may be an example of this shifting circumstance.

In this qualitative interview study, we explore the ex-perience of periprosthetic knee infection and its impact on patients' lives and draw on the concept of biographical disruption to sensitise us to the meanings of significance and consequences of this major health event for individ-uals in the context of their social worlds.

Methods
Study design
The study was a qualitative, interview study comprising in-depth interviews and thematic analysis.

Eligibility and recruitment
Eligible participants were people aged 18 years and over, with periprosthetic knee infection and experience of one-stage or two-stage revision surgery. They were all patients who had received treatment at one of six partici-pating UK National Health Service (NHS) orthopaedic de-partments in the 12 months before recruitment.

Between January 2016 and September 2016, 33 patients were invited to participate. A research nurse at each centre reviewed outpatient clinic lists. All eligible patients were provided with information packs and asked to complete and return a reply form to the research team indicating if they were interested in discussing participation. The re-search team then contacted those patients who expressed interest and arranged a mutually convenient visit to discuss the study and to conduct an interview if they agreed to par-ticipate. At that visit, patients had the opportunity to ask any further questions and were asked to provide their writ-ten, informed consent, including consent to audio-record-ing the interview and to publication of anonymised quotations. Once consent was provided, interviews took place at the same visit.

Sample size
Final sample size was intended to depend on the achieve-ment of saturation, evidenced by no new themes arising from the data [30, 31]. Saturation was achieved once 16 participants had been interviewed, and at this point data collection ceased.

Interview process
Interviews were conducted in participants' homes, by one of the research team's two experienced qualitative researchers (CM and AM). The interviewers were not previously known to the participants. Topic guides were developed in collaboration with the research unit's patient and public involvement forum [32]. Topic guides included key questions, with probes and prompts used where appro-priate to allow for flexibility and to ensure that participants had the opportunity to discuss subjects they deemed

important. Questions covered experience of periprosthetic infection, revision surgery and post-operative care, impact of infection and subsequent treatment, and concerns and expectations for the future. Interviews lasted from 33 to 95 min (mean 67 min).

Data analysis

A team science approach was used to ensure robust analysis, whereby our research was collaboratively conducted by a small team of researchers [33]. Interviews were transcribed, anonymised, with all identifying information removed or replaced with pseudonyms, and imported into the qualitative data management software QSR NVivo [34]. Using a thematic approach' the researcher (CM) read and re-read the transcripts, inductively and deductively coded them and sorted coded data into themes. Deductive coding involved working "down" from pre-existing understandings from previous research, which sensitised us to the data [35]. A second researcher (AM) double-coded four of the 16 transcripts, and the study team met to discuss and agree codes and themes [36]. Bury describes three aspects of disruption which we have used to frame our analysis: onset and the problem of recognition; emerging disability and the problem of uncertainty, and chronic illness and the mobilisation of resources [19]. Within this framework, we also consider both the meaning as consequence and the meaning as significance, for the symptoms and treatment of periprosthetic infection [29].

Ethical approval was granted by NRES Committee South West - Exeter (14/SW/0072).

Results

The sample consisted of 9 patients who received one-stage revision treatment, and 7 patients who received two-stage revision treatment; 9 men and 7 women, aged 59–80 years (mean age 72 years) (Table 1).

For 14 patients, this was their first revision surgery. One had received a previous two-stage revision. With the exception of one participant whose primary knee replacement was the result of a fracture, participants' primary replacements had been elective procedures to relieve pain associated with osteoarthritis.

The results highlighted participants' varied experiences, in particular regarding infection onset and subsequent treatment. Infection onset occurred over periods ranging from immediately to 19 years after their primary surgery. All participants felt that infection was life-changing, describing it as "devastating", "traumatic" and causing a "considerably restricted life". Patients' narratives suggest that the experience of infection can be understood as a temporal situation, which can be mapped onto Bury's three aspects of disruption: Onset and the problem of recognition; emerging disability and the problem of uncertainty; and chronic illness and the mobilisation of resources.

Table 1 Sample characteristics

Pseudonym	Sex	Age range	Revision Procedure
Winston	Male	71–80	Two-stage
Delia	Female	61–70	Two-stage
Harry	Male	71–80	One-stage
Shirley	Female	71–80	Two-stage
Hilary	Female	71–80	Two-stage
Margaret	Female	71–80	Two-stage
Brian	Male	71–80	Two-stage
Louisa	Female	61–70	One-stage
Peter	Male	61–70	Two-stage
Terry	Male	71–80	One-stage
Derek	Male	71–80	One-stage
Hazel	Female	51–60	One-stage
Pam	Female	71–80	One-stage
Doug	Male	61–70	One-stage
Lloyd	Male	61–70	One-stage
Jimmy	Male	61–70	One-stage

Participants discussed the ways in which infection and its treatment impacted on, and disrupted the life course within each aspect.

Our analysis suggests that the experience of infection and its treatment causes patients to negotiate major change brought about by this illness event, and to redefine their biographies. Participants described the disruption of taken-for-granted daily routines, uncertainty about the impact and course of infection and treatment, and anxiety and fear about the future. Illustrative quotations are referred to throughout the text and are presented in Tables 2, 3 and 4.

Onset and the problem of recognition (Table 2)

The onset of infection marked a biographical shift from an expected normal course of recovery after knee replacement, to one which was abnormal. Participants described the onset of infection in terms of length of time after surgery, diverse sensations and impact. The onset of infection did not appear to follow a predictable path, and varied from "immediately" after primary replacement (participants felt it never got better) to 19 years afterwards. Although some participants recalled discussing the risk of infection before they had their primary replacement, most did not recollect such conversations. Those participants who could recollect a discussion reported being informed that along with many other factors, infection was a "risk" of joint replacement, however despite this, they still felt largely unprepared for infection.

One participant reported having no indication that anything was wrong until she was suddenly unable to place her foot on the floor. Two patients felt so ill after their infection

Table 2 "Onset and the problem of recognition" quotations and themes

Recognition of infection	"I was annoyed, I was annoyed more than anything that I told so many people that I didn't think it was right and I trusted that they knew better than me because I'm not a doctor or a surgeon" Hazel (1)
	"Every time the answer was 'it can take up to two years to get better'…so all this wonderful Nirvana I were expecting never came about" Hazel (1)
	"Well just want to get right, get right, but um, it was gradually getting worse and worse and worse and at a different stage I thought 'I'm not gonna get out of here' I thought 'I've come to my end' cos that's how I felt" Delia (2)
	He said, "'I'm not giving antibiotics. We give too much of that out.' So anyway it got worse…and then the knee became very painful. I went back over the surgery and, I asked to see a different doctor, who took one look at it and said, 'It's very badly infected.'" Jimmy (1)
	The professionals in there appeared to not take the infection seriously enough, and the GPs also – which are normally your first point of call, didn't take it seriously. Jimmy (1)
Infection onset	"I can't believe it just because I had no, during the day no inclination that anything was wrong with my knee at all… Really, really strange but I mean I don't know if that's how infections happen I don't know, or if you have a build up to an illness, I never had a cold, I wasn't ill." Delia (2)
	"…it was very painful. In fact, it was so painful, I couldn't even walk for many months and it was decided I got an electric scooter." Harry (1)
	"I didn't really know what was happening, because I just thought it was the poison coming out and I'd be better, you see, so I was wrapping it up and wrapping it up, and in the end I thought, 'Well, you know, it's not stopping. I better go and speak to the doctor…'" Derek (1)
	"I was in horrendous pain and my knee was literally twice the size of my other one. [hmm] And I knew that couldn't be right. And no amount of icepacks was making any difference. [no] And the painkillers. I was on about five different painkillers and I mean I've got a high pain threshold but I, I just, I just couldn't get the pain, you know, I was climbing the walls, really." Louisa (1)
	I got out the bed one morning…went to walk to the bathroom and my knee just went, just let me down. Brian (2)
Preparing for diagnosis	"Well, I've always been very active and worked all my life, you can say, and I'm - I get up and go and I like to do things. I never thought I'd be wrong. I thought, 'I'll do the physio and I'll do …' you know. It didn't' occur to me that it would go wrong." Pam (1)
	"They did (mention the possibility of infection). Yes, they did say that, but, they sort of, did it so gently and so lightly, 'There's always that risk, but, you know, things will be expected to run normally. We're not expecting any problems,' so this came as a bit of a shock to me, actually." Margaret (2)
	"Well, yeah, it was. I mean, I was really annoyed with [surgeon], because, when I went up to theatre to have it manipulated I was on the trolley, coming out of the lift into the theatre area, and he came to me and said, 'If you'd put more effort in with the physios, there'd be no need for this.'" Peter (2)
	I just thought, 'This is nearly two years out of my life and at my age [yeah] it, it's not on.' After everything I'd been through as well previously with, you know, different operations [hmm]. I was fuming. I thought, 'If I see the guy I shall hit him.' Louisa (1)
	"Well, you see, it seems like they're in denial because they have this knowledge, they know how serious the infections are … some terrible stories…. But it seems like they let it get to such a bad state first of all before they do any of that. Whereas after, erm, joint surgery, if that's how serious an infection can be, it ought to be acted on earlier on, really." Jimmy (1)
	"I paid privately to have a private consultation to see him … I needed to have some sort of answers fairly soon for my own peace of mind and, er, he arranged for aspiration and it came back fairly quickly, 'You've got a, an infection'. So at least then to some extent I was quite happy because I knew what the problem was."

had manifested, they thought that they would die: one of these participants reported sudden onset at 19 years afterwards, the other described how she never reached her expected "Nirvana" of two years to fully recover after the primary replacement, and despite questioning clinicians, was eventually admitted to hospital by emergency ambulance after collapsing at home. Some participants described more obvious signs that something was wrong, such as red, warm and leaking wounds or scars; others described swelling or the presence of sinus tracts or lumps. Although some described severe pain, others did not.

The process of recognising and reporting the illness to a healthcare professional was problematic for all participants, and routes to diagnosis varied. The length of time between first reporting that there was a problem, and treatment at one of the six orthopaedic departments, ranged from immediately to five years. Some healthcare professionals recognised that participants' symptoms might indicate infection, and made a diagnosis quickly. For some participants diagnosis was prolonged as their symptoms were not immediately thought to be indicative of infection. Participants who experienced a slower route to diagnosis

Table 3 "Emerging disability and the problem of uncertainty" quotations and themes

Burden	"I got down a lot as well because I had to have so long off work it was six months. So I was on statutory sick pay and having to claim rent rebate and stuff, it were a nightmare to me … it's statutory sick pay 29 pound a week so I mean what's that when your rent's 96? So the finances things got me. I had to go into my overdraft and that's something I just don't, you know that's your rainy day money. Because living on your own you do live hand to mouth, you don't have savings, but I can still stand on my own two feet, pay all my bills and buy all my stuff what I need, so that's why I work every Sunday, to make sure I can do that but of course, for six months there were none of that." Hazel (1)
	"Well you have to rely on other people don't you? [Yeah] When you're stuck with a brace on your leg, it's like having a broken leg in a, in a cast for a year isn't it? [Yep] Yeah, you are dependent on everyone really." Delia (2)
	"As you can imagine, lots of things you can't do, for one thing I couldn't drive a car for a year" Delia (2)
Antibiotic therapy	"Actually I wasn't too bad, I mean some people have lots of side effects but I was, I was alright." Delia (2)
	"I think I lost about a stone and a half in weight [laughter] [mmm]. I really felt ill [yeah, yeah]. Erm, that was the thing I didn't like about it and erm… but it did the trick" Shirley (2)
	"When this doctor came in and said you should be able to go home tomorrow he came back to tell me I couldn't because I had to stay on these antibiotics again. Now this was three weeks and I was actually crying and saying I really can't deal with this diarrhoea and stuff and nobody would tell me 'why have I got to keep having them?'." Hazel (1)
Trust	"When he [surgeon], when he said, 'I think I might have to go in and have another look,' I knew what he meant. It's going to be a revision. [hmm] And I thought, 'He's, he's not going to do this. If it's - if I've got to have it done again I'm not letting him touch me.'" Louisa (1)
	"Trust them? [Yeah] Because we think they know, don't we? We think they're wise." Pam (1)
	"I have been through it over the last seven years, believe you, me but this last knee, so far, has been brilliant. [Surgeon] knows what he's doing." Harry (1)
	"I really felt that he was doing his best for me, I really did, you know, I thought so much of him, I had so much confidence in him, the way he dealt with everything … it was quite incredible actually, he was so good on that, erm, that, er, that I didn't query anything. I was just in his hands, I put myself in his hands." Derek (1)
	"I found an absolutely brilliant surgeon and I wouldn't go anywhere else, wouldn't go anywhere else, if he won't do I'll stick without [yeah] because I trust him." Winston (1)
Two-stage revision	"Well film someone who's – who's had that surgery in – in its – in its different stages, when you've just had it in, the first time you get up and use it and – and show you how his body is a bit wobbly and you know, and all this type of thing. Because if people can see for themselves that it's possible and it's good, because you don't know it is, because there's nothing, I was given no information on how I should react to it" Winston (2)
	"I spent … March, April, May, June, [mmm] not being able to do anything" Shirley (2)
	"Well, I thought it was gonna be a nightmare but, I mean, I was on crutches [yeah]. I'm still on crutches, on one crutch, and, er, I'm still wearing a, a brace on my leg, when I'm outside walking round. Erm, but, obviously, the wife's had to drive all the, all the time [yeah]. Erm, I haven't been able to do things I want to do. Erm, I'm retired, but I did intend to carry on doing a few jobs for, you know, people that I know well [yeah]. Erm, so, basically, you know, it has stopped me doing a lot of the things that … I mean, I'd just retired two months before the operation, so I've not really enjoyed retirement, because I've been restricted in what I can do." Peter (2)
	"Oh the whole thing's quite frightening but I mean I can be negative but my husband's so negative I'm determined to not to be negative you know what I mean, I think I can't put up with all of this." Hilary (2)

were dissatisfied and felt that their concerns had not been taken seriously enough by healthcare professionals. Although some patients were insistent with healthcare professionals that there was a problem, others felt frustrated with themselves for not "speaking up" when they had intuitively felt that something was wrong. Patients' reasoning for not challenging healthcare professionals about their symptoms included viewing surgeons as expert and therefore trusting, or having "faith" in their abilities, not wanting to be perceived as "bolshie or rude or pedantic", not knowing appropriate questions to ask, and fearing they would "hold everything up" by challenging decisions. Consequently, some participants felt that their pursuit of referral had been considerably delayed, and that if their infection had been diagnosed sooner, the impact on their life may have been less severe.

Participants described conflicting reactions to their diagnoses. The diagnosis of infection was a shock to some participants. Despite a late diagnosis some participants reported feeling "pleased" and "relief" that treatment was imminent. Others felt "disappointed", "unlucky" or "annoyed". One patient described feeling vindicated, and described how he had felt the surgeon who conducted his primary knee replacement "blamed" him for a lack of improvement after surgery. At the point of diagnosis, some patients felt uncertain about how the infection might progress, and what the subsequent treatment might entail. Despite a firm diagnosis the cause of the infection was often unknown, and participants reported feeling shocked,

Table 4 "Response to infection and treatment, and the mobilisation of resources" quotations and themes

Social support	"But, as I say, it's, err – and of course it means you don't go off to see your parents and your family and your children half as much as you normally would. They come to you, which is wonderful, but, I mean, it's putting them at difficulties sometimes, when on many occasion we go to visit them, you know." Margaret (2)
	"What was going to happen after I came out of hospital? Hubby's useless, absolutely useless, I'm there for him he isn't there for anybody else." Hilary (2)
Changing the physical environment	"I were frightened when I were left on my own and there were nobody in, I don't know what I was frightened of but I was frightened of irrational things. What if house catches fire downstairs?" Hazel (1)
	"I have trouble with my bath but that's not their fault. It's a, a shower bath and I can't have a seat on or anything because it's too wide. But it's a big corner and I sit on there and I swing my legs." Pam (1)
	"I try and go up to my daughter, she's got a walk-in shower" Brian (2)
Clinical support	"It's just that to start with I think I was feeling so low and so very unwell, I really felt neglected." Margaret (2)
	"One would tell you one thing, one would tell you another and I think again this all contributed to my feeling quite low and when I got home I came home thinking right I will get myself better now, I'm home now." Hazel (1)
	"No, I've not had any physio, no. It was, erm, before I came out it was a matter of, let me think, before I came out." Doug (1)
	"Yeah, they [physiotherapists] were around every day while I was in the hospital." Brian (2)
	"They [physiotherapists] didn't come to me. In fact, they never came to me. All they brought was that ice bucket thing … and I didn't actually know how to do it." Pam (1)
	"Six weeks it was before I could see a physio. Well, luckily, they gave me some exercise sheets at the hospital and luckily, I'm the sort that would do it." Shirley (2)
Life after periprosthetic infection	"I had discomfort, I couldn't walk very well so I went to see [surgeon] and err, he said I think you ought to have a knee replacement so that's what happened" Terry (1)
	"But I, I just thought, 'This is nearly two years out of my life and at my age it's not on" Louisa (1)
	"I'm 80 in September, and I'm not young, and I can't expect to be playing football and cricket and running around, and the only thing I wish I could get on the floor and play with the grandchildren and their games sometimes, but that's not the point, the point is that I've accepted my age, and I don't look for people running around after me" Derek (1)
	"What's the next stage, what's going to happen … am I going to get infection back, you know, there's only so much your knee can take" Delia (2)

and a mixture of fear and relief at the point of diagnosis, but also concerned and uncertain about their future.

For the participants in this study, the onset of infection was not perceived as a "normal" part of their biography. It was a shock, and a source of uncertainty and anxiety, about its cause, the treatment and the prognosis. The onset and diagnosis of infection was traumatic for many participants, and something for which they were unprepared.

Emerging disability and the problem of uncertainty (Table 3)

Surgical and antibiotic treatment for infection profoundly disrupted participants' everyday lives in multiple ways, reinforcing a biographical shift from a perceived normal to an altered situation and sense of self. Participants' responses to antibiotic therapy varied. Not all patients felt unwell during antibiotic treatment and most did not experience any adverse effects. However, some patients experienced unpleasant and distressing side effects, including nausea, sickness, loss of appetite, diarrhoea and weight loss. Describing her low mood and distress after three weeks of unpleasant side-effects, one patient felt that she could no longer cope with her treatment regimen.

Surgical treatment for infection impacted on patients' physical mobility and function, and some participants experienced associated social, psychological and financial burdens. Participants lived with mobility and lifestyle limitations including being unable to drive, work, sleep, carry out domestic duties, or walk without pain. Leisure activities, social engagements and visits to family were often cancelled, and participants were unable to continue their previous lifestyle as a result of severe immobility. Infection also had a financial impact on participants. One participant cancelled her holiday, losing money on flights and accommodation; another felt "lucky" that he had completed all of his mortgage payments in the same month as his operation, believing that he would have been forced to sell his house otherwise as he could no longer work. This profound physical, social, psychological and financial disruption led to participants describing their lives as "on hold".

Participants spoke of the trust and faith they placed in their surgeon. Some patients retained a trust in their surgeon especially if the same surgeon that performed their primary knee replacement also performed the revision operation. However, others lost trust in the surgeon who conducted their primary replacement. One participant described how she did not "trust" her original surgeon to perform a revision operation, because she felt that her insistence that something was wrong had not been taken seriously enough. Additionally, she described an initial conversation with her surgeon in which she was assured she would be able to walk, and engage in sporting activity after knee replacement: activities she was unable to do. In contrast, one participant insisted the same surgeon who had performed his primary replacement also performed his subsequent three revisions.

Participants expressed a sense of uncertainty about the eradication or the return of infection. Many patients reported that a recurrence of infection was their main concern for the future: some patients sought post-operative assurances from their surgeons about the "percentage" or "likelihood" of eradicating infection completely; other patients described their hopes that the infection would not return. This sense of uncertainty led to patients feeling "terrified" and "very anxious" of the impact that a recurrent infection and further surgery would have on their lives.

The significance of participants' treatment was neither downplayed, nor thought to be a "normal" part of their biography. For the participants in this study, the treatment of infection was a complex, and often lengthy process. In line with this, the consequences of participants' treatment for infection were severe for all participants, with profound physical, social, psychological and financial disruption, which profoundly changed their daily lives. Participants described withdrawal from their valued activities and relationships as a result of treatment, which prevented them from doing things they had previously enjoyed.

Response to infection and treatment, and the mobilisation of resources (Table 4)

Participants' responses to the disruption of infection and treatment involved a restructuring of their personal and social involvements. Participants experienced a sense of hopelessness, and felt that their personal identity had changed over the course of the infection and treatment: from a dependent, capable self to an uncertain, increasingly dependent self for whom the infection "takes over". Participants found that taken-for-granted activities they were once easily able to undertake were no longer possible. Most participants felt that their relationships with family and friends had been disrupted, either because of mobility restrictions, tiredness, or embarrassment in social situations. One participant described how he felt he placed an unfair burden on his wife who missed out on social and leisure opportunities. Another participant described how she felt she was a burden to her older children and had tried to avoid socialising with them.

In terms of mobilising resources to face a new and unexpected situation, participants relied mostly on support from social networks including family, friends and neighbours in relation to cooking meals, shopping for food, undertaking domestic duties, and accessing their own home. The presence of a supportive social network was fundamental to all participants' recovery, and participants described how maintaining their social network was of great concern.

Participants described how they made adaptations to their physical home environment, in order to manage their recovery after revision treatment. Some moved out of their home to live with others during their recovery. One patient moved in with her daughter, during her post-operative recovery, but became anxious when left alone in the house due to her immobility. As self-care became difficult, participants' spouses or children helped them to maintain their personal hygiene. Participants also discussed being unable to shower, or creating complex routines to enable them to do so, including travelling to a family member's home to use a walk-in shower.

In terms of medical support and resources, some participants reported needing more care and support with their post-operative and long-term recovery from Primary Care doctors and allied health professionals, in the period after surgical revision treatment. One participant felt that the lack of psychological support after her discharge from hospital had led to her low moods. Another patient described an absence of support from both clinicians and her spouse led to her being unable to manage her medication once discharged. Post-operative physiotherapy varied between treatment centres. Some participants reported having minimal physiotherapy input, or none at all, whilst others reported satisfactory post-operative physiotherapy. However, patients' experiences varied. Only one patient received a course of hydrotherapy. Another described having only one physiotherapy appointment in her eight-day recovery in hospital, at which she was shown how to use cold therapy ice pads, but still felt uncertain of how to use them.

There was a stark contrast between participants' expectations of primary knee replacement, and the reality of life after periprosthetic infection. Many participants described their altered life course in ways that inferred an acceptance of their situation as a new normal, rather than an illness event. Participants discussed feelings of uncertainty, about the recurrence of infection, or requiring lifelong antibiotic medication. When asked about their original preconceptions of primary knee replacement, participants largely spoke of reduced pain, walking without discomfort, and a return to being "fit and active". In contrast to their preconceptions, one patient had experienced a "superb" recovery after his primary replacement until his infection four years later, however at the time of interview was unable to walk without discomfort, and described a painful and stiff joint: he was fearful that his infection had not cleared. One patient had experienced a "terrible" and lengthy recovery after her primary replacement, and despite feeling satisfied with the revision operation, felt that she had lost two years of her life.

The frustration of coping with either pain or immobility in their daily lives contributed to patients' low mood. The impact of both infection and treatment on wider family and significant relationships was profound, with some participants acknowledging a fear of dependency. Participants' responses to the infection and treatment also expressed a sense of fragility, using phrases such as "I'm hopeless now", "I do need answers now because I can't carry on", and "It makes me feel useless."

Participants' narratives suggest that both the meanings as significance and consequence of symptoms and treatment for periprosthetic infection create a biographically abnormal and profoundly disruptive experience for patients, wherein social identities are challenged and redefined.

Discussion

People diagnosed with periprosthetic infection faced an altered and unexpected situation, in which they experienced profound disruption to their life course according to Bury's theory [19]. Infection and treatment appeared to derail people's sense of a planned or anticipated biographical trajectory, which they found distressing. Their distress was particularly related to difficulties in getting a diagnosis of infection; a relatively sudden lack of mobility from onset of infection and throughout treatment; an uncertainty about their future; and a forced withdrawal from their social worlds. Bury's theory provides a useful framework through which to view the narratives of patients, through each of the three aspects of disruption that take place in patients' experience of chronic illness.

Participants made sense of their experiences of infection through the narratives that they shared, giving meaning to the events of infection that disrupted the structures of their everyday lives, and the foundations that underpin these structures [19]. Narratives often began with an uncertain, difficult or traumatic diagnosis during which some patients felt that signs of infection were "not taken seriously enough" and should have been acted upon earlier. This was followed by a disruption of taken-for-granted behaviours, and persistent uncertainty during their treatment and rehabilitation, for which they were largely unprepared. Not all participants could recall discussing the risks of infection with their doctor, or receiving information about infection, before their primary joint replacement. While this apparent lack of information may have enabled patients to remain calm and positive about their primary joint replacement, it may also have increased the likelihood of patients' lack of preparedness when infection was later diagnosed. However, it is also possible that patients did not expect to be one of the 1% of primary knee replacement patients who develop an infection.

Periprosthetic infection can be life-changing, both physically and psychologically, and placing pressure on patients' social and supportive relationships. The impact on participants' mobility and physical function restricted their ability to participate in social roles and events as they had previously, subsequently affecting their sense of personal identity. Some participants were forced to adapt their home environments or move home entirely to cope with their recovery. Participants described disruption to their personal identity and relationships with others, in a context where infection and treatment precluded their former positive experiences and meanings [19, 22]. Withdrawal from social relationships as well as increasing social isolation are important features of chronic illness [37]. Increasing social isolation and dependency on their families and wider social networks, led participants to describe how they felt they were being a burden to those who cared for them. Throughout participants' narratives uncertainty is evident - at diagnosis, treatment, rehabilitation and in concerns about eradication or return of infection. In their narratives, participants incorporated this difficult and traumatic illness event into their biography, but they often remained uncertain regarding their future. The patients in this study described a persistent need for support throughout diagnosis, treatment and recovery. Despite the relatively small number of cases of periprosthetic infection each year, the impact on patients' lives is disproportionately adverse.

Despite its widespread application, biographical disruption has been debated [24, 25]. Yet notwithstanding these alternate views, it remains a powerful sensitising concept to the meanings of significance and consequences of periprosthetic infection for individuals in the context of their social worlds. In understanding the significance and consequence of periprosthetic infection, we suggest that its onset and treatment represents a completely unexpected and anomalous event which profoundly disrupts the lifecourse. This is the first study to explore the impact of one-stage and two-stage revision treatment for periprosthetic knee infection. Previous qualitative work has explored periprosthetic hip infection [18] and surgical site infection [38]. Our study also indicates that infection impacts on all aspects of patients' lives [16–18], but also explored the relationship between the experience of infection and treatment, and biographical disruption. Bury's work on biographical disruption focuses on the onset and the perception of illness [19]: our work extends this by also focusing on the treatment of, and recovery from illness, which in the context of prosthetic joint infection arguably has the greatest impact on patients. While we acknowledge that the onset of periprosthetic infection is distressing and impactful for patients, they remain largely unprepared for the potentially lengthy and complex treatment process and recovery period. This impacts on patients' ability to mobilise resources in order to cope with their treatment and recovery, and the participants in this study described feeling irrational, anxious and in low mood, and very aware of the burden they placed on their supportive networks. Our findings draw parallels with work describing how feelings of hopelessness are reported among patients with surgical site infections [38]. Both the loss of identity and independence established in this study are similar to those found in other chronic illnesses [39, 40]. The unpredictability and uncertainty of diagnosis and treatment of periprosthetic infection draw parallels with patients' perceptions of multiple sclerosis [41], HIV [42–44], and cancer [45]. The disruption to the life course that patients in this study experienced is similar to those experiencing HIV and cancer diagnoses [46–48]. Uncertainty is widely recognised in qualitative studies of illness experience literature, and patients' uncertainty is greatest during the diagnosis phase and when outcomes are unknown or unpredictable [49].

This study provides new information about patients' experiences of periprosthetic knee infection. Saturation was achieved in the sample of 16 patients from six UK NHS orthopaedic centres, and we took care to ensure rigour in analysis through a double coding and team science approach. We acknowledge that it is possible that the inclusion of more patients from additional study centres may have elicited supplementary findings. We also acknowledge that a study limitation, common to all research which employs opt-in consent is that there is an inherent self-selection bias, however, achievement of saturation gives us confidence that the sampling was appropriate in quantity and breadth. The study was conducted in the UK context, but we suggest that the experience of infection after knee replacement resonates with other contexts, including social impact and need for care. Interviewing participants between two and 10 months after revision surgery may have introduced recall bias but this approach gave the study the opportunity to explore the longer-term impact of infection, treatment and recovery.

Conclusions

The impact of periprosthetic infection is wide-ranging, and research to date has not paid sufficient attention to the experiences of people who have this complication after knee replacement. Participants within this study described a disruption to their everyday behaviours, a loss of identity, growing dependency on families and social support networks, as well as uncertainty about their futures. As such we suggest that periprosthetic knee infection may be described as an assault on patients' physical self, sense of self and life course. Further research into the impact of infection might take a longitudinal, prospective approach to explore recovery and change over time in

more detail. Our findings lead us to suggest that clinicians in primary, secondary and community care should be supported to provide consistency in care, not only through conveying the importance and urgency of infection diagnosis, but also by being vigilant to the early warning signs and symptoms of periprosthetic infection. Indeed, early diagnosis of periprosthetic infection maximises the chance of prosthesis retention [50]. Future research could focus on patient preparedness for adverse outcomes after joint replacement, help-seeking in the event of periprosthetic infection, and clinician support in the early recognition of periprosthetic infection.

Acknowledgements
The authors would like to thank those patients who gave their time to be involved in this study and the study administration and management team: Simon Strange, Makita Werrett and Beverley Evanson for their support.

Funding
This paper presents independent research funded by the National Institute for Health Research Programme Grants for Applied Research (NIHR PGfAR) programme (grant number: RP-PG-1210-12005) and supported by the NIHR Comprehensive Clinical Research Network (CRN). This study was supported by the NIHR Biomedical Research Centre at the University Hospitals Bristol NHS Foundation Trust and the University of Bristol. The views expressed in this publication are those of the author(s) and not necessarily those of the NHS, the National Institute for Health Research or the Department of Health.

Authors' contributions
RGH and AJM were involved in the conception and design of the study. CM conducted the interviews. All authors contributed to the analysis and interpretation of data. CM and AM drafted the article and all authors revised it critically for important intellectual content. All authors gave final approval of the version to be published.

Competing interests
AJM and RG-H are members of the Editorial Board of BMC Musculoskeletal Disorders.

Author details
Bristol Medical School, University of Bristol, Bristol, UK. [2]National Institute for Health Research Bristol Biomedical Research Centre, University of Bristol, Bristol, UK.

References
1. Cram P, Lu X, Kates SL, Singh JA, Li Y, Wolf BR. Total knee arthroplasty volume, utilization, and outcomes among Medicare beneficiaries, 1991-2010. JAMA. 2012;308:1227–36.
2. National Joint Registry Reports. National Joint Registry for England, Wales and Northern Ireland, 13th annual report. 2016. http://www.njrcentre.org.uk/njrcentre/Reports,PublicationsandMinutes/Annualreports/tabid/86/Default.aspx. Accessed 25 Jan 2016.
3. Dieppe P, Basler HD, Chard J, Croft P, Dixon J, Hurley M, et al. Knee replacement surgery for osteoarthritis: effectiveness, practice variations, indications and possible determinants of utilization. Rheumatology. 1999;38:73–83.
4. Beswick A, Wylde V, Gooberman-Hill RJS, Blom AW, Dieppe P. What proportion of patients report long-term pain after total hip or knee replacement for osteoarthritis? A systematic review of prospective studies in unselected patients. BMJ. 2012. https://doi.org/10.1136/bmjopen-2011-000435.
5. Whitehouse MR, Mehendale S. Periprosthetic fractures around the knee: current concepts and advances in management. Curr Rev Musculoskelet Med. 2014;7:136–44.
6. Blom AW, Brown J, Taylor AH, Pattison G, Whitehouse S, Bannister GC. Infection after total knee arthroplasty. Bone & Joint J. 2004;86:688–91.

7. Bozic KJ, Kurtz SM, Lau E, et al. The epidemiology of revision total knee arthroplasty in the United States. Clin Orthop Relat Res. 2010;468:45–51.
8. Kurtz SM, Ong KL, Lau E, Bozic KJ, Berry D, Parvizi J. Prosthetic joint infection risk after TKA in the Medicare population. Clin Orthop Relat Res. 2010;468:52–6.
9. Poss R, Thornhill TS, Ewald FC, Thomas WH, Batte NJ, Sledge CB. Factors influencing the incidence and outcome of infection following total joint arthroplasty. Clin Orth Rel Res. 1983;182:117–26.
10. Nazarian DG, de Jesus D, McGuigan F, Booth RE., Jr a two-stage approach to primary knee arthroplasty in the infected arthritic knee. J Arthroplast 2003;7 Suppl 1:16–21.
11. Kapadia BH. Periprosthetic joint infection. Lancet. 2016;387:386–94.
12. Kapadia BH, McElroy MJ, Issa K, Johnson AJ, Bozic KJ, Mont MA. The economic impact of periprosthetic infections following total knee arthroplasty at a specialized tertiary-care center. J Arthroplast. 2014;29:929–32.
13. Kallala RF, Vanhegan IS, Ibrahim MS, Sarmah S, Haddad FS. Financial analysis of revision knee surgery based on NHS tariffs and hospital costs: does it pay to provide a revision service? Bone Joint J. 2015; https://doi.org/10.1302/0301-620X.97B2.33707.
14. Parkinson RW, Kay PR, Rawal A. A case for one-stage revision in infected total knee arthroplasty? Knee. 2011;18:1–4.
15. Kunutsor SK, Whitehouse MR, Lenguerrand E, Blom AW, Beswick AD, INFORM Team. Re-infection outcomes following one and two-stage surgical revision of infected knee prosthesis: a systematic review and meta-analysis. PLoS One. 2016. https://doi.org/10.1371/journal.pone.0151537.
16. Cahill JL, Shadbolt B, Scarvell JM, Smith PN. Quality of life after infection in total joint replacement. J Orthop Surg. 2008;16:58–65.
17. Kunutsor SK, Beswick AD, Peters TJ, Gooberman-Hill R, Whitehouse MR, Blom AW, et al. Health care needs and support for patients undergoing treatment for prosthetic joint infection following hip or knee arthroplasty: a systematic review. PLoS One. 2017;12. https://doi.org/10.1371/journal.pone.0169068.
18. Moore AJ, Blom AW, Whitehouse MR & Gooberman-Hill R. Deep prosthetic joint infection: A qualitative study of the impact on patients and their experiences of revision surgery. BMJ Open. 2015; https://doi.org/10.1136/bmjopen-2015-009495.
19. Bury M. Chronic illness as biographical disruption. Sociol Health Illn. 1982;4:167–82.
20. Williams S. Chronic illness as biographical disruption or biographical disruption as chronic illness? Reflections on a core concept. Sociol Health Illn. 2000;22:40–67.
21. Bury M. The sociology of chronic illness: a review of research and prospects. Sociol Health Illn. 1991;13:451–68.
22. Charmaz K. Loss of self: a fundamental form of suffering in the chronically ill. Sociol Health Illn. 1983;5:168–95.
23. Morden A, Jinks C, Ong BN. Temporally divergent significant meanings, biographical disruption and self-management for chronic joint pain. Health (London). 2015;21:357–74.
24. Sanders C, Donovan J, Dieppe P. The significance and consequences of having painful and disabled joints in older age: co-existing accounts of normal and disrupted biographies. Sociol Health Illn. 2002;24:227–53.
25. Larsson AT, Grassman EJ. Bodily changes among people living with physical impairments and chronic illnesses: biographical disruption or normal illness? Sociol Health Illn. 2012;34:1156–69.
26. Bell SL, Tyrrell J, Phoenix C. Ménière's disease and biographical disruption: where family transitions collide. Soc Sci Med. 2016;166:177–85.
27. Leveälahti H, Tishelman C, Öhlén J. Framing the onset of lung cancer biographically: narratives of continuity and disruption. Psychoncology. 2007;16:466–73.
28. Hannum SM, Rubinstein RL. The meaningfulness of time; narratives of cancer among chronically ill older adults. J Aging Stud. 2016;36:17–25.
29. Bury M. Meaning at risk: the experience of arthritis. In: Anderson R, Bury M, editors. Living with chronic illness. The experience of patients and their families. London: Unwin Hyman; 1988. p. 89–116.
30. Glaser BG, Strauss AL. The discovery of grounded theory: strategies for qualitative research. Chicago: Aldine Pub. Co.; 1967.
31. Guest G, Bunce A, Johnson L. How many interviews are enough? : An experiment with data saturation and variability. Field Methods. 2006;18:59–82.
32. Gooberman-Hill R, Burston A, Clark E, Johnson E, Nolan S, Wells V et al. Involving patients in research: considering good practice. Musculoskeletal Care 2013; https://doi.org/10.1002/msc.1060.
33. National Research Council. In: Cooke NJ, Hilton ML, editors. Enhancing the effectiveness of team science. Washington, DC: The National Academies Press; 2015.
34. NVivo qualitative data analysis Software. QSR international Pty ltd. Version. 2012:10.
35. Ezzy D. Qualitative analysis. Practice and innovation. London: Routledge; 2002.
36. Barry CA, Britten N, Barber N, Bradley C, Stevenson F. Using reflexivity to optimize teamwork in qualitative research. Qual Health Res. 1999;9:26–44.
37. Strauss A, Glaser B. Chronic illness and the quality of life. St Louis: Mosby; 1975.
38. Andersson AE, Bergh I, Karlsson J, Nilsson K. Patients' experiences of acquiring a deep surgical site infection: an interview study. Am J Control. 2010;38:711–7.
39. Lempp H, Scott D, Kingsley G. The personal impact of rheumatoid arthritis on patients' identity: a qualitative study. Chronic Illn. 2006;2:109–20.
40. Sutanto B, Singh-Grewal D, McNeil HP, O'Neill S, Craig JC, Jones J, Tong A. Experiences and perspectives of adults living with systemic lupus erythematosus: thematic synthesis of qualitative studies. Arthritis Care Res. 2013;65:1752–65.
41. Dennison L, McCloy Smith E, Bradbury K, Galea I. How Do People with Multiple Sclerosis Experience Prognostic Uncertainty and Prognosis Communication? A Qualitative Study. PLoS One. 2016; https://doi.org/10.1371/journal.pone.0158982.
42. Burchardt M. "Life in brackets": biographical uncertainties of HIV-positive women in South Africa. Forum Qual Soc Res. 2010;11:1–18.
43. Davies ML. Shattered assumptions: time and the experience of long-term HIV positivity. Soc Sci Med. 1997;44:561–71.
44. Weitz R. Uncertainty and the lives of persons with AIDS. J Health Soc Behav. 1989;30:270–81.
45. Nanton V, Munday D, Dale J, Mason B, Kendall M, Murray S. The threatened self: considerations of time, place, and uncertainty in advanced illness. Br J Health Psychol. 2016;21:351–73.
46. Ciambrone D. Illness and other assaults on self: the relative impact of HIV/AIDS on women's lives. Sociol Health Illn. 2001;23:517–40.
47. Reeve J, Lloyd-Williams M, Payne S, Dowrick C. Revisiting biographical disruption: exploring individual embodied illness experience in people with terminal cancer. Health (London). 2010;14:178–95.
48. Navon L, Morag A. Liminality as biographical disruption: unclassifiability following hormonal therapy for advanced prostate cancer. Soc Sci Med. 2004;58:2337–47.
49. Mishel M. Uncertainty in Illness. J Nurs Schol. 1988;20:225–32.
50. Schoifet SD, Morrey BF. Treatment of infection after total knee arthroplasty by debridement with retention of the components. J Bone Joint Surg Am. 1990;72:1383–90.

18

Surface damage of bovine articular cartilage-off-bone: the effect of variations in underlying substrate and frequency

Humaira Mahmood[*] [ID], Duncan E. T. Shepherd and Daniel M. Espino

Abstract

Background: Changes in bone mineral density have been implicated with the onset of osteoarthritis, but its role in inducing failure of articular cartilage mechanically is unclear. This study aimed to determine the effect of substrate density, as the underlying bone, on the surface damage of cartilage-off-bone, at frequencies associated with gait, and above.

Methods: Bovine articular cartilage samples were tested off-bone to assess induced damage with an indenter under a compressive sinusoidal load range of 5–50 N at frequencies of 1, 10 and 50 Hz, corresponding to normal and above normal gait respectively, for up to 10,000 cycles. Cartilage samples were tested on four underlying substrates with densities of 0.1556, 0.3222, 0.5667 and 0.6000 g/cm^3. India ink was applied to identify damage as cracks, measured across their length using ImageJ software. Linear regression was performed to identify if statistical significance existed between substrate density, and surface damage of articular cartilage-off-bone, at all three frequencies investigated ($p < 0.05$).

Results: Surface damage significantly increased ($p < 0.05$) with substrate density at 10 Hz of applied frequency. Crack length at this frequency reached the maximum of 10.95 ± 9.12 mm (mean ± standard deviation), across all four substrates tested. Frequencies applied at 1 and 50 Hz failed to show a significant increase ($p > 0.05$) in surface damage with an increase in substrate density, at which the maximum mean crack length were 3.01 ± 3.41 mm and 5.65 ± 6.54 mm, respectively. Crack formation at all frequencies tended to form at the periphery of the cartilage specimen, with multiple straight-line cracking observed at 10 Hz, in comparison to single straight-line configurations produced at 1 and 50 Hz.

Conclusions: The effect of substrate density on the surface damage of articular cartilage-off-bone is multi-factorial, with an above-normal gait frequency. At 1 Hz cartilage damage is not associated with substrate density, however at 10 Hz, it is. This study has implications on the effects of the factors that contribute to the onset of osteoarthritis.

Keywords: Articular cartilage, Bone mineral density, Damage, Frequency, Mechanical loading, Osteoarthritis

Background

The principal function of articular cartilage is to allow for ease in the kinetics of two connecting ends of the bones in contact [1, 2]. Cartilage prevents high stress concentrations which would be expected to occur through bone to bone contact and provides low friction articulation, aided by a surface roughness of 80–170 nm [3]. Osteoarthritis (OA) involves articular cartilage deficit and is progressive, such that joint motion becomes more painful with time [4]. Globally, OA is reported as the highest occurring joint health condition [5]. Alterations in the underlying bone are key to diagnosing OA, illustrated by the concept of an enhanced subchondral bone stiffness being associated with advances in cartilage impairment [6]. However, the link between destruction of cartilage and changes in subchondral bone are less clear, focusing on associating the relationship between a high bone mineral density (BMD) and cartilage degradation [7, 8]. This relationship

* Correspondence: HXM624@student.bham.ac.uk
Department of Mechanical Engineering, University of Birmingham, B15 2TT, Birmingham, UK

is further associated by the development of radiographic knee OA [9], and with increased cartilage volume [10] and cartilage thickness [11] during the early stages of OA.

The mechanical behaviour of articular cartilage appears to differ when off-bone and on-bone. For example, off-bone articular cartilage is more capable of dissipating energy than on-bone articular cartilage [12, 13], with the restrictive behaviour of the underlying bone constraining articular cartilage [12–14]. However, there may be a direct effect by the underlying bone on the mechanical characteristics of the overlying articular cartilage [15]. This has been recently shown by the correlation between BMD and the loss modulus of articular cartilage [16]. Further, the correlation between the effective cartilage tangent modulus and the Young's modulus of its underlying substrate, such that damage to cartilage via impact loading has occurred at a decline in effective cartilage and substrate modulus, representing cartilage damage at a lowered BMD [17].

Damage experienced by articular cartilage has been linked to the mechanism of loading, such as the effects of loading rates [13, 18], impact loading [17, 19], and frequency independent of load [2, 20, 21]. Further, the effects of hydration [22] as well as rapid heel-strike [2, 13, 20, 21] have also been associated with cartilage damage. However, it is unknown whether there is a direct mechanical link of a variation in frequency, between the damage experienced by articular cartilage and the density of its underlying subchondral bone.

Therefore, the aim of this current investigation was to assess, experimentally, whether substrate density affects the surface damage of bovine articular cartilage-off-bone, with a variation in applied frequency associated with normal gait; 1 Hz, and above normal gait; 10 and 50 Hz [2, 23, 24]. Surface damage was evaluated as total crack length, identified with the application of India ink, following on from comparison to the cartilage-off-bone specimen photographed prior to testing, for clear damage detection.

Methods
Preparation of specimens
Twelve bovine humeral heads were obtained from a supplier (Dissect Supplies, Kings Heath, Birmingham, UK) from animals of maximum 30 months old at slaughter. Bovine articular cartilage was selected based on the previously established relationship of the frequency-dependent viscoelastic properties, consistent with that of human articular cartilage [25]. The humeral heads were covered in tissue paper, coated with Ringer's solution prepared to a full strength mass concentration by dissolving 4.83 g of Ringer's tablets (Oxoid Ltd., Hampshire, UK), per 500 ml of distilled water, and separately stored in double

heat-sealed plastic at − 40 °C [13, 23]. Bovine humeral heads were thawed at room temperature for testing preparation [25]. The freeze-thaw process does not affect the mechanical properties of articular cartilage [26]. India ink (Daler-Rowney, Bracknell, UK) was used to ensure that humeral head cartilage surfaces were free from lesions ahead of testing [13, 21, 27]. For this procedure, the entire humeral head surface was covered with India ink so that on removal (rinsing) any defects could be identified; a commonly employed technique [13, 21, 27]. This allowed the coring procedure to take place at intact regions only. Further, on harvesting of each cartilage core, India ink was applied to each specimen, rinsed off, and an image captured for comparing damage post-testing. A representative image of a specimen captured before testing (but following application/removal of India ink) is displayed in Fig. 1.

Cartilage-off-bone specimens
To prepare off-bone cartilage cores, a hand cork-borer with an *on face* diameter of 10.5 mm was used to create circular dents on the surface of the articular cartilage, and through to the underlying bone. Following on from confirmation with the use of India ink of undamaged regions for coring, caution was taken during the harvesting process to attain undamaged cartilage specimens. Further, the absence of damage was confirmed via

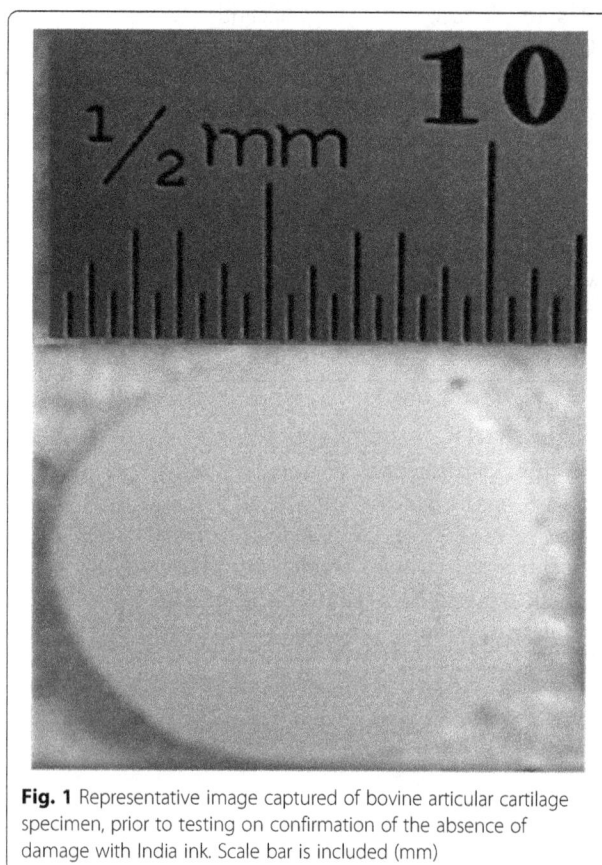

Fig. 1 Representative image captured of bovine articular cartilage specimen, prior to testing on confirmation of the absence of damage with India ink. Scale bar is included (mm)

observation following the use of India ink post-harvesting. The locations selected were identical for all specimens, namely at the central region, ensuring the cartilage surface was complete and undamaged [25]. A surgical scalpel with blade size 10A (Swann-Morton, Sheffield, UK) was used to isolate the cartilage core from the underlying subchondral bone [12, 13, 17, 25, 28]. On harvesting of the cartilage cores from the underlying bone, they were immediately immersed in Ringer's solution to prevent dehydration. Furthermore, the specimens were extracted on the day of testing; curling was not observed on any tissue harvested. To measure thickness, the cartilage core was held with a Vernier calliper at its centre; care was taken to avoid compression of the cartilage specimen. The thickness of the cartilage specimens measured prior to testing was 0.99 ± 0.004 mm (mean ± standard deviation), and the diameter was 10.9 ± 0.210 mm, as measured using a Vernier calliper (Draper Tools Ltd., Hampshire, UK). Six off-bone bovine articular cartilage cores were removed from each of twelve humeral heads, resulting in 72 individual specimens of off-bone cartilage. The specimens were immersed in Ringer's solution for 30 min [29] prior to testing [25].

Substrate design and mechanical loading

Specimens were positioned on the substrate blocks (Sawbones, Washington, USA) for testing. Four Sawbone densities were tested, which were 0.1556, 0.3222, 0.5667 and 0.6000 g/cm^3. The substrate with the lowest density, substrate one, was used as an osteoporotic representation of bone [30, 31] whereas the highest density, substrate four, was closer to that of cancellous bone [32]. The Sawbone was prepared with a vertical bandsaw (Startrite Volant 24, UK) into blocks with dimensions 30 mm × 30 mm × 10 mm. The Young's modulus of each substrate was obtained from compression tests using a Bose Electroforce 3300 testing machine run using Bose WinTest software (Bose Corporation, ElectroForce Systems Group, Minnesota, USA; updated to: TA Instruments, New Castle, DE, USA), derived from the slope of the stress-strain curve calculated from the force-displacement plot, at 0.02 mm/s with compression from a metal plate, 81 mm in diameter onto the substrate block (Table 1).

A square aluminium test rig was designed with dimensions 41 mm × 41 mm × 16 mm into which the Sawbone substrate was placed. A stainless-steel flat circular faced indenter, with a 0.5 mm bevelled edge to avoid stress concentration at its edges, 5.2 mm in diameter [2] was fixed to the actuator of the testing machine and used to induce damage through indentation to the surface of the cartilage-off-bone specimen. This procedure was similar to a previous study for on-bone cartilage [2]. A Bose ElectroForce 3200 testing machine controlled via the Bose WinTest 4.1 software (Bose Corporation, ElectroForce Systems Group, Minnesota, USA; updated to: TA Instruments, New Castle, DE, USA) was used for testing. The stainless-steel indenter was descended onto the cartilage specimen at the point of testing (Fig. 2).

Six cartilage specimens were tested per substrate, at a given frequency. The cartilage specimens were manually positioned on the underlying substrate, without the use of adhesive treatment prior to testing. Specimens were not observed to move during testing. This placement replicates the effect of the soft-on-hard construct but may not replicate the restriction of collagen at the cartilage calcified zone, due to the removal of the underlying bone [12]. A sinusoidally varying force under unconfined compression between 5 and 50 N was applied to the specimens for 10,000 cycles [2]. Repeated loading has previously been found to induce disruption to the articular cartilage surface [1, 2, 33]. Frequencies of 1, 10 and 50 Hz were applied to the specimens, for a completion of 72 individual tests. At 5000 cycles, the halfway point during testing, the articular cartilage-off-bone specimens were irrigated with Ringer's solution [20, 21], to ensure hydration of the cartilage. Further, recent work has also confirmed the absence of a significant difference on the dynamic viscoelastic behaviour of articular cartilage, when tested for short periods in either air or Ringer's solution [13].

Quantification of changes to the cartilage surface

Pictures were taken of each specimen before and after testing for clear observation of the damage induced after testing. India ink was used to identify alterations to the cartilage-off-bone specimen following testing, in addition to the sample prior to testing for damage

Table 1 Material properties of the four underlying substrates utilised to represent varied bone mineral densities positioned beneath each cartilage-off-bone core during testing, allowing for investigation of the effect of substrate density on the damage to articular cartilage

Substrate	Density (g/cm^3)	Mass (g)	Young's Modulus (E) (MPa)	Volume (cm^3)	Poisson's ratio
1	0.1556	1.4	435	9	0.30
2	0.3222	2.9	810	9	0.30
3	0.5667	5.1	1238	9	0.30
4	0.6000	5.4	2861	9	0.30

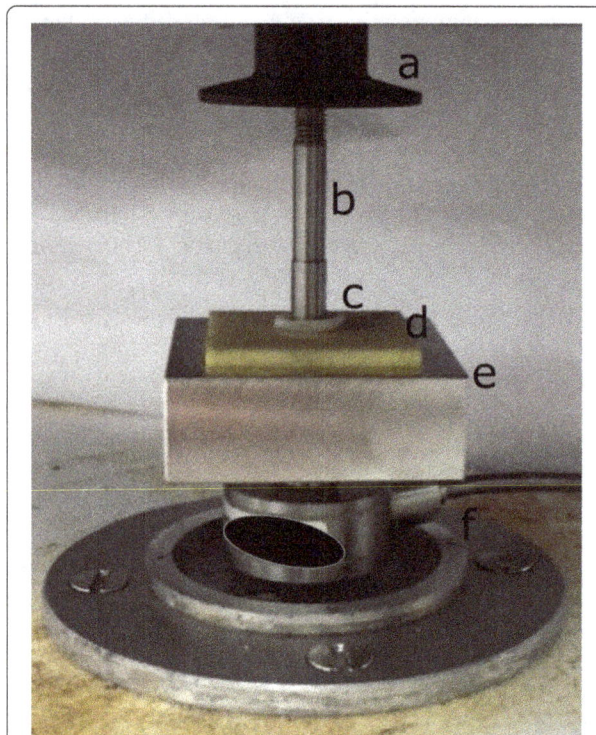

Fig. 2 Example set-up at actuator (**a**) for mechanical testing with stainless-steel indenter (**b**) at off-bone cartilage specimen (**c**) and lowest density underlying substrate (**d**), within customised test rig (**e**). Cartilage off-bone specimen is positioned above the substrate. Stainless-steel indenter is lowered onto the cartilage-off-bone specimen for testing, movement operated with testing machine. Load cell component (**f**) for experimental load control

absence confirmation [2, 27, 33]. For evaluation of the damage present, ImageJ software (version 1.48, Rasband, W.S., U.S. National Institutes of Health, Bethesda, Maryland, USA) was used with calibration of the image via a scale bar. The area of indentation (mm^2) and crack length (mm) were analysed as two separate conditions for each specimen. Image measurements were repeated twice per sample and the mean value reported. Firstly, the area indented following testing with the indenter was highlighted (i.e. a non-damaged measurement), with use of the free-hand tool on the ImageJ software. Secondly, the length of cracks was measured using an existing method, and this was considered as a damage measurement [2].

Data analysis

Sigmaplot Version 12.0 (Systat Software Inc., London, UK) was used to perform regression analysis on the relationship between the four substrates of varying densities and the following parameters: the area of indentation; crack length; damage, at all frequencies tested; 1, 10 and 50 Hz. A linear regression fit was assessed as the most appropriate representation of the empirical relationships derived ($p < 0.05$).

Results

Surface assessment

Representative images of cartilage specimens after testing are shown for 1, 10 and 50 Hz, in Fig. 3, Fig. 4 and Fig. 5, respectively, at all four substrates investigated. The damage observed as crack formation is clearly indicated with a black outlined ellipse. Figure. 6 and Fig. 7 display the relationship between substrate density and the mean crack length and mean indented area, respectively, at all three frequencies investigated.

Crack length was significantly correlated to substrate density at 10 Hz ($p < 0.05$) (Fig. 6, Table 2), however, it was not significantly associated with substrate density at 1 or 50 Hz ($p > 0.05$) (Fig. 6, Table 2). The combined variables of frequency at 10 Hz with substrate density led to an increase in crack length with density ($p < 0.05$) (Fig. 6, Table 2). This relationship between the effects of frequency and substrate density, on the crack length of off-bone articular cartilage is best described by a linear curve as represented by eq. (1):

$$c = D + AB \tag{1}$$

where c is the crack length mean total, A is the gradient of the slope, B is substrate density and D is the intercept; D and A are empirically derived constants. The associated details are summarised in Table 2, at all three frequencies tested.

Frequency of loading in combination with substrate density had no effect on the area of indentation when samples were tested at 1, 10 and 50 Hz ($p > 0.05$) (Fig. 7). The effect of frequency alone, on the area of indentation, however, did demonstrate a negative correlation between an increase in frequency from 1 to 50 Hz, and the indented area (Fig. 7). The post-test recovery following the testing of the cartilage specimens varied for each frequency. Testing at 1 Hz of frequency resulted in the least recovery of the articular cartilage specimen; with a larger indented area observed. This is represented by the observations where the indented area, as clearly highlighted by the black circular staining of India ink, extended to the majority of the cartilage specimen surface at 1 Hz (Fig. 3), in comparison to the lesser surface indented at 10 (Fig. 4) and 50 Hz (Fig. 5).

Sample images displayed at 1 Hz (Fig. 3) illustrate cracks that were of a single-line configuration, notably through the specimen periphery, parallel to the specimen circumference, observed at a maximum mean of 3.01 mm (Fig. 6; Table 3). As the applied frequency at testing increased to 10 Hz, mean crack length at this frequency increased to its maximum by 7.94 mm (Fig. 6; Table 3).

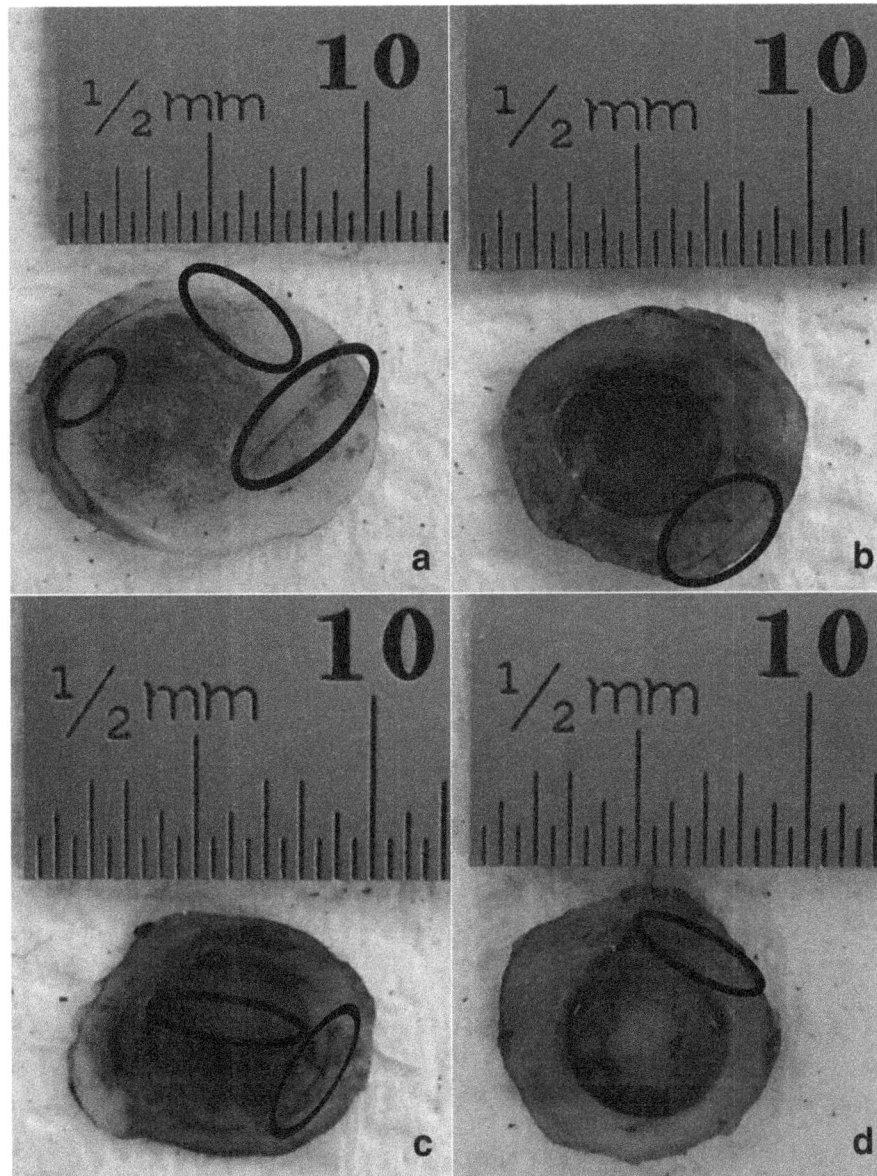

Fig. 3 Representative images of bovine articular cartilage-off-bone samples after testing, at 1 Hz frequency of loading. Image **a-d** display a sample result at substrates 1–4, respectively. Damage as cracks and indentation were identified with application of India ink. Cracks formed are highlighted with the black ellipse for clear observation. Indentation can be observed across most of the cartilage-off-bone specimen surface, at this frequency of loading. Scale bar (mm) included for quantifying results

Representative images of 10 Hz in applied frequency at each substrate (Fig. 4), illustrate crack formation predominantly observed as multiple parallel straight-line arrangements, of various lengths, similar to previous studies [1, 2], commonly observed at the periphery of the cartilage specimen. At 50 Hz, the maximum mean crack length reduced by 5.30 mm from 10 Hz (Fig. 6; Table 3), where crack formation was primarily located across the diameter of the sample of single-line conformations, of various lengths, parallel to the specimen circumference (Fig. 5).

Discussion

In this study the measured surface damage experienced by articular cartilage was independent of substrate density, as a single variable. Increased damage due to greater energy absorption is expected with a stiffer substrate, however, this was not observed statistically, for substrate density alone, using our experimental protocol (with articular cartilage off-bone). Instead, it was demonstrated that a combined effect of substrate density, and a specific loading frequency of 10 Hz, led to an increase in surface damage (total crack length) in the cartilage.

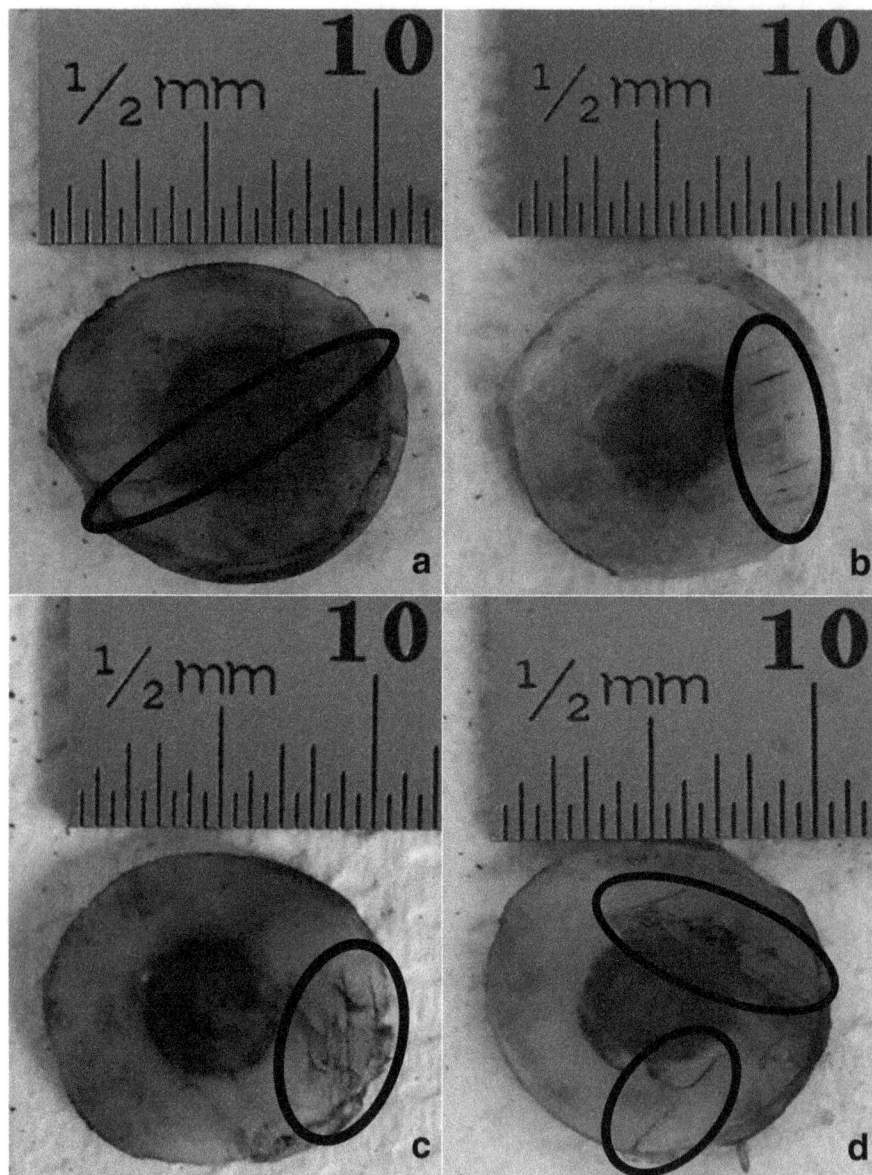

Fig. 4 Representative images of bovine articular cartilage-off-bone samples after testing, at 10 Hz frequency of loading. Image **a-d** display a sample result at substrates 1–4, respectively. Damage as cracks and indentation were identified with application of India ink. Cracks formed are highlighted with the black ellipse for clear observation, notably of multiple parallel straight-lines. Scale bar (mm) included for quantifying results

Thus, it is suggested that the combination of BMD and above normal gait frequencies (e.g. 10 Hz), predisposes articular cartilage to damage.

It is worth highlighting the importance of the particular application of 10 Hz in frequency. Within the region of, and beyond, 10 Hz, it is thought that cartilage enters a glass transition phase [21]. Therefore, a change in cartilage material properties is noticed from behaving as a deformable ('soft') material to one which is hard but brittle [24]. Due to this alteration in the physical behaviour of articular cartilage, it may affect the extent of damage. This is supported by the results shown in this study, as maximum cartilage damage is observed at 10 Hz, in comparison to 1 and 50 Hz. The reduction in damage observed above the application of 10 Hz, such as 50 Hz as in this study, could be due to the recently established relationship such that the loss stiffness of off-bone articular cartilage is dependent upon frequency [13]. Thus, articular cartilage may be better able to disspiate energy at 50 Hz which might explain why, off-bone, the extent of damage to the tissue is reduced as compared to 10 Hz of loading.

The multi-factorial finding from this study that an increase in substrate density combined with 10 Hz

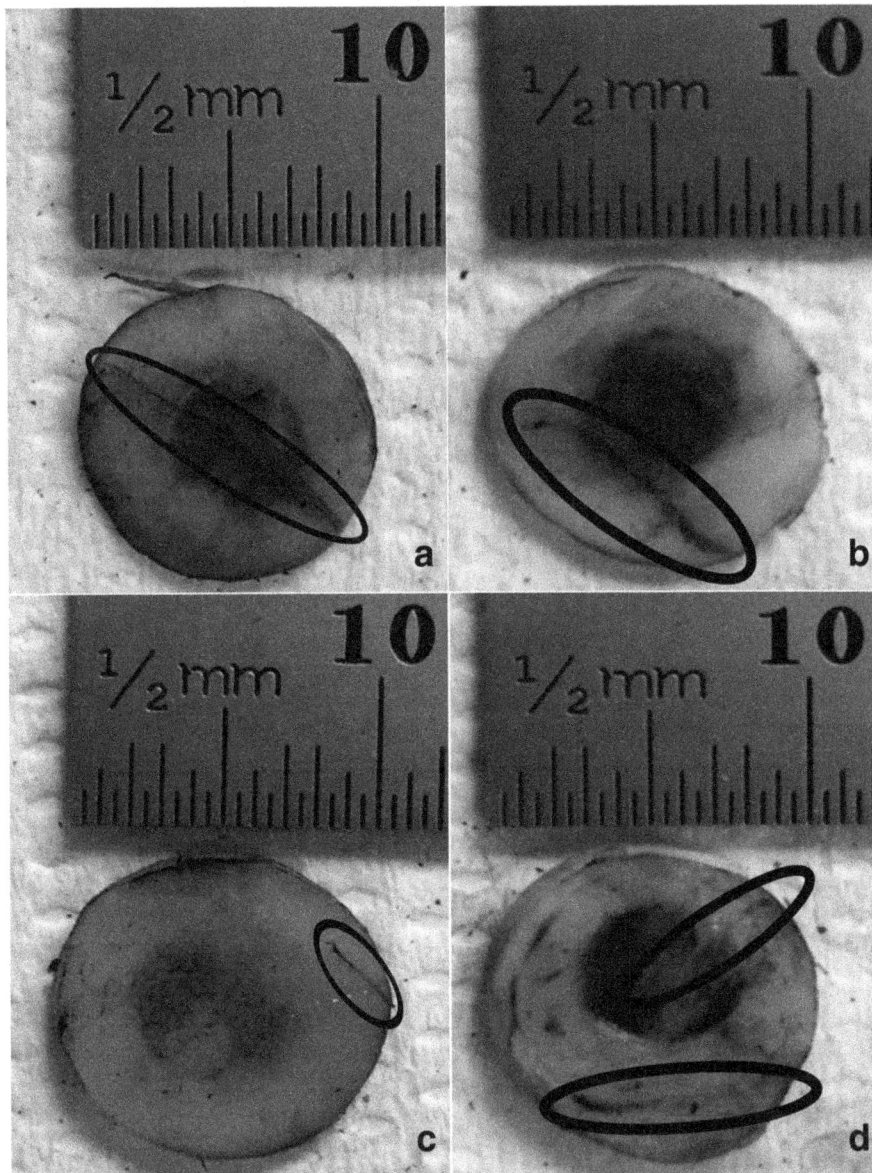

Fig. 5 Representative images of bovine articular cartilage-off-bone samples after testing, at 50 Hz frequency of loading. Image **a-d** display a sample result at substrates 1–4, respectively. Damage as cracks and indentation were identified with application of India ink. Cracks formed are highlighted with the black ellipse for clear observation, notably of single-line configurations of varying lengths. Scale bar (mm) included for quantifying results

increases surface damage, corresponds to the advancement in damage of cartilage during OA which may progressively worsen during a remodelling process [6]. Further, damage of cartilage during OA may relate to the remodelling process directly, rather than purely due to alterations in the stress distribution between cartilage and its underlying subchondral bone following a change in bone density. Bone remodelling is defined by the hypothesised relationship between impulse loading of the bone at the joint experiencing fracture to result in a stiffened base for the cartilage, therefore, exposing the cartilage to greater stress and enhancing its rate of damage development [6]. The process of remodelling weakens cartilage [34], so that per load it would degrade with the influence of an above normal gait frequency, independent of the effect of a high BMD alone to induce cartilage damage at 10 Hz. Therefore, in the case where an individual experiences the combined effect of an above gait-heel strike with a high BMD, this collective relationship per load may enforce the process of bone remodelling to mechanically become self-propagating as regards damage. It is also worth noting there are

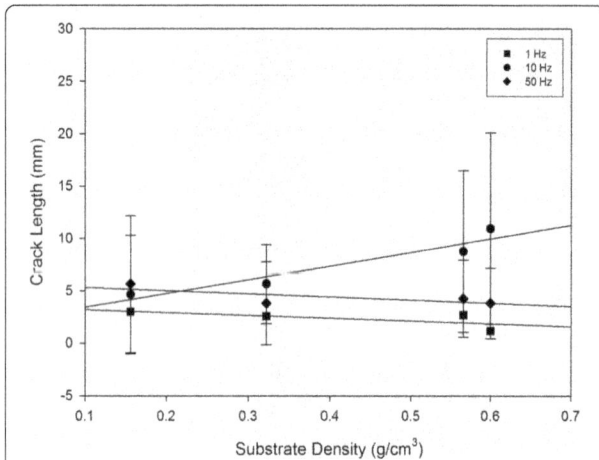

Fig. 6 Mean crack length plotted with substrate density at 1, 10 and 50 Hz for off-bone articular cartilage, represented by the square, circle and diamond, respectively. Linear regression displayed by eq. (1) fit the data at R^2 values of 0.485, 0.909 and 0.524 at 1, 10 and 50 Hz, respectively. Error bars represent standard deviations

Table 2 Statistical details derived from mean crack length and substrate density plots of Fig. 6, at frequencies 1, 10 and 50 Hz. A and D are the constants from the curve fits. R^2, the squared correlation coefficient indicates the extent of the data and regression line fit. A *P*-value less than 0.05 confirms statistically significant data, as displayed at 10 Hz of loading frequency

Frequency (Hz)	Total crack length linear fit details			
	A	D	R^2	*P*
1	(−)2.652	3.454	0.485	0.304
10	(+)13.077	2.124	0.909	0.047
50	(−)2.999	5.612	0.524	0.276

density, the data shows mean crack length of off-bone articular cartilage increased from 1 to 10 Hz. These findings are consistent with a previous study for on-bone articular cartilage, with an increase in frequency [2, 20, 21]. However, in our current study for off-bone cartilage there was no increase in damage when loading at 50 Hz, unlike for the on-bone study of loading [2, 20, 21]. Thus, it is worth noting the differences in the behaviour of cartilage on- and off-bone, as a result of the presence or absence, respectively, of the restraining effect provided by the underlying bone [12]. This may be due to the loss stiffness being frequency-dependent for off-bone articular cartilage [13], but not for on-bone cartilage [24]. Therefore, off-bone articular cartilage is more able to dissipate energy potentially preventing damage to the cartilage itself (i.e. via dissipating the energy through the formation of cracks); this ability to dissipate energy is greater at higher frequencies, particularly at 50 Hz, potentially reducing the extent to which cartilage undergoes damage at 50 Hz (which may not happen when cartilage is on-bone).

At 1 Hz, previous work demonstrates mean total crack length close to 1 mm at the highest tested load of 160 N for on-bone cartilage [2]. At 1 Hz in this study, for off-bone cartilage, with the peak tested load at 50 N, results show a maximum mean crack length at 3.01 mm. At 10 Hz, previous work determines a mean crack length close to 2.4 mm for on-bone cartilage at the maximum load [2], whilst this study has observed a maximum mean crack length at 10.95 mm. It is expected, however, that on-bone cartilage experiences greater

additional factors that relate to the development and progression of OA, including obesity [35, 36], the suggested effect of leptins on chondrocyte behaviour [37] and the role of leptins in Matrix metalloproteinases degrading collagen within the extracellular matrix [38, 39].

The peak stress induced in this study was 2.88 MPa, greater than the stress at approximately 1–1.7 MPa within the knee and hip while walking [40], thus, encouraging damage. Damage was induced on the surface of the articular cartilage at 1, 10 and 50 Hz, corresponding to frequencies associated with gait and above, consistent with previous studies [2, 20, 21]. With particular attention to the effects of frequency, excluding substrate

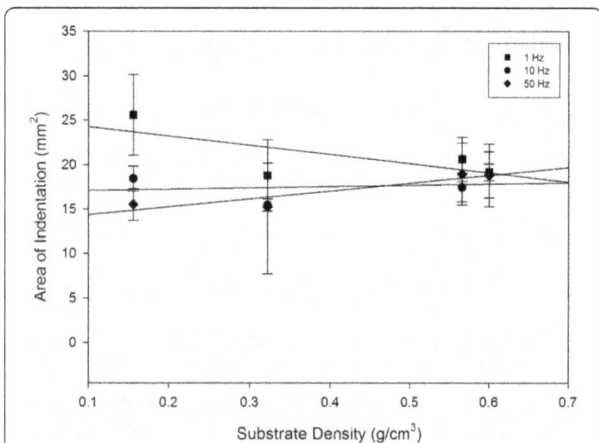

Fig. 7 Mean area of indentation plotted with substrate density at 1, 10 and 50 Hz for off-bone articular cartilage, represented by the square, circle and diamond, respectively. Linear regression displayed by eq. (1) fit the data at R^2 values of 0.487, 0.0386 and 0.851 at 1, 10 and 50 Hz, respectively. Error bars represent standard deviations

Table 3 Mean total crack length values with standard deviation for cartilage-off-bone samples, following testing, at all frequencies and substrates investigated, as a combined study

Frequency (Hz)	Mean total crack length (mm) ± SD			
	Substrate 1	Substrate 2	Substrate 3	Substrate 4
1	3.01 ± 3.41	2.57 ± 2.42	2.69 ± 2.66	1.19 ± 1.63
10	4.65 ± 5.66	5.65 ± 3.80	8.76 ± 7.70	10.95 ± 9.12
50	5.65 ± 6.54	3.80 ± 3.95	4.25 ± 3.68	3.82 ± 3.36

damage than off-bone cartilage; as previously hypothesised that the resulting energy may be released as cracks [13]. This is primarily as a result of the rationale of the presence of the underlying bone that provides constriction to the cartilage, increasing the induced stress [12–14]. This concept is further reinforced by the deep zone of articular cartilage restricted in its ability to deform laterally [41]. The ability of bone to dissipate more energy after an applied load than cartilage [42] is also in support of increased damage for on-bone cartilage.

Previous studies have identified the condition of "sclerotic subchondral bone" [43] at an increased BMD in volume associated with OA [44, 45]. Further, there is an established link of OA with a high BMD as reviewed [46] and extensively described elsewhere [7, 30, 47–56]. This study contributes to the outcome of these findings, such that it is not necessarily the change in BMD, alone that encourges cartilage damage, but that BMD interacts with other factors such as above normal-gait frequency. It is hypothesised that the remodelling process may account for further predisposition to damage [57].

The results indicate an increase in cartilage damage with substrate density, and therefore, the use of a softer substrate may redistribute stresses over a larger underlying area. Our study has modelled osteoarthritic to osteoporotic bone, using commercial grades of synthetic materials used to mimic bone as substrates, which has allowed assessment of cartilage failure across a range of substrate densities. This study is the first to illustrate the effects of the specific combination of BMD and an above-gait frequency, on cartilage damage, and therefore potentially to OA predisposition/progression. The resulting crack propagation through articular cartilage, may be worth investigating in future at 1 and 10 Hz.

Limitations

It is worth highlighting the potential limitation of testing off-bone cartilage, due to the absence of the restrictive attachment provided by the underlying subchondral bone that is found in the natural environment in-vivo [14]. The removal of the subchondral bone creates an alteration in the load transfer properties of the cartilage-off-bone specimen, notably the absence of the calcified cartilage layer with a stiffness in-between that of articular cartilage and the subchondral bone [15]. Despite this, however, the substrates used in this study have acted as the underlying bone of a controlled density, to allow for evaluation of the effects of the density of the underlying substrate alone, on associated cartilage damage.

While the results for off-bone cartilage failure in this study are larger than for on-bone data in the literature [2], there are limitations in directly comparing the on- and off-bone cartilage results from this study and the previous study [2]. Although identical joint locations i.e. the bovine humeral head have been assessed, load ranges applied during testing have differed, as well as specimen geometries [2]. In addition, in this study bovine articular cartilage cores have been removed from the adjacent regions of cartilage, therefore, weakening the cartilage due to the disruption of its extracellular matrix. The previous study [2], tested a select area of cartilage on a large joint sample with an undisrupted matrix [58]. However, the removal of the articular cartilage in this way was kept consistent throughout the investigation, thus specifically concerning the unknown relationship between underlying substrate density and cartilage, off-bone, at a varied frequency.

This study has used freeze-thaw cycles when preparing samples for testing. Although this process may have limitations, a recent study has concluded "multiple freeze-thaw cycles cannot be explicitly or statistically linked to mechanical changes within the cartilage" [59]. Previous studies have utilised bovine humeral heads [22], bovine knee joints [23], as well as bovine femoral heads [25]; each study referring to the absence of a freeze-thaw effect on the mechanical properties of cartilage [26]. Additionally, the storage of tissue at -40 °C is a previously established protocol utilised by several studies [20–25], and therefore was the approach taken for tissue storage in this study. Regardless, the results and conclusions obtained from this study on the effect of frequency and substrate on surface failure of cartilage are based upon a controlled testing protocol, and so findings are unlikely to be biased due to the freeze-thaw process used.

The use of an indentation test with articular cartilage is an established method previously developed to closely represent the physiological loading conditions of articular cartilage in vivo [60], as well as for damage inducing to the surface of articular cartilage [2]; having the advantage of being highly repeatable. Despite the hardness as well as the smaller diameter of the indenter in comparison to the cartilage specimen, a 0.5 mm radius bevelled edge was used to prevent artificial damage induced through stress concentrations at the edge. Further, the use of an indenter with a diameter smaller than the cartilage specimen, enables the deformation behaviour by the collagen matrix of the surrounding cartilage specimen [61] outside of the indentation area. Ultimately, this protocol has enabled a controlled evaluation of the effect of substrate density on cartilage failure.

Conclusions

The effect of substrate density on the surface damage of articular cartilage-off-bone is multi-factorial. The significant increases in cartilage damage with increased substrate density, additionally requires the application of loading at 10 Hz in frequency. Peak surface damage was observed at 10 Hz, detected as multiple parallel lines of varying lengths; in contrast to single straight-line profiles produced at 1 and 50 Hz. Thus, the effect of bone mineral density on the onset of osteoarthritis, should also be considered with additional damage inducing factors, including an above-normal gait of frequency at loading.

Abbreviations
BMD: Bone mineral density; OA: Osteoarthritis

Acknowledgements
The authors would like to thank Dr. Hamid Sadeghi for technical advice.

Funding
The equipment used in this project was funded by Arthritis Research UK (Grant Number: H0671).

Authors' contributions
HM carried out the experimental work, design of the study, data analysis and drafted the manuscript. DETS and DME participated in design of the study, data analysis and critically revising the manuscript. All authors have read and approved the final manuscript.

Competing interests
The authors declare that they have no competing interests.

References
1. Kerin AJ, Coleman A, Wisnom MR, Adams MA. Propagation of surface fissures in articular cartilage in response to cyclic loading in vitro. Clin Biomech. 2003. https://doi.org/10.1016/j.clinbiomech.2003.07.001.
2. Sadeghi H, Shepherd DET, Espino DM. Effect of the variation of loading frequency on surface failure of bovine articular cartilage. Osteoarthritis Cartilage. 2015. https://doi.org/10.1016/j.joca.2015.06.002.
3. Ghosh S, Bowen J, Jiang K, Espino DM, DET S. Investigation of techniques for the measurement of articular cartilage surface roughness. Micron. 2013. https://doi.org/10.1016/j.micron.2012.06.007.
4. Creamer P, Hochberg MC. Osteoarthritis. Lancet. 1997. https://doi.org/10.1016/S0140-6736(97)07226-7.
5. Philp AM, Davis ET, Jones SW. Developing anti-inflammatory therapeutics for patients with osteoarthritis. Rheumatology. 2017. https://doi.org/10.1093/rheumatology/kew278.
6. Radin EL, Paul IL, Rose RM. Role of Mechanical Factors in Pathogenesis of Primary Osteoarthritis. Lancet. 1972. https://doi.org/10.1016/S0140-6736(72)90179-1.
7. Dequeker J, Aerssens J, Luyten FP. Osteoarthritis and osteoporosis: Clinical and research evidence of inverse relationship. Aging Clin Exp Res. 2003. https://doi.org/10.1007/BF03327364.
8. Teichtahl AJ, Wang Y, Wluka AE, Strauss BJ, Proietto J, Dixon JB, Jones G, Cicuttini FM. Associations between systemic bone mineral density and early knee cartilage changes in middle-aged adults without clinical knee disease: a prospective cohort study. Arthritis Res Ther. 2017. https://doi.org/10.1186/s13075-017-1314-0.
9. Zhang Y, Hannan MT, Chaisson CE, McAlindon TE, Evans SR, Aliabadi P, Levy D, Felson DT. Bone mineral density and risk of incident and progressive radiographic knee osteoarthritis in women: the Framingham study. J Rheumatol. 2000;27:1032–7.
10. Brennan SL, Pasco JA, Cicuttini FM, Henry MJ, Kotowicz MA, Nicholson GC, Wluka AE. Bone mineral density is cross sectionally associated with cartilage volume in healthy, asymptomatic adult females: Geelong Osteoporosis Study. Bone. 2011. https://doi.org/10.1016/j.bone.2011.06.015.
11. Cao Y, Stannus OP, Aitken D, Cicuttini F, Antony B, Jones G, Ding C. Cross-sectional and longitudinal associations between systemic, subchondral bone mineral density and knee cartilage thickness in older adults with or without radiographic osteoarthritis. Ann Rheum Dis. 2014. https://doi.org/10.1136/annrheumdis-2013-203691.
12. Edelsten L, Jeffrey JE, Burgin LV, Aspden RM. Viscoelastic deformation of articular cartilage during impact loading. Soft Matter. 2010. https://doi.org/10.1039/c0sm00097c.
13. Lawless BM, Sadeghi H, Temple DK, Dhaliwal H, Espino DM, Hukins DWL. Viscoelasticity of articular cartilage: Analysing the effect of induced stress and the restraint of bone in a dynamic environment. J Mech Behav Biomed Mater. 2017. https://doi.org/10.1016/j.jmbbm.2017.07.040.
14. Aspden RM. Constraining the lateral dimensions of uniaxially loaded materials increases the calculated strength and stiffness: application to muscle and bone. J Mater Sci-Mater M. 1990. https://doi.org/10.1007/BF00839075.
15. Radin EL, Rose RM. Role of subchondral bone in the initiation and progression of cartilage damage. Clin Orthop Relat Res. 1986;213:34–40.
16. Fell NLA, Lawless BM, Cox SC, Cooke ME, Neil M, Espino DM. The role of subchondral bone and its histomorphology on the dynamic viscoelasticity of osteochondral tissues. 2017. unpublished results.
17. Burgin LV, Aspden RM. Impact testing to determine the mechanical properties of articular cartilage in isolation and on bone. J Mater Sci-Mater M. 2008. https://doi.org/10.1007/s10856-007-3187-2.
18. DET S, Seedhom BB. A technique for measuring the compressive modulus of articular cartilage under physiological loading rates with preliminary results. Proc IMechE Part H: J Engineering in Medicine. 1997. https://doi.org/10.1243/0954411971534278.
19. Jeffrey JE, Aspden RM. The biophysical effects of a single impact load on human and bovine articular cartilage. Proc IMechE Part H: J Engineering in Medicine. 2006. https://doi.org/10.1243/09544119JEIM31.
20. Sadeghi H, Espino DM, Shepherd DET. Fatigue strength of bovine articular cartilage-on-bone under three-point bending: the effect of loading frequency. BMC Musculoskelet Disord. 2017. https://doi.org/10.1186/s12891-017-1510-8.
21. Sadeghi H, Lawless BM, Espino DM, Shepherd DET. Effect of frequency on crack growth in articular cartilage. J Mech Behav Biomed Mater. 2017. https://doi.org/10.1016/j.jmbbm.2017.08.036.
22. Pearson B, Espino DM. Effect of hydration on the frequency-dependent viscoelastic properties of articular cartilage. Proc IMechE Part H: J Engineering in Medicine. 2013. https://doi.org/10.1177/0954411913501294.
23. Espino DM, Shepherd DET, Hukins DWL. Viscoelastic properties of bovine knee joint articular cartilage: dependency on thickness and loading frequency. BMC Musculoskelet Disord. 2014. https://doi.org/10.1186/1471-2474-15-205.
24. Fulcher GR, Hukins DWL, Shepherd DET. Viscoelastic properties of bovine articular cartilage attached to subchondral bone at high frequencies. BMC Musculoskelet Disord. 2009. https://doi.org/10.1186/1471-2474-10-61.
25. Temple DK, Cederlund AA, Lawless BM, Aspden RM, Espino DM. Viscoelastic properties of human and bovine articular cartilage: a comparison of frequency-dependent trends. BMC Musculoskelet Disord. 2016. https://doi.org/10.1186/s12891-016-1279-1.
26. Szarko M, Muldrew K, Bertram JEA. Freeze-thaw treatment effects on the dynamic mechanical properties of articular cartilage. BMC Musculoskelet Disord. 2010. https://doi.org/10.1186/1471-2474-11-231.
27. Meachim G. Light microscopy of Indian ink preparations of fibrillated cartilage. Ann Rheum Dis. 1972. https://doi.org/10.1136/ard.31.6.457.
28. Lewis RJ, MacFarland AK, Anandavijayan S, Aspden RM. Material properties and biosynthetic activity of articular cartilage from the bovine carpo-metacarpal joint. Osteoarthritis Cartilage. 1998. https://doi.org/10.1053/joca.1998.0142.
29. Barker MK, Seedhom BB. The relationship of the compressive modulus of articular cartilage with its deformation response to cyclic loading: does cartilage optimize its modulus so as to minimize the strains arising in it due to the prevalent loading regime? Rheumatology. 2001. https://doi.org/10.1093/rheumatology/40.3.274.
30. Li B, Aspden RM. Composition and mechanical properties of cancellous bone from the femoral head of patients with osteoporosis or osteoarthritis. J Bone Miner Res. 1997. https://doi.org/10.1359/jbmr.1997.12.4.641.
31. Patel PSD, Shepherd DET, Hukins DWL. Compressive properties of commercially available polyurethane foams as mechanical models for osteoporotic human cancellous bone. BMC Musculoskelet Disord. 2008. https://doi.org/10.1186/1471-2474-9-137.
32. Haba Y, Skripitz R, Lindner T, Kockerling M, Fritsche A, Mittelmeier W, Bader R. Bone mineral densities and mechanical properties of retrieved femoral bone samples in relation to bone mineral densities measured in the respective patients. TSWJ. 2012. https://doi.org/10.1100/2012/242403.

33. Weightman BO, Freeman MAR, Swanson SAV. Fatigue of articular cartilage. Nature. 1973. https://doi.org/10.1038/244303a0.

34. Radin EL, Paul IL, Tolkoff MJ. Subchondral bone changes in patients with early degenerative joint disease. Arthritis Rheumatol. 1970;13:400–5.

35. Bliddal H, Leeds AR, Christensen R. Osteoarthritis, obesity and weight loss: evidence, hypotheses and horizons - a scoping review. Obes Rev. 2014. https://doi.org/10.1111/obr.12173.

36. King LK, March L, Anandacoomarasamy A. Obesity & osteoarthritis. Indian J Med Res. 2013;138:185–93.

37. Dumond H, Presle N, Terlain B, Mainard D, Loeuille D, Netter P, Pottie P. Evidence for a key role of leptin in osteoarthritis. Arthritis Rheumatol. 2003. https://doi.org/10.1002/art.11303.

38. Aspden RM. Obesity punches above its weight in osteoarthritis. Nat Rev Rheumatol. 2011. https://doi.org/10.1038/nrrheum.2010.123.

39. Koskinen A, Vuolteenaho K, Nieminen R, Moilanen T, Moilanen E. Leptin enhances MMP-1, MMP-3 and MMP-13 production in human osteoarthritic cartilage and correlates with MMP-1 and MMP-3 in synovial fluid from OA patients. Clin Exp Rheumatol. 2011;29:57–64.

40. Yao JQ, Seedhom BB. Mechanical conditioning of articular cartilage to prevalent stresses. Br J Rheumatol. 1993;32:956–65.

41. Park S, Hung CT, Ateshian GA. Mechanical response of bovine articular cartilage under dynamic unconfined compression loading at physiological stress levels. Osteoarthritis Cartilage. 2004. https://doi.org/10.1016/j.joca.2003.08.005.

42. Malekipour F, Whitton C, Oetomo D, Lee PV. Shock absorbing ability of articular cartilage and subchondral bone under impact compression. J Mech Behav Biomed Mater. 2013. https://doi.org/10.1016/j.jmbbm.2013.05.005.

43. Li G, Yin J, Gao J, Cheng TS, Pavlos NJ, Zhang C, Zheng MH. Subchondral bone in osteoarthritis: insight into risk factors and microstructural changes. Arthritis Res Ther. 2013. https://doi.org/10.1186/ar4405.

44. McCrae F, Shouls J, Dieppe P, Watt I. Scintigraphic assessment of osteoarthritis of the knee joint. Ann Rheum Dis. 1992. https://doi.org/10.1136/ard.51.8.938.

45. Radin EL, Parker HG, Pugh JW, Steinberg RS, Paul IL, Rose RM. Response of joints to impact loading - III. Relationship between trabecular microfractures and cartilage degeneration. J Biomech. 1973. https://doi.org/10.1016/0021-9290(73)90037-7.

46. Hardcastle SA, Dieppe P, Gregson CL, Smith GD, Tobias JH. Osteoarthritis and bone mineral density: are strong bones bad for joints? Bonekey Rep. 2015. https://doi.org/10.1038/bonekey.2014.119.

47. Bergink AP, Uitterlinden AG, Van Leeuwen JPTM, Hofman A, Verhaar JAN, Pols HAP. Bone mineral density and vertebral fracture history are associated with incident and progressive radiographic knee osteoarthritis in elderly men and women: The Rotterdam Study. Bone. 2005. https://doi.org/10.1016/j.bone.2005.05.001.

48. Burger H, van Daele PLA, Odding E, Valkenburg HA, Hofman A, Grobbee DE, Schutte HE, Birkenhager JC, Pols HAP. Association of radiographically evident osteoarthritis with higher bone mineral density and increased bone loss with age. The Rotterdam Study. Arthritis Rheumatol. 1996. https://doi.org/10.1002/art.1780390111.

49. Dequeker J, Mbuyi-Muamba JM. Bone mineral density and bone turnover in spinal osteoarthritis. Ann Rheum Dis. 1996;55:331–4.

50. Foss MVL, Byers PD. Bone density, osteoarthrosis of the hip, and fracture of the upper end of the femur. Ann Rheum Dis. 1972;31:259–64.

51. Haugen IK, Slatkowsky-Christensen B, Orstavik R, Kvien TK. Bone mineral density in patients with hand osteoarthritis compared to population controls and patients with rheumatoid arthritis. Ann Rheum Dis. 2007. https://doi.org/10.1136/ard.2006.068940.

52. Hart DJ, Mootoosamy I, Doyle DV, Spector TD. The relationship between osteoarthritis and osteoporosis in the general population: the Chingford study. Ann Rheum Dis. 1994;53:158–62.

53. Lane NE, Nevitt MC. Osteoarthritis, bone mass and fractures: how are they related? Arthritis Rheumatol. 2002;46:1–4.

54. Nevitt MC, Lane NE, Scott JC, Hochberg MC, Pressman AR, Genant HK, Cummings SR. Radiographic osteoarthritis of the hip and bone mineral density. Arthritis Rheumatol. 1995;38:907–16.

55. Sowers MF, Lachance L, Jamadar D, Hochberg MC, Hollis B, Crutchfield M, Jannausch ML. The associations of bone mineral density and bone turnover markers with osteoarthritis of the hand and knee in pre-and perimenopausal women. Arthritis Rheumatol. 1999;42:483–9.

56. Sowers MF, Hochberg M, Crabbe JP, Muhich A, Crutchfield M, Updike S. Association of bone mineral density and sex hormone levels with osteoarthritis of the hand and knee in premenopausal women. Am J Epidemiol. 1996. https://doi.org/10.1093/oxfordjournals.aje.a008655.

57. Hunter DJ, Guermazi A, Roemer F, Zhang Y, Neogi T. Structural correlates of pain in joints with osteoarthritis. Osteoarthritis Cartilage. 2013. https://doi.org/10.1016/j.joca.2013.05.017.

58. Loeser RF, Goldring SR, Scanzello CR, Goldring MB. Osteoarthritis. A disease of the joint as an organ. Arthritis Rheumatol. 2012. https://doi.org/10.1002/art.34453.

59. Peters AE, Comerford EJ, Macaulay S, Bates KT, Akhtar R. Micromechanical properties of canine femoral articular cartilage following multiple freeze-thaw cycles. J Mech Behav Biomed Mater. 2017. https://doi.org/10.1016/j.jmbbm.2017.03.006.

60. Lu XL, Sun DDN, Guo XE, Chen FH, Lai WM, Mow VC. Indentation determined mechanoelectrochemical properties and fixed charge density of articular cartilage. Ann Biomed Eng. 2004;32:370–9.

61. Korhonen RK, Laasanen MS, Toyras J, Rieppo J, Hirvonen J, Helminen HJ, Jurvelin JS. Comparison of the equilibrium response of articular cartilage in unconfined compression, confined compression and indentation. J Biomech. 2002; doi.org/https://doi.org/10.1016/S0021-9290(02)00052-0.

19

Modified Robert Jones bandage can not reduce postoperative swelling in enhanced-recovery after primary total knee arthroplasty without intraoperative tourniquet

Haoda Yu[†], Haoyang Wang[†], Kai Zhou, Xiao Rong, Shunyu Yao, Fuxing Pei and Zongke Zhou[*]

Abstract

Background: Compression therapy is commonly used to reduce lower limb swelling and blood loss after knee surgery. This study was performed to investigate whether modified Robert Jones bandage (MRJB) as a postoperative compression therapy is necessary for enhanced-recovery primary total knee arthroplasty without the tourniquet application.

Methods: In this prospective randomized controlled trial, 90 patients were grouped into 2 groups randomly. The experimental group received compression therapy with MRJB from toes to thigh for 24 h and the control group received no compression therapy. Knee swelling, blood loss, range of motion (ROM), pain, patient reported comfort level and complications were recorded.

Results: No significant differences were observed between the two groups when we compared knee swelling. Similarly, no significant difference on postoperative blood loss, pain, ROM, complications was found. However, patients in control group had significantly higher comfort ratings than compression group during the first 24 h.

Conclusions: MRJB is not routinely indicated in enhanced-recovery primary total knee arthroplasty without tourniquet application.

Keywords: Total knee arthroplasty, Swelling, Modified Robert jones bandage, Compression

Background

Total knee arthroplasty (TKA) is a common and highly successful orthopedic operation to relieve pain and improve knee function in people with end-stage knee osteoarthritis [1]. However, TKA is associated with the high prevalence of postoperative knee swelling, which results in decreased knee-extension strength and impaired functional performance [2]. Knee swelling is due to intra-articular bleeding and peri-articular inflammation. Postoperative compression therapy with Modified Robert Jones bandage (MRJB) from toes to mid-thigh is commonly performed in patients who underwent arthroplasty with the hypothesis that it could reduce intra-articular bleeding by providing tamponade effect in the knee and reduce soft tissue edema by increasing intra-tissular pressure, aiding venous return in the lower limb [3, 4]. However, if the bandage is too tight, the excessive external pressure could lead to tissue ischemia by obliterating blood flow to subcutaneous tissue [5]. Compression-related complications including bruises, blisters, peroneal nerve palsy and discomforts

* Correspondence: zongkezhou@126.com
[†]Haoda Yu and Haoyang Wang contributed equally to this work.
Department of Orthopedics, West China Hospital, Sichuan University, Chengdu 610041, China

complaint from patients have been reported by various researchers [6–8].

Recently, the growing trend of quicker recovery following orthopedic procedures has stimulated the development of the techniques focused on reducing post-operative knee swelling. In addition to compression, various postoperative methods including surgery without intraoperative tourniquet use, administration of tranexamic acid (TXA) and corticosteroid medication have been reported to be effective to reduce hemarthrosis and soft tissue edema [9, 10], as this multi-modal swelling management could effectively reduce post-operative hidden blood loss and limit inflammation. However, few studies have adequately investigated and demonstrated the benefits of MRJB when applied together with this multi-modal swelling management, resulting in a knowledge gap and inability to determine if MRJB is still necessary for patients undergoing primary TKA in an enhanced recovery after surgery (ERAS) program. Therefore, we conducted this prospective randomized controlled trial (RCT) to evaluate the effect of using MRJB on knee swelling, blood loss, pain, complications and patient-reported knee function after TKA. We hypothesized that MRJB is not necessary when this multi-modal swelling management is utilized in enhanced-recovery after primary total knee arthroplasty.

Methods

Study design

This prospective, randomized controlled study was approved by the institutional review board of West China Hospital of Sichuan University (no. 201302009) and registered in the Chinese Clinical Trial Registry (ChiCTR-INR-16010177). All patients, aged 18 years or older, who were scheduled for a primary total knee arthroplasty for end-stage osteoarthritis were eligible for inclusion. Exclusion criteria included simultaneously bilateral total knee arthroplasty or revision case, surgical history of the knee joint, peripheral vascular disease, ankle brachial pressure index, ABPI< 0.8, peripheral neuropathy, blood coagulation disorders, history of deep venous thrombosis, BMI > 35, knee stiffness characterized as flexion deformity of ≥30°. Informed consent was obtained from all participants.

Treatment groups

Recruited patients were randomly allocated to either the MRJB or the conventional wound dressing group according to a computerized random sequence generator. After wound closure, sequentially numbered, sealed envelopes were opened in the operating room. In the MRJB group, the sterile adhesive wound dressing Cosmopor®E (Paul Hartmann AG, Heidenheim, Germany) was placed over the wound followed by a soft inner layer thick cotton padding Winner (Chengdu Wenjian Likang Medical Products Ltd., Sichuan, China) which was applied from toes to thigh. The outer layer was composed of elastic bandage Coban™ (3 M Deutschland GmbH, Neuss, Germany). To enhance venous return, more tension was applied distally than proximally (Fig. 1). The MRJB retained for 24 h postoperatively, while the conventional wound dressing group was treated with sterile adhesive wound dressing over the wound only (Fig. 2). The surgeons were blinded to the treatment assignment until wound closure, and data collector were blinded during the entire study.

Surgical procedures

All TKAs were performed by the same surgical team by using a midline skin incision, a standard medial parapatellar approach, and a measured resection technique. A cemented posterior-stabilized prosthetic total knee prosthesis (PFC, Johnson & Johnson/DePuy, Warsaw, IN, USA) was used. All of the patients received an intravenous administration of TXA 5 to 10 min before the skin incision (20 mg/kg) and 3, 6 h later (1 g) along with 1 g of topical TXA in 50 mL of normal saline solution. No tourniquet or wound drainage was used in any patient and no blood salvage system was used. Electrocautery and routine hemostasis were performed during the surgery. Surgical time, intraoperative blood loss volume was recorded. All patients had adductor canal block (20 ml 5 g/L ropivacaine and 0.1 mg adrenaline) performed before surgery and periarticular infiltration analgesia (70 ml 2.5 g/L ropivacaine and 0.1 mg adrenaline) during surgery.

Postoperative care protocol

After the operation, the patients were transferred to the anesthesia recovery unit, where they remained for 1 h, and then to the bed-ward. A cold pack was used on the surgical site and a single dose of 10 mg intravenous

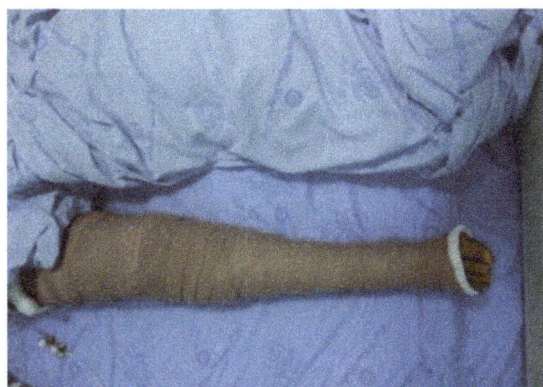

Fig. 1 A MRJB is shown on a patient

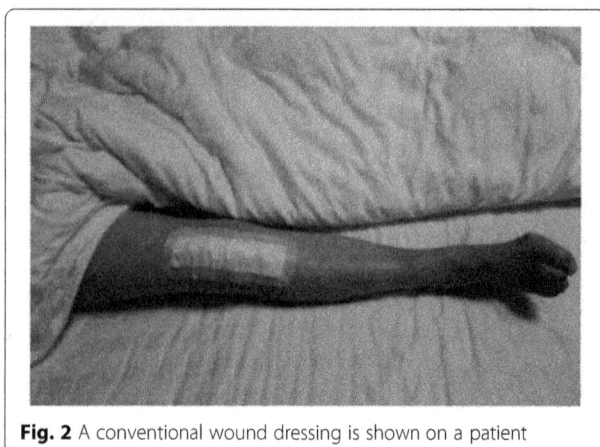

Fig. 2 A conventional wound dressing is shown on a patient

dexamethasone was administered when patients arrived inpatient unit [9, 11]. Postoperative oral Loxoprofen sodium (Loxonin; 60 mg three times daily) and Pregabalin (Lyrica; 75 mg twice daily) were administered for pain [12, 13]. A standard venous thromboembolism prophylaxis protocol combined mechanical and chemical prophylaxis was adopted for all patients [9]. An intermittent inflatable lower-extremity pump was used as a routine practice to prevent deep venous thrombosis (DVT) before the patient began walking. Low-molecular-weight heparin (LMWH; Clexane, Sanofi-Aventis, France, 2000 IU) was administered subcutaneously 8 h postoperatively, and a full dose (0.4 mL containing 4000 IU) was given at 24-h intervals during hospitalization. After discharge, rivaroxaban (10 mg, Xarelto, Bayer, Germany) was administered orally for 10 days if no bleeding events occurred.

Criteria for transfusion included a Hb level less than 7 g/dL or symptomatic anemia (light-headedness, palpitation, or shortness of breath not due to other causes) in a patient with an Hb level of 7 to 10 g/dL [9].

Outcome measurements

The primary outcome was swelling, which was measured as circumference of superior pole of patella, inferior pole of patella, mid-line of patella, thigh (10 cm above superior pole of the patella) and calf (10 cm below to inferior pole of the patella) at postoperative day (POD) 1, POD3 and 3 weeks after surgery. The secondary outcomes included range of motion (ROM), hospital for special surgery knee score, visual analog scale (VAS) at rest and at walking, reduction in Hb concentration, postoperative calculated blood loss, complications and patient satisfaction. The blood volume of each patient was calculated according to a formula published by Nadler et al. that considers patients' weight, height and gender [14, 15]. Complications such as nerve palsy, bruises, blisters were recorded. Doppler ultrasound was used to evaluate for DVT when a patient has any suspicious symptom of

DVT, including severe pain, swelling, tenderness, superficial venous engorgement and Homan's sign. Pulmonary embolism (PE) was diagnosed by clinical symptoms and an enhanced chest computed tomography (CT) scan. All adverse events were recorded during the first 3 weeks after surgery (Fig. 3). All of the patients completed a comfort level questionnaire regarding the feeling of the operated lower limb that asked them to rate their comfort on a 5-point scale ranging from very uncomfortable to very comfortable.

Statistical analysis

Quantitative data were presented as mean and standard deviation, qualitative data were presented as size number. Differences in continuous variables between the two groups were evaluated using Student's t-test or Mann–Whitney U test, depending on the distribution characteristics of the data. A chi-square test or Fisher's exact test for difference in proportions was used to estimate differences between groups in categorical variables. The sample size estimate was based on the difference in the primary outcome (i.e., reduction in mean knee circumference) and calculation was performed using G*Power Version 3.1.9.2 (Franz Faul, Uni Kiel, Germany) software with an unpaired t test of variance design assuming a standard effect size (d) = 0.67, an alpha level (two-tailed) = 0.05, and power = 0.90. We took 2 cm as clinical minimal relevance in circumference based on a previous study [16], and assumed standard deviation within each group to be 3 cm. Based on the information mentioned above, 39 patients each arm were needed. Allowing for a 15% loss to follow up, a total of 90 patients were planned to include in this study.

Results

Patients' demographics

During recruitment from December 2016 to May 2018, a total of 453 patients scheduled to take a primary

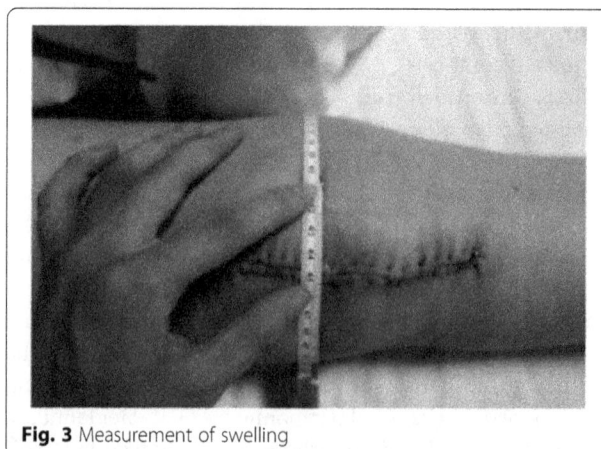

Fig. 3 Measurement of swelling

unilateral TKA were screened. Of them all, 143 patients were ineligible, 220 declined to participate, and the remaining 90 participants were enrolled. Each group lost 1 patient during follow-up. Baseline demographic data were comparable between the 2 groups (Table 1).

Primary outcome
No significant differences were observed between the two groups when we compared knee circumference at superior margin of patella, inferior margin of patella, mid-line of patella at any measurement point (Table 2).

Secondary outcome
No significant differences were observed in the total blood loss between the 2 groups. Similarly, transfusion rate showed no significant difference. As to the postoperative general assessments, no significant difference on Pain, ROM, HSS was found (Table 3). However, patients in control group had significantly higher comfort ratings than the experimental group during the first 24 h (Table 4). No nerve palsy, PE or DVT was observed in the 2 groups. Superficial skin complications including bruises and blisters also showed no significant difference.

Discussion
Hidden blood loss and inflammation are believed to be main factors that caused post-operative swelling. Based on this mechanism, various methods have been introduced to reduce post-operative knee swelling.

Table 1 Demographic characteristic of patients

	Compression group	Control group	P value
Age (yr)	69.32 ± 8.29	69.11 ± 8.66	0.91
[a]Gender (Male/Female)	10/34	10/34	1
Height (m)	1.58 ± 0.09	1.59 ± 0.08	0.64
Weight (kg)	64.39 ± 9.47	64.67 ± 10.82	0.90
BMI (kg/m^2)	25.80 ± 2.88	25.60 ± 3.24	0.76
Circumference (cm)			
Superior pole of patella	39.53 ± 2.91	39.47 ± 3.64	0.93
Mid-line of patella	38.31 ± 2.71	38.13 ± 3.28	0.78
Inferior pole of patella	36.31 ± 2.85	36.18 ± 3.15	0.83
Thigh	44.83 ± 36.59	44.64 ± 4.30	0.82
Calf	34.07 ± 2.43	33.79 ± 2.52	0.60
Hemoglobin (g/dL)	132.23 ± 12.55	134.09 ± 12.84	0.49
Hematocrit (%)	40.25 ± 3.25	40.11 ± 3.38	0.85
ROM	96.55 ± 14.22	92.91 ± 14.04	0.23
Pain at walking(VAS)	6.23 ± 1.27	6.34 ± 1.20	0.59
Pain at rest(VAS)	1.39 ± 1.71	1.14 ± 1.49	0.55

BMI body mass index, ROM range of motion, VAS visual analogue scale
[a]Presented as number and percent, and P-values were calculated by chi-square and Fisher exact test

Table 2 Postoperative primary outcomes

Variable	Compression group	Control group	P value
Mean circumference (cm)			
Superior pole of patella			
POD1	41.75 ± 2.90	41.61 ± 3.46	0.84
POD3	42.64 ± 2.88	42.56 ± 3.50	0.91
3w	40.19 ± 2.89	40.11 ± 3.57	0.91
POD1 change	2.22 ± 1.01	2.14 ± 0.86	0.71
POD3 change	3.10 ± 1.31	3.08 ± 1.12	0.95
3w change	0.66 ± 0.26	0.64 ± 0.25	0.80
Mid-line of patella			
POD1	40.40 ± 2.66	40.26 ± 3.28	0.84
POD3	41.31 ± 2.62	41.03 ± 3.37	0.67
3w	38.97 ± 2.62	38.82 ± 3.25	0.82
POD1 change	2.09 ± 0.96	2.13 ± 0.93	0.81
POD3 change	3.00 ± 1.32	2.90 ± 1.27	0.73
3w change	0.66 ± 0.31	0.69 ± 0.26	0.56
Inferior pole of patella			
POD1	38.08 ± 2.71	37.97 ± 3.22	0.87
POD3	38.88 ± 3.11	38.53 ± 3.54	0.63
3w	36.92 ± 2.81	36.73 ± 3.17	0.77
POD1 change	1.76 ± 1.14	1.79 ± 0.98	0.90
POD3 change	2.57 ± 1.63	2.35 ± 1.46	0.52
3w change	0.61 ± 0.36	0.56 ± 0.31	0.48
Thigh			
POD1	46.23 ± 3.49	45.90 ± 4.19	0.68
POD3	46.87 ± 3.68	46.57 ± 4.22	0.72
3w	45.79 ± 3.46	45.53 ± 4.14	0.74
POD1 change	1.40 ± 0.71	1.26 ± 0.66	0.35
POD3 change	2.03 ± 0.96	1.93 ± 0.90	0.61
3w change	0.96 ± 0.61	0.89 ± 0.58	0.58
Calf			
POD1	35.20 ± 2.44	34.95 ± 2.63	0.65
POD3	35.30 ± 2.52	35.07 ± 2.67	0.68
3w	34.82 ± 2.39	34.54 ± 2.46	0.60
POD1 change	1.12 ± 0.66	1.16 ± 0.62	0.83
POD3 change	1.22 ± 0.78	1.27 ± 0.70	0.75
3w change	0.74 ± 0.56	0.75 ± 0.43	0.95

POD postoperative day, 3w 3 weeks after surgery

Tourniquet-induced ischemia could increase fibrinolytic activity and induce local reactive hyperemia, resulting in more hidden blood loss [17]. Thus, abandoning tourniquet could lead to less hidden blood loss and a lower ratio of postoperative knee swelling [9]. Ishida et al. reported that the intra-articular administration of TXA reduced knee swelling by diminishing the hidden blood loss [18]. Furthermore, both TXA and corticosteroid

Table 3 Postoperative secondary outcomes

Variable	Compression group	Control group	P value
Postoperative Hb drop (g/dL)			
POD1 drop	18.91 ± 7.68	18.45 ± 8.17	0.79
POD3 drop	28.75 ± 10.01	29.27 ± 12.21	0.83
Postoperative blood loss (mL)			
POD1 drop	252.48 ± 124.92	250.75 ± 106.60	0.94
POD3 drop	529.30 ± 232.62	558.94 ± 252.74	0.57
Intraoperative blood loss (mL)	188.70 ± 80.33	178.14 ± 77.65	0.53
VAS at walking			
*POD1	6.23 ± 1.89	5.89 ± 1.62	0.37
*POD3	2.16 ± 0.94	1.98 ± 0.93	0.46
VAS at rest			
*POD1	2.39 ± 1.91	1.91 ± 1.60	0.28
*POD3	0.39 ± 0.72	0.41 ± 0.62	0.59
ROM (°)			
POD1	77.50 ± 20.00	78.30 ± 17.39	0.84
POD3	99.16 ± 9.36	97.68 ± 10.43	0.49
HSS	80.55 ± 5.36	79.34 ± 4.66	0.26
Complications			
†DVT	0	0	–
†PE	0	0	–
†Transfusion	0	0	–
†Bruises	1	1	1
†Blisters	1	1	1
†Nerve palsy	0	0	–

POD postoperative day, VAS visual analogue scale, ROM range of motion, HSS hospital for special surgery knee score, DVT deep vein thrombosis, PE pulmonary embolism
*P values calculated using the Mann–Whitney U test
†presented as number and the P-values were calculated by chi-square and Fisher exact test

have anti-inflammatory effects which could also contribute to reduction of swelling [19, 20]. All of the methods mentioned above are now routinely used in our institution for enhanced recovery.

Modified Robert Jones bandage, which was introduced by Brodell, is one of the most common compressive dressing following orthopedics surgery during the last 30 years, with the benefits of reducing tissue bleeding and edema by increasing intramuscular and intraarticular pressures [21]. However, Concerns about the complications such as peroneal nerve palsy, bruises and patient-reported discomforts still remain [6–8]. Due to the effective modern multi-modal swelling management, modified Robert Jones bandage use after total knee arthroplasty may now be unnecessary. To our best

Table 4 Comfort level at different time points

Comfort level	Compression group	Control group	P value
*Postoperative 24 h			0.03
Very comfortable	0	0	
Somewhat comfortable	2	4	
Fair	6	12	
Somewhat uncomfortable	27	24	
Very uncomfortable	9	4	
*Postoperative 72 h			0.58
Very comfortable	1	1	
Somewhat comfortable	7	8	
Fair	20	21	
Somewhat uncomfortable	13	13	
Very uncomfortable	3	1	

*P values calculated using the Mann–Whitney U test

knowledge, the present study was the first to evaluate the effect of MRJB in an ERAS program after TKA without use of a tourniquet and post-operative drains.

In this study, we found significantly lower patient comfort level in the compression group during the first 24 h, but no significant difference between the 2 groups at POD3, when MRJB had been removed for patients in the compression group. This was in accord with the previous study, compression therapy was with poor patients' compliance [4]. One of the reasons was reported to be the compression induced discomfort factors, including obliteration of circulation, "too hot" to wear, limb soreness, dermatitis or itching [22]. Moreover, low-pressure compression therapy was determined to be more comfortable than the high-pressure compression therapy [23].

Another finding of our study was that there was no difference in swelling, ROM and total blood loss between the 2 groups, and this was similar with a RCT performed by Pinsornsak et al. In their study, MRJB were placed for 24 h after TKA in the compression group, while patients in the control group received no compression but conventional wound dressing with sterile gauze pads only [6]. The difference between their study and ours was that they performed with routine tourniquet, no administration of intra-articular TXA or post-operative corticoids. In contrast, Charalambides et al. reported that compression bandage could control intra-articular bleeding effectively and few patients with compression bandaging experienced post-operative lower limb swelling [3]. However, the study was not in an enhanced recovery setup and the swelling was not evaluated by knee circumference. One of the possible reasons for the positive result of Charalambides et al.'s study may be the bandages were maintained for 48 h, which was at twice the time of ours. And this may be too long for patients to achieve early mobilization and may be conflict to the idea of ERAS, as this bandage is bulky and hard for patients to do flexion exercise.

Furthermore, we found no differences in pain relief between the two groups. However, in a study evaluating the effect of compression bandage on pain control, Andersen et al. found patients with compression bandage experienced less pain than those with non-compression bandage [24]. This might be due to the cooling effect of cryotherapy in our study was partly affected by MRJB because of its thick layer [25], as cryotherapy was reported to reduce pain by slowing the conduction of nerve signals [26].

There are several limitations in our study. First, we did not measure the inflammatory markers before surgery, so the level of inflammation could be confounding issue and may have effect on knee swelling. However, the effect may be negligible due to the randomization design. Second, sub-bandage pressure measurement was not performed in each patient with the MRJB dressing, so the interface pressures might differ with each application. However, measurement of sub-bandage pressure is not practical and a pressure-guided application method of MRJB was not routinely used in clinical practice. Third, patients were not blinded in this study, as it was difficult to prevent patients from noticing if they received compression or not. Fourth, during our clinical practice, we found intraoperative tourniquet was still necessary for patients with severe obesity because of their greater surgical difficulty, so we excluded patients with a BMI > 35. Therefore, our conclusion may not be applicable for patients with severe obesity.

Conclusions

In conclusion, we found avoidance of MRJB use could provide higher patients' reported comfort level, without increasing swelling, blood loss, severity of pain or damaging knee function. Therefore, MRJB after primary TKA without tourniquet and drainage may not be routinely indicated in common clinical use.

Abbreviations

CT: Computed tomography; DVT: Deep venous thrombosis; MRJB: Modified Robert Jones bandage; PE: Pulmonary embolism; POD: Postoperative day; ROM: Range of motion; TKA: Total knee arthroplasty; VAS: Visual analog scale

Acknowledgements

This study adheres to CONSORT guidelines. We would like to thank the relevant staff for guidance and assistance for their support and collaboration in our hospital.

Authors' contributions

ZKZ, FXP conceived and designed this study; HDY, HYW XR and SYY collected the data; HDY, HYW performed the statistical analysis; HYW and HDY prepared Tables 1–4; HDY, KZ and HYW wrote the manuscript; HDY and ZKZ revised this manuscript. All authors reviewed the final manuscript. All authors agree to be accountable for all aspects of the work.

Competing interests

The authors declare that they have no competing interests.

References

1. Carr AJ, Robertsson O, Graves S, Price AJ, Arden NK, Judge A, Beard DJ. Knee replacement. Lancet. 2012;379(9823):1331–40.
2. Holm B, Kristensen MT, Bencke J, Husted H, Kehlet H, Bandholm T. Loss of knee-extension strength is related to knee swelling after total knee arthroplasty. Arch Phys Med Rehabil. 2010;91(11):1770–6.
3. Charalambides C, Beer M, Melhuish J, Williams RJ, Cobb AG. Bandaging technique after knee replacement. Acta Orthop. 2005;76(1):89–94.
4. Ramelet AA. Compression therapy. Dermatol Surg. 2002;28(1):6–10.
5. Ogata K, Whiteside LA. Effects of external compression on blood flow to muscle and skin. Clin Orthop Relat Res. 1982;(168):105–7.
6. Pinsornsak P, Chumchuen S. Can a modified Robert Jones bandage after knee arthroplasty reduce blood loss? A prospective randomized controlled trial. Clin Orthop Relat Res. 2013;471(5):1677–81.
7. Idusuyi OB, Morrey BF. Peroneal nerve palsy after total knee arthroplasty. Assessment of predisposing and prognostic factors. J Bone Joint Surg Am. 1996;78(2):177–84.
8. Hughes DL, Crosby AC. Treatment of knee sprains: modified Robert Jones or elastic support bandage? J Accid Emerg Med. 1995;12(2):115–8.
9. Huang Z, Xie X, Li L, Huang Q, Ma J, Shen B, Kraus VB, Pei F. Intravenous and topical tranexamic acid alone are superior to tourniquet use for primary Total knee arthroplasty: a prospective, randomized controlled trial. J Bone Joint Surg Am. 2017;99(24):2053–61.
10. Rytter S, Stilling M, Munk S, Hansen TB. Methylprednisolone reduces pain and decreases knee swelling in the first 24 h after fast-track unicompartmental knee arthroplasty. Knee Surg Sports Traumatol Arthrosc. 2017;25(1):284–90.
11. Richardson AB, Bala A, Wellman SS, Attarian DE, Bolognesi MP, Grant SA. Perioperative dexamethasone administration does not increase the incidence of postoperative infection in Total hip and knee arthroplasty: a retrospective analysis. J Arthroplast. 2016;31(8):1784–7.
12. Han C, Kuang MJ, Ma JX, Ma XL. Is pregabalin effective and safe in total knee arthroplasty? A PRISMA-compliant meta-analysis of randomized-controlled trials. Medicine. 2017;96(26):e6947.
13. Onda A, Ogoshi A, Itoh M, Nakagawa T, Kimura M. Comparison of the effects of treatment with celecoxib, loxoprofen, and acetaminophen on postoperative acute pain after arthroscopic knee surgery: a randomized, parallel-group trial. J Orthop Science. 2016;21(2):172–7.
14. Nadler SB, Hidalgo JH, Bloch T. Prediction of blood volume in normal human adults. Surgery. 1962;51(2):224–32.
15. Gross JB. Estimating allowable blood loss: corrected for dilution. Anesthesiology. 1983;58(3):277–80.
16. Munk S, Jensen NJ, Andersen I, Kehlet H, Hansen TB. Effect of compression therapy on knee swelling and pain after total knee arthroplasty. Knee Surg Sports Traumatol Arthrosc. 2013;21(2):388–92.
17. Li B, Wen Y, Wu H, Qian Q, Lin X, Zhao H. The effect of tourniquet use on hidden blood loss in total knee arthroplasty. Int Orthop. 2009;33(5):1263–8.
18. Ishida K, Tsumura N, Kitagawa A, Hamamura S, Fukuda K, Dogaki Y, Kubo S, Matsumoto T, Matsushita T, Chin T, et al. Intra-articular injection of tranexamic acid reduces not only blood loss but also knee joint swelling after total knee arthroplasty. Int Orthop. 2011;35(11):1639–45.
19. Godier A, Roberts I, Hunt BJ. Tranexamic acid: less bleeding and less thrombosis? Crit Care. 2012;16(3):135.
20. Yue C, Wei R, Liu Y. Perioperative systemic steroid for rapid recovery in total knee and hip arthroplasty: a systematic review and meta-analysis of randomized trials. J Orthop Surg Res. 2017;12(1):100.

21. Brodell JD, Axon DL, Evarts CM. The Robert Jones bandage. J Bone Joint Surg Bri. 1986;68(5):776–9.
22. Raju S, Hollis K, Neglen P. Use of compression stockings in chronic venous disease: patient compliance and efficacy. Ann Vasc Surg. 2007;21(6):790–5.
23. Ayhan H, Iyigun E, Ince S, Can MF, Hatipoglu S, Saglam M. A randomised clinical trial comparing the patient comfort and efficacy of three different graduated compression stockings in the prevention of postoperative deep vein thrombosis. J Clin Nurs. 2015;24(15–16):2247–57.
24. Andersen LO, Husted H, Otte KS, Kristensen BB, Kehlet H. A compression bandage improves local infiltration analgesia in total knee arthroplasty. Acta Orthop. 2008;79(6):806–11.
25. Weresh MJ, Bennett GL, Njus G. Analysis of cryotherapy penetration: a comparison of the plaster cast, synthetic cast, ace wrap dressing, and Robert-Jones dressing. Foot Ankle Int. 1996;17(1):37–40.
26. Algafly AA, George KP. The effect of cryotherapy on nerve conduction velocity, pain threshold and pain tolerance. Br J Sports Med. 2007;41(6):365–9 discussion 369.

20

Influence of the site of acromioplasty on reduction of the critical shoulder angle (CSA) – an anatomical study

Dominik Kaiser[1*], Elias Bachmann[2], Christian Gerber[1] and Dominik C. Meyer[1]

Abstract

Background: A large critical shoulder angle (CSA) >35° is associated with the development of rotator cuff tearing. Lateral acromioplasty (AP) has the theoretical potential to prevent rotator cuff tearing and/ or to reduce the risk of re-tears after repair. It is, however unclear which part of the lateral acromion has to be reduced to obtain the desired CSA. It was the purpose of this study to determine which part of the lateral acromion has to be resected to achieve a desired reduction of the CSA in a given individual.

Methods: First, the influence of the exact radiographic projection on the CSA was examined. Second, the influence of anterolateral versus strict lateral AP on the CSA was studied in eight scapulae with different anatomic characteristics. Differences in CSA reduction were investigated using paired t-test or Wilcoxon test.

Results: Scapular rotation in the sagittal and axial plane had a marked influence on the radiologically measured CSA ranging from -6 to +16°. Overall, lateral AP of 5/10mm reduced the CSA significantly greater than anterolateral AP of 5mm/10mm [5mm: 2.3° (range: 0.7°-3.6°) SD±0.8° vs. 1.2° (range: 0°-3.3°) SD±1.1°, $p=0.0002$]/[10mm: 4.8° (range: 2.1°-7°) SD±1.3° vs. 2.7° (range: 0°-5.3°) SD±1.7°, $p=0.0001$]. Depending on scapular anatomy anterolateral AP did not alter CSA at all.

Conclusions: For comparison of pre- and postoperative CSA, the exact orientation of the X-ray and the spatial orientation of the scapula must be as identical as possible. Anterolateral AP may not sufficiently correct CSA in scapulae with great acromial slopes and smaller relative external rotation of the acromion as the critical acromial point (CAP) may be located too posteriorly and thus is not addressed by anterolateral acromioplasty. Consistent reduction of the CSA could be achieved by lateral AP in all eight scapulae.

Keywords: Rotator cuff tear, Acromioplasty, Critical shoulder angle, Rotator cuff retear, Digitally reconstructed radiograph, Computed tomography

Background

The morphology of the scapula shows great differences between individuals. Its variable radiographic appearance has led Bigliani et al. to distinguish three different forms of the acromion as early as 1986 [1]. Later reports focused on different acromial spurs, acromial slope (AS), acromial tilt (AT), lateral acromial angle (LAA), acromion index (AI) and critical shoulder angle (CSA) [2–7]. The interest of these studies is to understand how the scapular anatomy is related to clinical shoulder pathologies and how it might be altered in order to possibly reduce the incidence of degenerative rotator cuff tears or their recurrence after repair [8]. Other reports found a highly relevant impact of a presumably "faulty" body posture on rotator cuff tears, as differences in posture alter the position of the scapula in space [9].

While Moor et al. noted little variation of the radiographic appearance and the CSA in different scapular rotation [10], a newer study has shown a greater susceptibility of the CSA to malposition especially in ante- and retroversion [11].

* Correspondence: dominik14k@gmail.com
[1]Department of Orthopaedics, University of Zurich, Balgrist University Hospital, Uniklinik Balgrist, Forchstrasse 340, 8008 Zürich, Switzerland
Full list of author information is available at the end of the article

At our institution all standard AP shoulder radiographs are obtained with the x-ray beam angled 15 degrees caudally in the sagittal plane and vertically in the axial plane, independent of the patient specific scapular morphology especially regarding the acromion, the position in space or the patient's posture. Using the above-mentioned protocol, it has been shown that a CSA of <28 is highly predictive (odds-ratio >10) for the development of osteoarthritis and a CSA > 35° is highly predictive of rotator cuff tears (RCT) [6]. Consequently, we assume that normalization of a very high (>35°) CSA may be helpful in preventing rotator cuff re-tears and we therefore seek to achieve this goal with acromioplasty in these patients.

We made however the observation that a small resection of an anterolateral acromial spur relevantly decreases the CSA in some patients (Fig. 1), whereas extensive trimming of the whole lateral acromion reduces the CSA only minimally in others. This observation led us to the hypothesis that similar acromioplasties may lead to different corrections of the CSA in different scapular anatomies. Consequently, the first goal of this experimental study was to understand how anterolateral and lateral acromioplasties can have a profoundly different effect on the postoperative radiologically measured CSA as recently described by Katthagen et al. [12]. The second goal was to understand the behavior of the critical acromial point (CAP) in scapulae with different anatomies and in different spatial position [13]. This should help the surgeon achieve a predictable and sufficient correction of a large CSA as defined by Moor et al. [6], while minimizing possible detrimental effects of over- resection of the acromion.

Methods
Step 1- Variation of the CSA in three anatomically different scapulae
In a first step, we assessed which point forms the most inferolateral part of the acromion (CAP) on the radiograph. We selected three patients (p1-p3) with distinctly different scapular anatomy regarding acromial slope and relative external rotation of the acromion.

All the shoulders of the studied scapulae had a symptomatic rotator cuff tear, operated at our institution and treated with an additional lateral acromioplasty. The MRI Dicom data of these scapulae were segmented using Mimics (Materialise, Leuven, Belgium) and improvement of the models mesh was performed using Meshlab (visual Computing Lab-ISTI-CNR). The segmented scapulae were positioned according to the preoperative true anteroposterior and true lateral view radiographs according to Moor et al. [10] using Blender 2.78 (Amsterdam, Netherlands), a professional open-source 3D computer graphics toolset used for interactive 3D applications. The scapular position was then changed in steps of ±10°, ±20°, ±30°, ±40° flexion/extension and combined with internal/ external rotation up to 10° each. The CSA was measured using Blender 2.78. The relative external rotation of the acromion was defined as the angle between a tangent to the lateral border of the acromion and a line parallel to the scapular body, as seen on an axial radiograph. Posterior acromial slope was defined as the angle of a line connecting the posteroinferior and anteroinferior acromial border and a line parallel to the scapular body as seen on a true lateral view radiograph (Fig. 2), measurements were confirmed by the segmented 3D models.

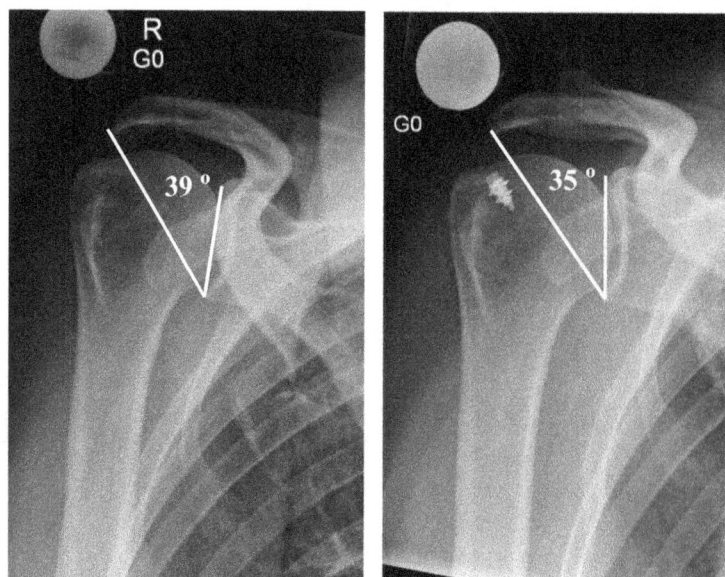

Fig. 1 Pre- and postoperative x-ray (*p1 scapula*) reducing CSA from 39° to 35° by anterolateral acromioplasty

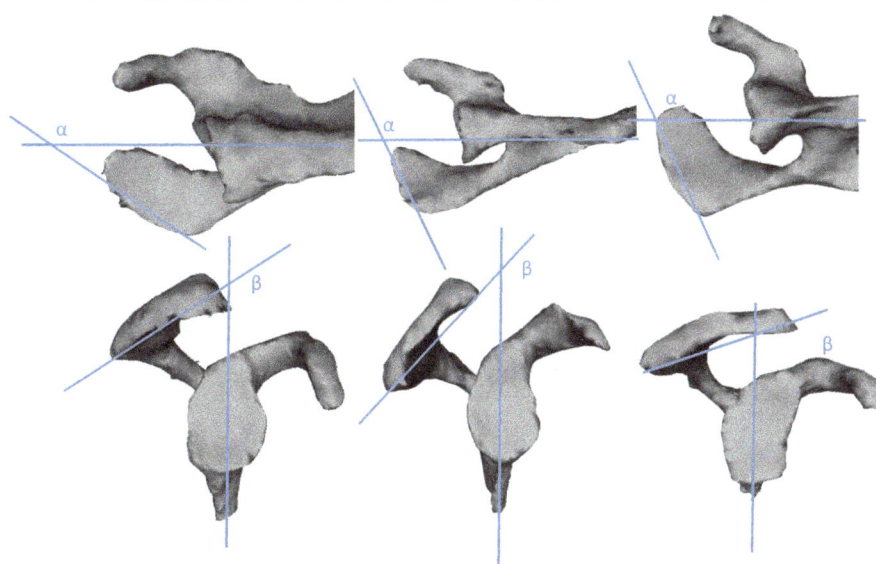

Fig. 2 3-D reconstruction of the segmented scapulae showing distinct differences regarding relative external acromial rotation (α – angle between a tangent to the lateral acromial border and a line parallel to the scapular body) and posterior acromial slope (β- angle between a line *connecting the posteroinferior* and the anteroinferior acromion and a line parallel to the scapular body). From left to right *"p1"* scapula, *"p2"* scapula, *"p3"* scapula

Step 2- Effect of lateral vs. anterolateral acromioplasty

In a second step lateral and anterolateral acromioplasty of 5mm and 10mm were simulated on the 3 segmented scapulae using Blender 2.78 (Fig. 3). Starting position was defined by the preoperative radiographs as well as the preoperative CSA of the unaltered scapula as measured on a true anteroposterior radiograph according to Moor et al. [10]. Each scapula was then rotated in steps of ±10° from -40° (extension) to +40° (flexion). The CSA was measured in every position as the angle between CAP, inferior glenoid rim and superior glenoid rim.

To increase the validity of the study five additional scapulae (p4-p8) were included. Segmentation of the scapulae from MRI Dicom data, simulation of

acromioplasty and CSA measurement were performed identically as described above.

Written informed consent was obtained from all eight patients and Ethic Committee Approval was obtained (KEK Nr.: ZH2016-000826).

Statistical analysis

Differences in reduction of CSA between anterolateral and lateral acromioplasty in different flexion angles were investigated using paired t-test (or Wilcoxon test, where applicable). *P*-values <0.05 were considered statistically significant. Results are reported with mean, standard deviation and associated p-values if not stated otherwise.

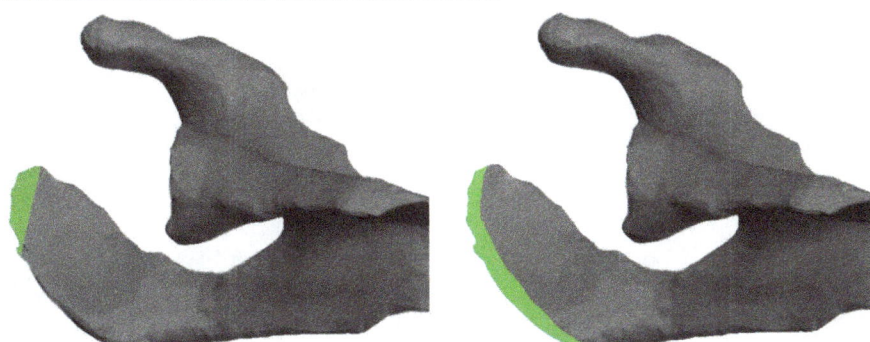

Fig. 3 Axial view of the p1 scapula schematically depicting the area of the acromion (green), which is surgically removed during anterolateral (left) and lateral (right) acromioplasty

Results

Step 1- Variation of the CSA in three anatomically different scapulae

The CSA varied markedly depending on the flexion/extension and internal or external rotation of the scapula as shown in Diagram 1.

Extreme scapular positions, especially ±30° and ±40° flexion/extension, were deliberately included, fully aware that these are unacceptable for clinical use. They were performed to help understand how extreme positions may become relevant for the CSA. In Diagram 1 these are highlighted gray while clinically more likely variations are highlighted white. In clinically likely variations,

the CSA varied from 33° to 54° in the "p1" scapula, from 34° to 52° in the "p2" scapula and from 35° to 45° in the "p3" scapula. Internal rotation consistently increases the CSA, while external rotation decreases the CSA in clinically likely variations.

Step 2- Effect of anterolateral vs. lateral acromioplasty

The first three scapulae were chosen for their distinct anatomical differences and labeled p1, p2 and p3. Five additional scapulae were included to increase validity of the study. These were chosen randomly, segmented and labeled p4-p8. The anatomical characteristics of the eight scapulae regarding preoperative CSA, posterior acromial slope and relative external rotation are summarized in Table 1.

Overall reduction of the CSA was significantly greater by lateral than by anterolateral acromioplasty of 5mm [2.3° (range: 0.7°-3.6°) SD±0.8° vs. 1.2° (range: 0°-3.3°) SD±1.1°, $p=0.0002$] and significantly greater by lateral than by anterolateral acomioplasty of 10mm [4.8° (range: 2.1°-7°) SD±1.3° vs. 2.7° (range: 0°-5.3°) SD±1.7°, $p=0.0001$].

In neutral position reduction of the CSA did not significantly differ between lateral and anterolateral acromioplasty of 5mm [2.0° (range: 0.7°-2.9°) SD±0.9° vs. 1.1° (range: 0-2.5°) SD±1.1°; $p=0.15$] and between lateral and anterolateral acromioplasty of 10mm [4.4° (range: 2.1°-6.2°) SD±1.5° vs. 2.6° (range: 0-4.5°) SD±1.8°; $p=0.06$].

In 10° flexion reduction of the CSA was significantly greater by lateral than by anterolateral acromioplasty of 5mm [2.5° (range: 1.2°-3.3°) SD± 0.7° vs. 1.6° (range: 0°-3.3°) SD± 1.1°; $p=0.02$] and significantly greater by lateral than by anterolateral acromioplasty of 10mm [5.3° (range: 3.5°-7°) SD± 1.1° vs. 3.3° (range: 0-5.3°) SD± 1.5°; $p=0.008$].

In 10° extension reduction of the CSA was significantly greater by lateral than by anterolateral acromioplasty of 5mm [2.3° (range: 1°-3.6°) SD± 0.8° vs. 1° (range: 0-2.4°) SD± 1.1°; $p=0.007$] and significantly greater by lateral than by anterolateral acromioplasty of 10mm [4.7° (range: 2.1°-6.3°) SD± 1.2° vs. 2.1° (range: 0-4.6°) SD± 1.7°; $p=0.006$].

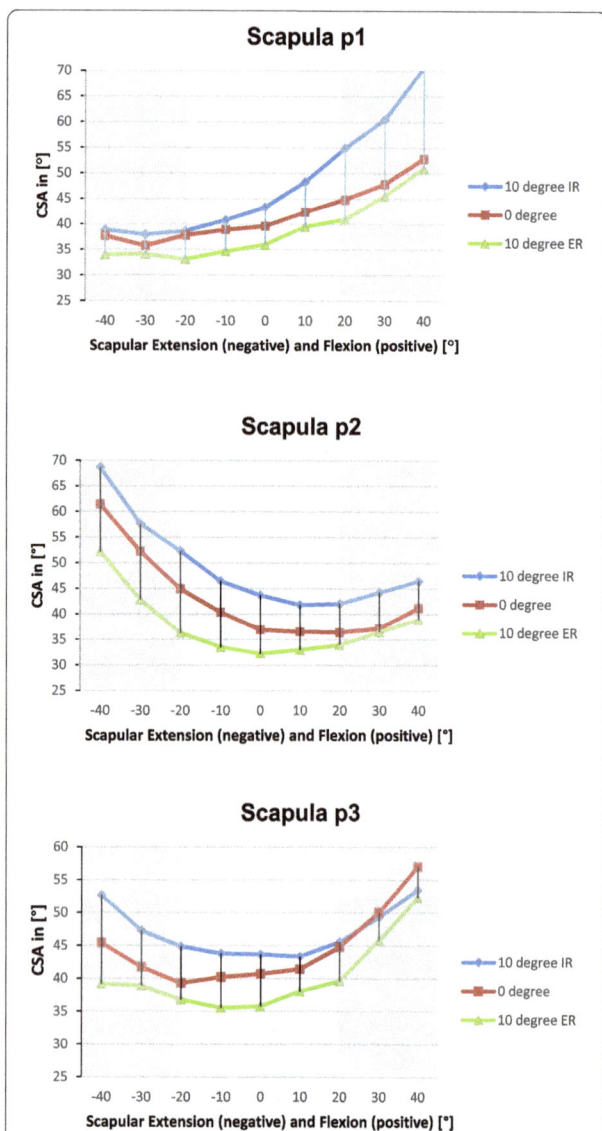

Diagram 1 CSA (y-axis) of the three scapulae "p1", "p2" and "p3" in relation to different extension (negative values) and flexion angles (positive values) (x-axis) in different internal and external rotation, clinically unacceptable rotations highlighted gray

Table 1 Anatomical characteristics regarding preoperative CSA, posterior acromial slope and relative external rotation of the 8 examined scapulae (p1-8)

	p1	p2	p3	p4	p5	p6	p7	p8
Preoperative CSA [°]	40	37	40	31	29	37	35	42
Posterior acromial slope [°]	133	145	116	136	117	110	128	102
Relative external rotation [°]	133	114	108	123	132	128	130	111

Anterolateral acromioplasty had no effect on the CSA in 10° extension to 10° flexion in scapulae p2 and a partial effect on p3 (0- 3.3°) and p7 (0-2.8°) (Diagrams 2 and 3).

Anterolateral acromioplasty had a notable effect on the CSA in 10° extension to 10° flexion in the other scapulae with the greatest reduction in scapulae p1 (2.1°-4.6°) and p7 (2°-5.3°). (Diagrams 4 and 5).

The average correction achieved by lateral acromioplasty of 5mm (10mm) was 2.3° (4.7°) in 10° extension, 1.96° (4.44°) in neutral and 2.4° (5.3°) in 10° flexion.

The average correction achieved by anterolateral acromioplasty of 5mm (10mm) increased with increasing flexion of the scapula from 1.2° (2.3°) in 10° extension to 1.3° (2.95°) in neutral and 1.7° (3.70°) in 10° flexion.

Discussion

Multiple reports [3, 6, 7, 14–16] leave currently little doubt that the radiologically visible lateral extension of the acromion is a relevant predictor for either development of osteoarthritis ("small" acromion) or RCT ("large" acromion). The acromial extension may be measured either by the critical shoulder angle (CSA) or with the acromion index (AI) [7]. Altering these values by acromioplasty during rotator cuff repair may contribute to a lower rate of re-tears, as recently reported by Garcia et al. and Hong et al. [17, 18] even though this has not been widely verified in long-term follow up yet. For rotator cuff repair, the goal at our institution has been arbitrarily set to reduce the CSA to less than 35° in a

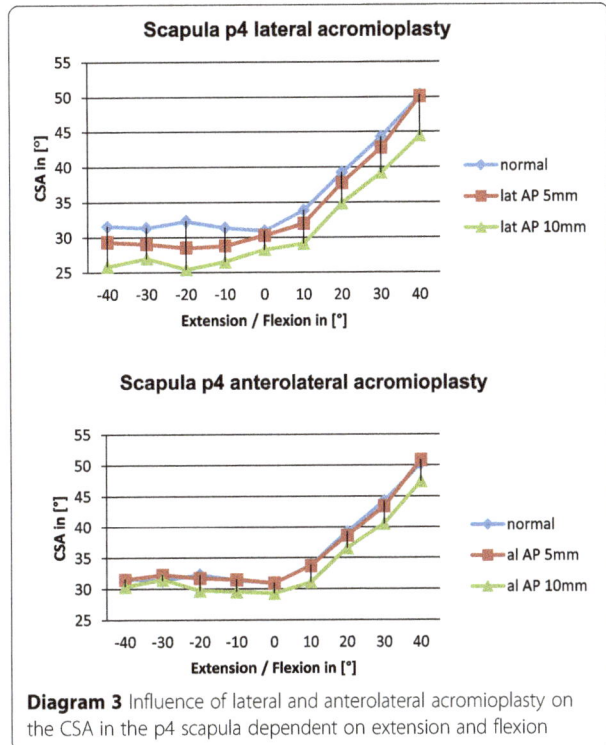

Diagram 3 Influence of lateral and anterolateral acromioplasty on the CSA in the p4 scapula dependent on extension and flexion

postoperative follow-up x-ray, as a CSA of greater than 35° has been associated with a higher risk of rotator cuff disease [6, 10].

In our surgical practice however, we made the surprising observation that similar surgical corrections show variable corrections of the CSA. We observed that in

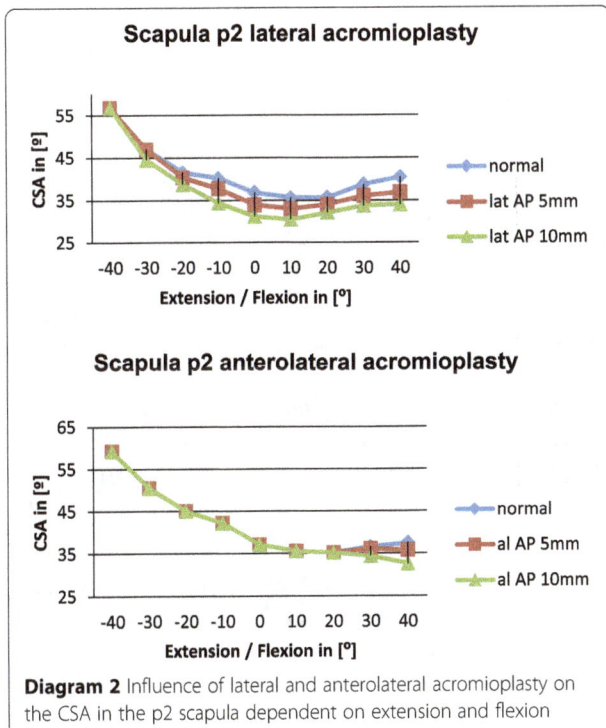

Diagram 2 Influence of lateral and anterolateral acromioplasty on the CSA in the p2 scapula dependent on extension and flexion

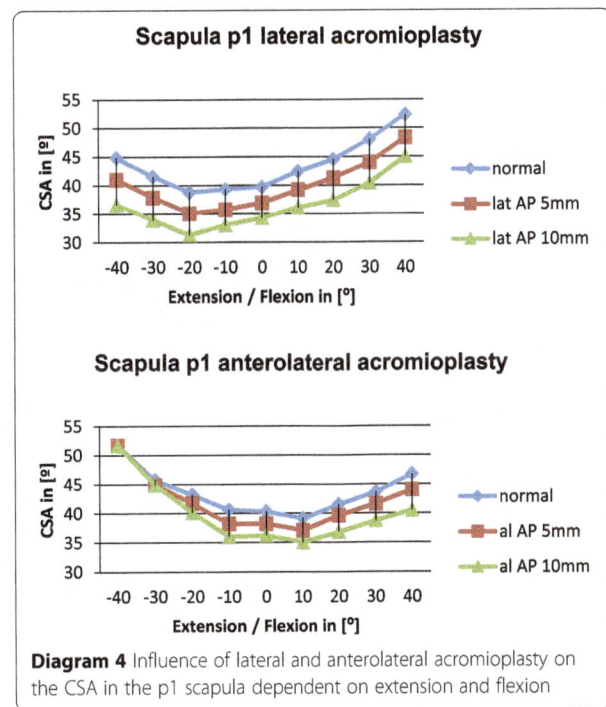

Diagram 4 Influence of lateral and anterolateral acromioplasty on the CSA in the p1 scapula dependent on extension and flexion

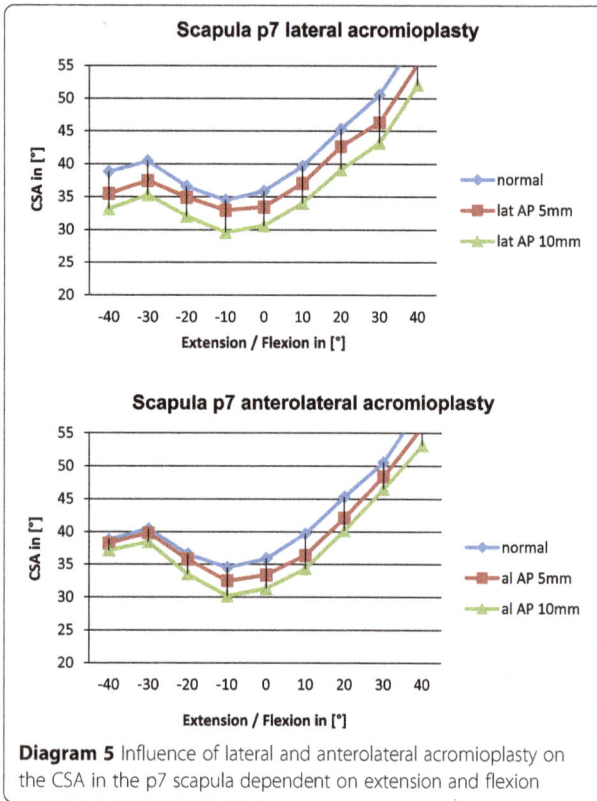

Diagram 5 Influence of lateral and anterolateral acromioplasty on the CSA in the p7 scapula dependent on extension and flexion

measured CSA by understanding how the CAP behaves in scapulae with different anatomies and in different spatial position.

The analyses of our experimental measurements confirmed our clinical observation in two regards:

1. Great external rotation of the acromion leads to prominence of the anterolateral acromion in defining the CSA. This prominence can be further increased by a bony spur in the AC ligament. The CAP is thus located anteriorly on the acromion and is medialized by strict anterolateral acromioplasty, profoundly reducing the CSA. This applies to our index patient's scapula where an isolated anterolateral acromioplasty resulted in a similar correction of the CSA as a lateral acromioplasty (Fig. 1, Fig. 4 (left side) and Diagram 4). 2. Anterolateral acromioplasty may lead to little or no change in the postoperative radiological CSA if the CAP is posterior to the site of correction (Fig. 4 (right side)) and therefore a dedicated lateral acromioplasty may be necessary. This seems to occur especially in acromia with greater acromial slope and smaller external rotation.

one patient (scapula p1) with a preoperative CSA of 39° a purely anterolateral acromioplasty led to a correction of the CSA by 4° to 35° (Fig. 1), while in other patients subjectively similar acromioplasties barely altered the CSA. It was therefore the purpose of this study to understand how lateral and anterolateral acromioplasties can have a profoundly different effect on the postoperatively

Direction of the x-ray beam

Corresponding to the recently published study on the dependency of the CSA of the radiographic viewing perspective of Suter et al. [11] the CSA of the scapulae p1-3 showed a certain positional susceptibility of this clinically valuable parameter even at low angular variations (Diagram 1).

In our second experimental array we did not alter scapular rotation as malrotated x- rays are easily identified at the glenoid and rejected in clinical practice.

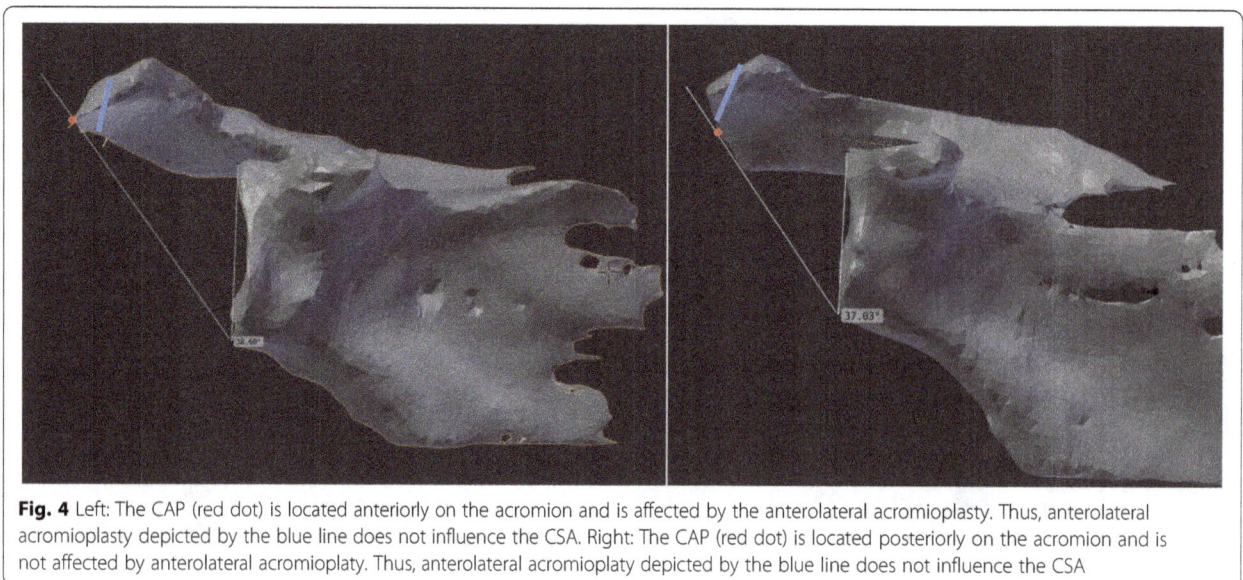

Fig. 4 Left: The CAP (red dot) is located anteriorly on the acromion and is affected by the anterolateral acromioplasty. Thus, anterolateral acromioplasty depicted by the blue line does not influence the CSA. Right: The CAP (red dot) is located posteriorly on the acromion and is not affected by anterolateral acromioplaty. Thus, anterolateral acromioplaty depicted by the blue line does not influence the CSA

Effect of anterolateral vs lateral acromioplasty

Overall lateral acromioplasty of 5mm and 10mm reduced the CSA significantly greater than anterolateral acromioplasty of 5mm and 10mm, respectively. We believe this is mainly due to the fact, that the CSA is reduced consistently by lateral acromioplasty in all of the included scapulae independent of acromial anatomy. The reduction of the CSA by lateral acromioplasty depends on the amount of bone which is resected (Diagrams 2, 3, 4, 5).

On the other hand anterolateral acromioplasties have a variable effect on the postoperative CSA ranging from no effect at all in scapula p2 (average reduction by lateral AP= 4.1° vs average reduction by anterolateral AP = 0°) to a comparable effect in scapula p1 (average reduction by lateral AP 4.6° vs average reduction by anterolateral AP 3.2°).

We noticed that the CAP seemed to move anteriorly in scapulae with greater external rotation and posteriorly with greater acromial slope. As the CSA is only reduced if the CAP is included in the osseous resection; a more anterior located CAP is more likely to be included by an anterolateral acromioplasty. We concluded that in acromia with greater external rotation and smaller acromial slope, an anterolateral acromioplasty is more likely to reduce CSA.

Further supporting this conclusion is the tendency of greater CSA reduction in increasing flexion of the scapula by anterolateral acromioplasty. Increasing flexion of the scapula relatively reduces the posterior slope, moving the CAP more anteriorly and as mentioned above making it more likely to be included in an anterolateral acromioplasty. Vice versa, increasing scapular extension moves the CAP more posteriorly potentially reducing the effect of anterolateral acromioplasty, which can be seen well in Diagram 4.

There are several limitations to this experimental study. Segmentation was performed by hand using a standardized MRI by the first author. Only eight different scapulae were used to test our hypothesis and simulate acromioplasty. A larger number of test scapulae may be useful to confirm the above mentioned findings, however will most likely not change the intuitively well understandable principal findings we have made. The greatest limitation appears, that we do not know what the real biomechanical effect is that we generate with each acromioplasty procedure.

In summary, a large lateral acromial extension with large CSA and AI may be the result of the projection of a possible anterolateral spur in the coracoacromial ligament especially in scapulae with a smaller posterior acromial slope and a larger relative external acromial rotation (Fig. 1). In such patients, the CAP is located anterior and pure anterolateral acromioplasty may

relevantly alter and "correct" the radiologically visible CSA. However, with greater posterior acromial slope and less relative external acromial rotation, the CAP moves further posterior and may exit the area affected by anterolateral acromioplasty. Therefore in those patients, only a lateral acromioplasty will lead to the currently desired reduction of the CSA.

Conclusion

For comparison of pre- and postoperative CSA, the exact orientation of the X-ray and the spatial orientation of the scapula must be as identical as possible. Anterolateral AP may not sufficiently correct CSA in scapulae with great acromial slopes and smaller relative external rotation of the acromion as the critical acromial point (CAP) may be located too posteriorly and thus is not addressed by anterolateral acromioplasty. Consistent reduction of the CSA was achieved by lateral AP in all eight scapulae.

Abbreviations
AP: Acromioplasty; CAP: Critical acromial point; RCT: Rotator cuff tears

Authors' contributions
DK and DM designed and carried out the study. EB participated in its design and the computer analysis. CG and DM contributed substantially to the manuscript. All authors read and approved the final manuscript.

Competing interests
The authors declare that they have no competing interests.

Author details
[1]Department of Orthopaedics, University of Zurich, Balgrist University Hospital, Uniklinik Balgrist, Forchstrasse 340, 8008 Zürich, Switzerland. [2]Department of Orthopaedics, Biomechanical Research Laboratory, Balgrist Campus, University of Zürich, Zürich, Switzerland.

References
1. Bigliani LU, Morrison DS, April EW. The morphology of the acromion and its relationship to rotator cuff tears. Orthop Trans. 1986;10:228.
2. Hamid N, Omid R, Yamaguchi K, Steger-May K, Stobbs G, Kenner JD. Relationship of radiographic acromial characteristics and rotator cuff disease: a prospective investigation of clinical, radiographic, and sonographic findings. J Shoulder Elbow Surg. 2012;2:1289–98.
3. Oh JH, Kim JY, Lee HK, Choi JA. Classification and clinical significance of acromial spur in rotator cuff tear. Clin Orthop Relat Res. 2010;468:1542–50.
4. Balke M, Liem D, Greshake O, et al. Differences in acromial morphology of shoulders in patients with degenerative and traumatic supraspinatus tendon tears. Knee Surg Sports Traumatol Arthrosc. 2016;24:2200–5.
5. Balke M, Schmidt C, Dedy N, Banerjee M, Bouillon B, Liem D. Correlation of acromial morphology with impingement syndrome and rotator cuff tears. Acta Orthop. 2013;84(2):178–83.
6. Moor BK, Wieser K, Slankamenac K, Gerber C, Bouaicha S. Relationship of individual scapular anatomy and degenerative rotator cuff tears. J Shoulder Elbow Surg. 2014;23:536–41.
7. Nyffeler RW, Werner CM, Sukthankar A, Schmid MR, Gerber C. Association of a large lateral extension of the acromion with rotator cuff tears. J Bone Joint Surg Am. 2006;88(4):800–5.
8. Yamamoto A, Takagishi K, Osawa T, Yanagawa T, Nakajima D, Shitara H, et al. Prevalence and risk factors of a rotator cuff tear in the general population. J Shoulder Elbow Surg. 2010;19(1):116–20.
9. Yamamoto A, Takagishi K, Kobayashi T, Shitara H, Ichinose T, Takasawa E, et al. The impact of faulty posture on rotator cuff tears with and without symptoms. J Shoulder Elbow Surg. 2014;24(3):446–52.

10. Moor BK, Bouaicha S, Rothenfluh DA, Sukthankar A, Gerber C. Is there an association between the individual anatomy of the scapula and the development of rotator cuff tears or osteoarthritis of the glenohumeral joint? A radiological study of the critical shoulder angle. Bone Joint J. 2013;95-B:935–41.

11. Suter T, Gerber Popp A, Zhang Y, Zhang C, Tashjian RZ, Henninger HB. The influence of radiographic viewing perspective and demographics on the critical shoulder angle. J Shoulder Elbow Surg. 2015;24:e149–58.

12. Katthagen JC, Marchetti DC, Tahal DS, Turnbull TL, Millett PJ. The effects of arthroscopic lateral acromioplasty on the critical shoulder angle and the anterolateral deltoid origin: an anatomic cadaveric study. Arthroscopy. 2016;32(4):569–75.

13. Karns MR, Jacxens M, Uffmann WJ, Todd DC, Henninger HB, Burks RT. The critical acromial point: the anatomic location of the lateral acromion in the critical shoulder angle. J Shoulder Elbow Surg. 2018;27(1):151–9.

14. Banas MP, Miller RJ, Totterman S. Relationship between the lateral acromion angle and rotator cuff disease. J Shoulder Elbow Surg. 1995;4(6):454–61.

15. Gerber C, Catanzaro S, Betz M, Ernstbrunner L. Arthroscopic Correction of the Critical Shoulder Angle Through Lateral Acromioplasty: A Safe Adjunct to Rotator Cuff Repair. Arthroscopy. 2018;34(3):771–80.

16. Beeler S, Hasler A, Götschi T, Meyer DC, Gerber C. The Critical Shoulder Angle: Acromial Coverage is More Relevant than Glenoid Inclination. J Orthop Res. 2018. https://doi.org/10.1002/jor.24053.

17. Garcia GH, Liu JN, Degen RM, Johnson CC, Wong A, Dines DM, Gulotta LW, Dines JS. Higher critical shoulder angle increases the risk of retear after rotator cuff repair. J Shoulder Elbow Surg. 2016;26(2):241–5.

18. Hong L, Chen Y, Chen J, Hua Y, Chen S. Large Critical Shoulder Angle Has Higher Risk of Tendon Retear After Arthroscopic Rotator Cuff Repair. Am J Sport Med. 2018;46(8):1892–900.

21

3D Markerless asymmetry analysis in the management of adolescent idiopathic scoliosis

Maliheh Ghaneei[1]* (iD), Amin Komeili[2], Yong Li[1], Eric C. Parent[3] and Samer Adeeb[1]

Abstract

Background: Three dimensional (3D) markerless asymmetry analysis was developed to assess and monitor the scoliotic curve. While the developed surface topography (ST) indices demonstrated a strong correlation with the *Cobb angle* and its change over time, it was reported that the method requires an expert for monitoring the procedure to prevent misclassification for some patients. Therefore, this study aimed at improving the user-independence level of the previously developed 3D markerless asymmetry analysis implementing a new asymmetry threshold without compromising its accuracy in identifying the progressive scoliotic curves.

Methods: A retrospective study was conducted on 128 patients with Adolescent Idiopathic Scoliosis (AIS), with baseline and follow-up radiograph and surface topography assessments. The suggested "cut point" which was used to separate the deformed surfaces of the torso from the undeformed regions, automatically generated deviation patches corresponding to scoliotic curves for all analyzed surface topography scans.

Results: By changing the "cut point" in the asymmetry analysis for monitoring scoliotic curves progression, the sensitivity for identifying curve progression was increased from 68 to 75%, while the specificity was decreased from 74 to 59%, compared with the original method with different "cut point".

Conclusions: These results lead to a more conservative approach in monitoring of scoliotic curves in clinical applications; smaller number of radiographs would be saved, however the risk of having non-measured curves with progression would be decreased.

Keywords: Scoliosis, Surface topography, 3D markerless asymmetry analysis, Monitoring, Curve progression

Background

Adolescent idiopathic scoliosis (AIS) is the most common form of three-dimensional (3D) spinal deformity. It affects 2–4% of the population, predominantly females [1]. The AIS spine deformity progresses rapidly during the adolescent growth period, resulting in a need for frequent follow-ups [2]. The gold standard for assessing the spine curve is measuring the *Cobb angle* on the full torso radiograph, defined as the angle between the two most tilted vertebrae in each curve [3].

The conventional monitoring of the scoliosis using the *Cobb Angle* has limitations recognized in the literature.

Firstly, the measurement is limited to 2D posterior-anterior radiographs, and thus the method fails to address the 3D characteristics of AIS [4]. In addition, the use of radiographs in scoliosis clinics has several pitfalls of growing concern, such as excessive X-ray radiation exposure, with their associated risk of developing cancers [5–9], and the contra-indication of radiograph acquisitions for pregnant women.

Surface topography (ST) was introduced as a new approach to improve the monitoring of the scoliosis [5, 10–12]. ST is a method for which non-invasive visible light is used for scanning the torso surface in order to assess cosmetic deformities often based on some landmarks placed on the patient's torso by trained clinicians and using related indices based on the coordinates of the landmarks with respect to each other and the

* Correspondence: ghaneei@ualberta.ca
[1]Department of Civil and Environmental Engineering, Donadeo-ICE, University of Alberta, 9203 116th St, Edmonton, AB T6G 1R1, Canada
Full list of author information is available at the end of the article

geometric properties of transverse cross section of the torso, such as the cosmetic score and Quantec spinal angle [13–17]. Measurements based on ST could possibly be used effectively in combination with the radiographs to decrease the radiation dose and risk of cancer resulting from the multiple X-ray acquisitions. At this point, the ST approach is by no means designed to fully replace the gold-standard radiograph measurements, because it is subject to validation with the radiograph measurements. Nevertheless, the development of accurate ST methods has significantly contributed to the management of scoliosis [12].

On the other hand, marker placements can be associated with human errors in collecting the raw data [14] and such methods fail to take into account the whole torso geometry in the analysis. In contrast, our team has developed a novel markerless ST asymmetry analysis approach, which is independent of human interactions, and considers the full 3D torso surface for the analysis [12]. This technique provides a deviation contour map

that visualizes the areas affected by AIS corresponding to the location of each curve, called deviation patch [12]. These patches are isolated to calculate ST parameters for such deviations. The method demonstrated the potential for reducing 44% of radiograph exposure in the monitoring of scoliosis [15].

In the study presented by Komeili et al. [12], areas with deviation less than 3 mm were considered normal while greater deviations were considered as a deformation and separated the deviation patches for further analysis. Further application of this proposed ST asymmetry analysis in over 250 AIS patients illustrated that in 30 cases the method failed to either locate the curve properly or to correlate to the corresponding scoliotic curve, and led to misclassification of the AIS severity or progression. For example, in the ST analysis of some patients with a double scoliotic curve, a single isolated deviation patch encompassed the entire back torso (see Fig. 1), and therefore did not reflect the double scoliotic

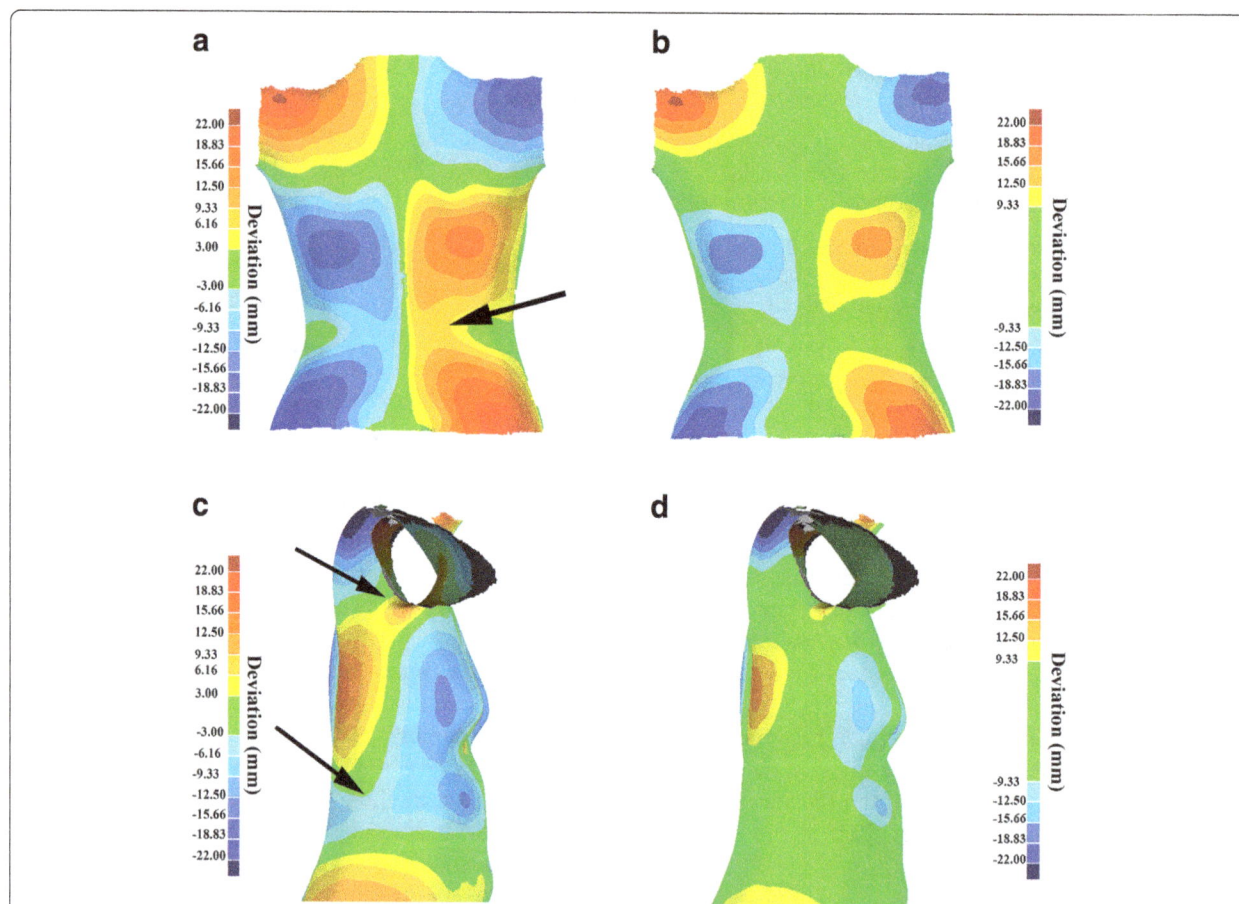

Fig. 1 a, c the deviation patches of two torsos analyzed by Komeili et al. [12], in which the 3 mm deviation was defined as the threshold between normal and deformed area, and b, d the deviation patches of the same torsos analyzed by the modified ST analysis proposed in this study with the threshold of 9.33 mm. The arrows point to the artifacts in deviation patches, such as continuous deviation patches on the back and side of the torso and deviation patches due to the folded skin near the armpits, which were resolved after using the suggested modifications in this study. The green regions of the torso are considered normal. The blue and red patches represent abnormal protruded and indented regions of the torso, respectively, due to the scoliosis condition curve in the corresponding radiograph. In some other cases, the deviation patch extended to the anterior part of the torso due to the asymmetry introduced by the breasts or axial rotation of the torso. Folded skin near the armpits and waist also introduced artifact in the ST analysis. The reasons for such lack of correspondence between the surface and the radiographic results were traced to the patch isolating stage where 3 mm was used as a "cut point". So far, these cases have been manually handled case by case by a scoliosis professional, which can introduce human errors in the measurements and decrease the correlation between the ST parameters and radiograph measurements.

This study aimed to eliminate patch overlaps by enhancing the patch isolation procedure, and to increase the accuracy of the analysis in identifying patients where we could prevent unnecessary X-ray exposure (mild patients and those who did not experience any progression from the last visit). Our hypothesis is that the modifications suggested in this study would isolate the deviation patches without compromising the accuracy of the method in monitoring the scoliotic curve severity or progression.

Method

Data collection

Full-torso surface topography scans of 128 AIS patients were collected from the Edmonton Scoliosis Clinic database between October 2009 and 2012. In the cohort, 95 patients (76 females, 19 males) had both baseline and follow-up ST and radiograph scans obtained with an interval of 12 ± 3 months. The inclusion criteria used were patients aged 10 to 18 years old (14.4 ± 1.8 years), with *Cobb angle* greater than 10° ($26.5° \pm 11.4°$) at baseline, with no spine operation.

To develop a classification tree in order to identify the curve severity, 128 baseline radiograph and ST scans were used. In this sample, 99 thoracic-thoracolumbar

(T-TL) curves and 98 lumbar (L) curves were measured, with double curves accounting for more curves than the number of patients.

To predict the progression of the scoliotic curve, a sample of 95 ST and radiograph scans with corresponding follow-up scans were used, in which the progression of 134 curves in total were analyzed. The data sets were randomly divided into two groups (i.e., the Training group and the Validation group) using common data splitting rules (80/20) [16] as illustrated in Fig. 2. The Training group included 80% of curves and was used in the derivation of the classification tree, whereas the validation group included the other 20% of curves and was used to examine the validity of the obtained classification tree.

Asymmetry analysis

The ST and radiograph scans were taken on the same day for each patient. The ST data was collected as described previously [12]. Briefly, four VIVID 910 3D laser scanners (KONICA MINOLTA Sensing Inc.) scanned the geometry of the patient's torso from each side, while the patient was positioned inside a custom designed frame with the torso in its natural posture. The accuracy of the scanning system was 1.8 ± 0.9 mm [17]. The outputs of scanners were four binary files including the spatial locations (i.e., x, y, z coordinates) of the torso surface, and they were imported as inputs to the Geomagic Control software (3D System Corporation, CA, USA) to be merged for the whole torso. Unneeded parts of the scan, namely those for the frame, the head, pants, and arms, were cropped off to isolate the torso [12]. After smoothing the scanning noises, the asymmetry analysis was performed on the torso. The torso was duplicated and reflected along the sagittal plane. Then, the torso and its reflection were aligned by minimizing the sum of squares of distances between these two geometries [18]. The misalignment between the torso and its reflection,

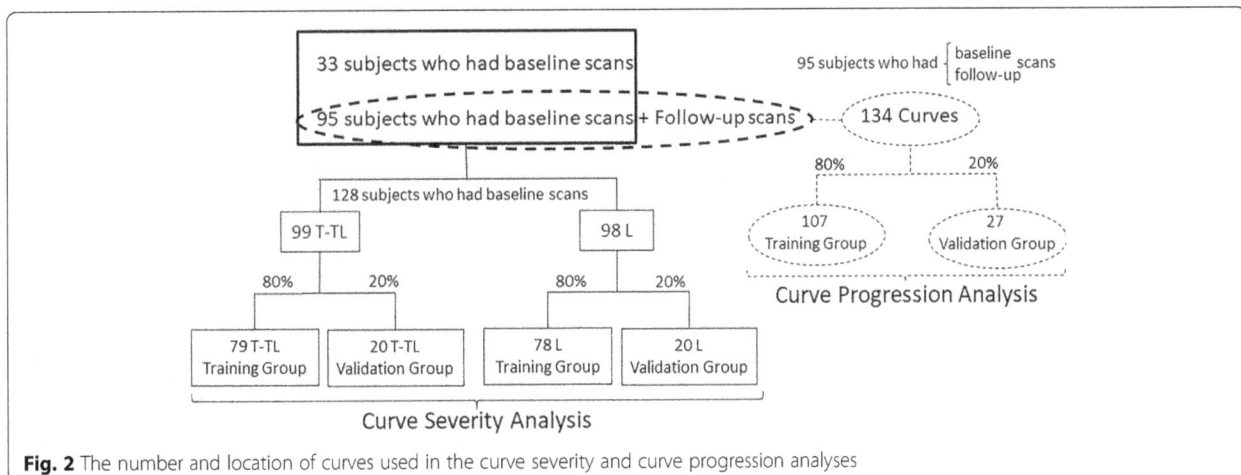

Fig. 2 The number and location of curves used in the curve severity and curve progression analyses

resulting from the asymmetry shape of the torso, was measured using the 3D Comparison function and visualized using the contour plot in the Geomagic Control software. In our earlier study [12], the threshold between normal and abnormal deviations was set to 3.0 mm. However, in this study, the threshold, beyond which the asymmetry of the torso was considered scoliotic deformation, was varied from 3 to 10 mm with a 0.33 mm step until the isolated patches matched the curves observed in the radiographs by the clinicians in all subjects. The optimum cut point, which defined the minimum deviation as a scoliotic deformation and avoided patch overlap, was found to be 9.33 mm (Fig. 1). This modification was applied only if the ST scan had a maximum deviation greater than 9.33 mm, otherwise the threshold of 3 mm was used as suggested by Komeili et al. [13, 19]. To measure the ST parameters, the scoliosis deformations were isolated from the other regions creating deformity patches. The macro, that was used by Komeili et al. [12], was modified to isolate the asymmetry patches from the other areas in the deviation contour map in Wolfram Mathematica (Wolfram Research, Inc., Mathematica 8.0.4.0). The process of isolating a deviation patch was as follows:

Step 1- Identify the point with the maximum absolute deviation in the cloud of points and set it as the centre point of a sphere with a radius of 5 mm.

Step 2- Collect all points inside the sphere with the deviation greater than 9.33 mm (the optimum cut point) and include them in the isolated deviation patch.

Step 3- Consider each selected point as the centre of a new sphere.

Step 4- Repeat Step 2 and 3 to progressively expand the boundary of deviation patch.

The maximum deviation (*MaxDev*) used in step 1 and the root mean square (*RMS*) of deviation patches were calculated, respectively, with the following equations:

$$MaxDev = Max(|Deviation_i|) \quad i = 1, 2, 3, ..., n$$

$$RMS = \sqrt{\frac{\sum_{i=1}^{n}(Deviation_i^2)}{n}} \quad i = 1, 2, 3, ..., n$$

where, *n* is the number of points representing the torso shape included in a given patch.

Figure 1 shows a contour-plot comparison between the deviation patches of a torso analyzed by Komeili et al. [12] (cut point 3.0 mm) and the deviation patches of the same torso analyzed by the modified ST analysis in this study (cut point 9.33 mm). In the contour plot shown in Fig. 1b, the green represents the area with

deviation smaller than 9.33 mm, and shades of blue/red (referred to as deviation patches) indicate the area that protruded/sunken more than 9.33 mm, respectively. The patient's torso in an ST scan was divided into two parts, namely the lower one-third part was considered the lumbar area (L) and the upper two-third was considered the thoracic / thoraco-lumbar area (T-TL). The asymmetry parameters were assigned to each section, accordingly. The same procedure was repeated for the follow-up ST scans to calculate the progression of *RMS* and *MaxDev*, i.e. *ΔRMS* and *ΔMaxDev*. From the corresponding radiographs, progressions of *Cobb angles* (*ΔCA*) were retrieved from the clinical database. During each patient clinic visit, *Cobb angles* are measured by the clinician and entered in the clinic database along with the end vertebra level and the apex for each curve.

Based on the *Cobb angle*, curve severity is classified into three groups in clinical practice: mild ($10° \leq Cobb$ $angle \leq 25°$), moderate ($25° < Cobb$ $angle \leq 40°$), and severe ($40° > Cobb$ $angle$) [20]. An increase of 5° or more in the *Cobb angle* during consecutive follow-up visits is recognized as a curve progression [21].

Classification analysis

The classification tree technique implemented in IBM SPSS Statistics 24.0 was employed to build a classification model, using the asymmetry parameters (referred to as independent variables) to classify the curve severity (dependent variable i.e., Mild or Moderate/Severe). On purpose, the criteria in the development of classification tree used in this study placed more weight for the false negative error in the cost function of the classification tree analysis. The underlying rationale for this preference was to prevent classification of moderate or severe scoliotic curves in the mild group as much as possible, which could lead to a late diagnosis or an ineffective treatment of the scoliotic curve in the clinical application.

A separate tree was developed to classify progression (i.e., Progression or Non-progression) of the radiographic curve measurement (dependent variable). Note that the deviation patches in the T-TL and L sections were analyzed together to build the classification tree for categorizing the progression of torso asymmetry. The underlying motivation was the fact that, if a curve progression is predicted by a classification system for a patient, a full vertebra radiograph scan is required regardless of its location and severity.

The classification analysis results were reported in the "Results" section including the tabulated results to show the accuracy, sensitivity, and specificity [19]. In the curve severity prediction, a positive test represents a moderate/severe curve and a negative test represents a mild severity. In the curve progression classification, a positive test represents the curve progression of 5° or more and a negative test represents any curve progression less than 5° (Non-progression).

The classification analysis mentioned above was conducted using the Training group. The obtained classification tree was used to classify the subjects in the Validation group. The resulting accuracy, sensitivity, and specificity of the classification for the Training and Validation groups were compared to assess the validity of the method.

Results

Curve severity classification
None of patients were excluded from the analysis. Figure 3 shows the severity classification trees for T-TL and L curves with the performance indices for the Training and Validation samples. Based on the statistical analysis, the *RMS* was a better independent variable (i.e., predictor) to be used in the classification of T-TL curves, i.e. deviation patches with *RMS* greater than 11 mm in the T-TL section represented a moderate/severe curve regardless of their *MaxDev* value. While the combination of *RMS* and *MaxDev* worked well for identifying the severity of L curves; a deviation patch with *RMS* < 9.6 mm and *MaxDev* < 9.6 mm represented a Mild curve in the L section, otherwise it represented a moderate/severe curve.

Out of 79 T-TL curves in the Training group, there were 35 curves with clinically moderate/severe curves, 34 of which were correctly identified with a sensitivity of 97%. Half of 44 mild curves were correctly classified in the mild group with a specificity of 50%. The majority of

patients (22 out of 23), who were classified in the mild T-TL group based on their deviation patches, had truly a *Cobb angle* less than 25° in the corresponding radiographs, resulting in false negative error of only 3%. The overall accuracy of the T-TL curve severity prediction was 71%. The classification of the 20 T-TL curves in the Validation group resulted in similar accuracy and sensitivity, with a maximum difference of ±7%, with respect to the Training group. No moderate/severe thoracic curves were misclassified by the ST analysis in the Validation sample.

In the Training group of 78 deviation patches analyzed for the L section, 39 (50%) had moderate/severe curves based on the *Cobb angle* measurements in radiographs. The ST analysis successfully identified 35 of them in the moderate/severe group, resulting in a sensitivity of 90%. The mild L curves were correctly identified in 31% of cases but only 4 of 39 (11%) moderate/severe curves were missed by the ST analysis. The overall accuracy of the ST analysis in classifying curve severity in the L section was 60%. The classification of the 20 L curves in the Validation group also resulted in the same level of accuracy and sensitivity compared with the Training group. Only one (10%) moderate/severe lumbar curve in the Validation group was misclassified by ST as mild.

Figure 4 shows the distribution of *RMS* and *MaxDev* of 79 T-TL and 78 L deviation patches and the thresholds for defining the severity of the curves in the Training group. The ST patches with *MaxDev* less than 9.33 mm were used in the Komeili et al. [12] classification tree to determine the severity of these deviation

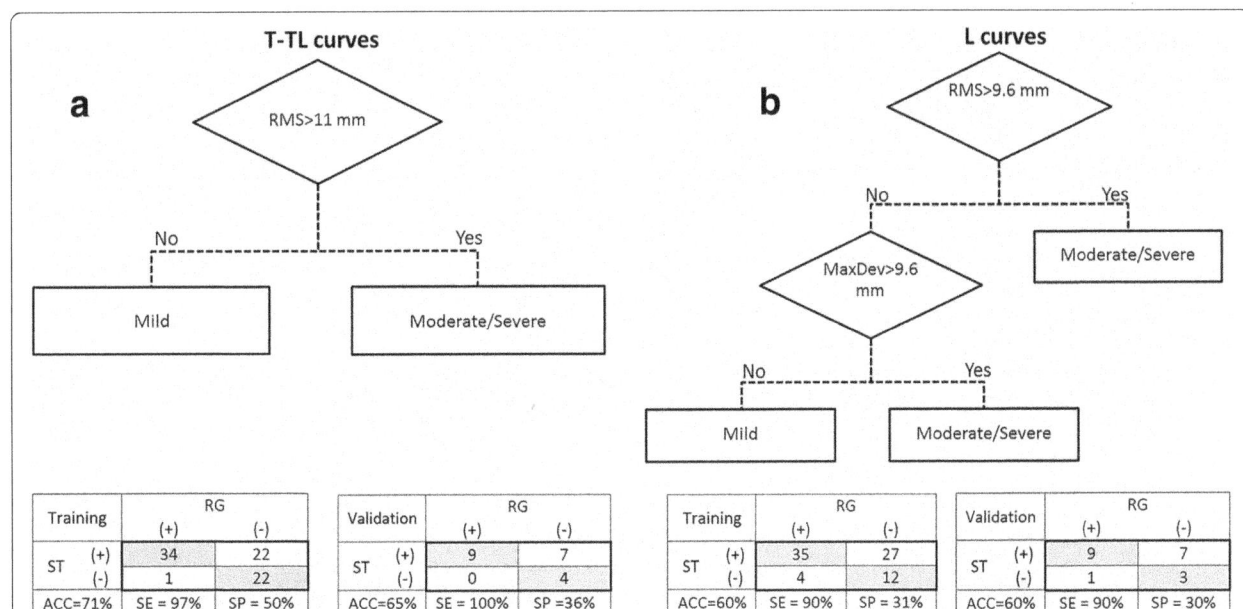

Fig. 3 The classification trees and the tabulated accuracy (ACC), sensitivity (SE), and specificity (SP) values for the curve severity classification of (**a**) T-TL curves and (**b**) L curves. The (+) and (−) illustrate the moderate/severe and mild groups, respectively. RG: radiograph, ST: surface topography

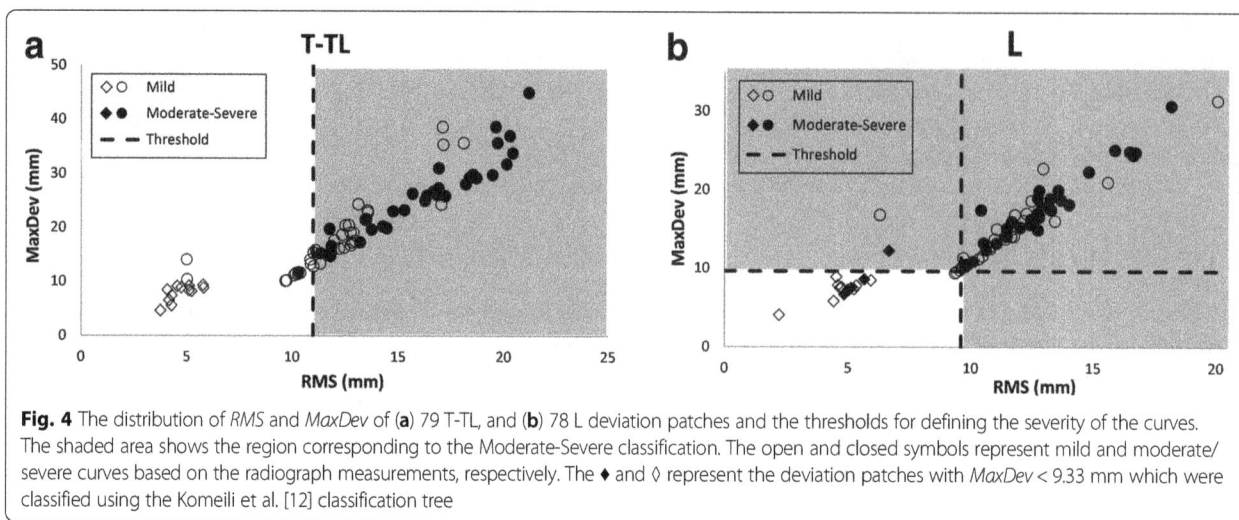

Fig. 4 The distribution of *RMS* and *MaxDev* of (**a**) 79 T-TL, and (**b**) 78 L deviation patches and the thresholds for defining the severity of the curves. The shaded area shows the region corresponding to the Moderate-Severe classification. The open and closed symbols represent mild and moderate/severe curves based on the radiograph measurements, respectively. The ◆ and ◊ represent the deviation patches with *MaxDev* < 9.33 mm which were classified using the Komeili et al. [12] classification tree

patches. Only one and four subjects with moderate/severe T-TL and L curves, respectively, were misclassified in the mild region, but their ST parameters were not far below the threshold.

The performance of the modified ST analysis in identifying the curve severity proposed in this study was compared with our previous work [19, 22] in Fig. 5a. The sensitivity in the prediction of curve severity was as high as the sensitivity in the work presented by Komeili et al. [22].

Curve progression prediction

Figure 6 shows the classification tree for the prediction of curve progression independent of the curve location, since the T-TL and L curves were mixed in the classification tree analysis. In the classification tree, a positive change of surface topography parameters between two consecutive visits correlated with more than 5° curve progression. In other word, if a curve has positive *MaxDev* and *RMS* changes in the

follow-up visit compared with the corresponding values in the baseline assessment, the curve is considered as progression and the patient needs radiography for further assessments. Out of 107 curves in the Training group, 22 curves increased at least by 5°, while there were no clinically important progressions for the other 85 curves. Based on the analysis, 17 out of 22 curves were accurately identified in the progression group (i.e., sensitivity 77%). Five (22%) of the cases with curve progression were missed. The percentage of the non-progressive curves that were detected by the asymmetry analysis was 59%. The diagnostic accuracy was 63%. The classification of deviation patches in the Validation group also resulted in an accuracy of 63% with a sensitivity of 67%, which are close to the corresponding values for the Training group. Figure 7 illustrates the variation of ST parameters in 107 deviation patches analyzed in baseline and follow-up visits, and the thresholds for identifying the scoliotic curves having progressed. There were four patients for whom both ST

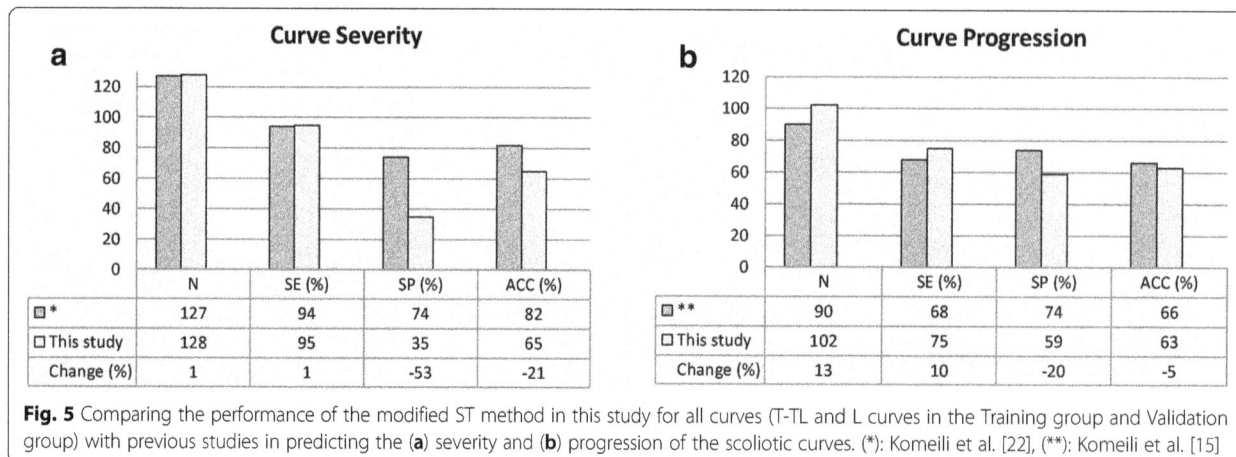

Fig. 5 Comparing the performance of the modified ST method in this study for all curves (T-TL and L curves in the Training group and Validation group) with previous studies in predicting the (**a**) severity and (**b**) progression of the scoliotic curves. (*): Komeili et al. [22], (**): Komeili et al. [15]

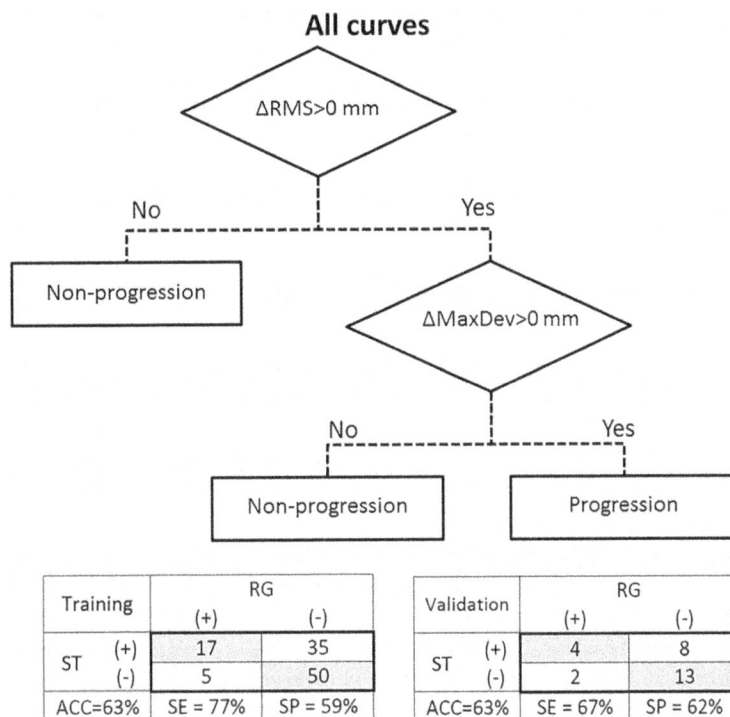

Fig. 6 The classification tree for categorizing patients in Progression and Non-progression groups using the Δ*RMS* and Δ*MaxDev* parameters. The (+) and (−) in the tables represent the Progression and Non-progression groups, respectively. ACC: accuracy, SE: sensitivity, SP: specificity, RG: radiograph, ST: surface topography

parameters improved, however their scoliotic curves progressed.

Compared with the sensitivity and accuracy obtained in Komeili et al. [15] study, the sensitivity of the ST method in monitoring curve progression in this study was improved by 10.3% (i.e., from 68 to 75%), while accuracy decreased by a relatively small percentage, 4.5%

(i.e., from 66% obtained in Komeili et al. [15] to 63%) (see Fig. 5b).

Discussion

The markerless asymmetry analysis developed previously [12] showed promising results in identifying curves with progression in the follow-up visits with the potential

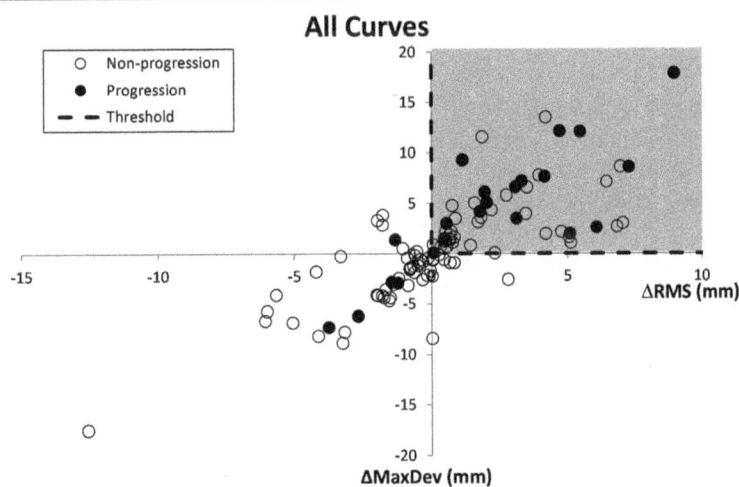

Fig. 7 The distribution of Δ*RMS* and Δ*MaxDev* parameters. The threshold of Δ*RMS* and Δ*MaxDev* are shown with the dashed lines. The shaded area shows the region that is considered as the Progression group. The close and open circles represent a progressed (Δ*CA* ≥ 5°) and Non-progressed (Δ*CA* < 5°) case based on the radiograph measurements, respectively

ability of reducing 44% of radiation exposure in the monitoring of AIS. The research presented in this study aimed at modifying the markerless asymmetry analysis by simplifying the application of the previously developed method while also improving the sensitivity and accuracy of the prediction in identifying the moderate/severe curves and the progression of the scoliotic curve. While the need for manual handling of deviation patches was resolved and the sensitivity in identifying the progressed curves improved by 10%, the overall accuracy of the method decreased by 5%. As a result, the applied modifications on the original method resulted in more conservative monitoring and curve severity assessment of scoliosis where fewer cases of moderate/severe curves and progression cases were missed (see Fig. 5).

In this study, the optimum threshold of deviation for isolating the deviation patches was found to be 9.33 mm. The isolated deviation patches were generally smaller in size than those obtained in Komeili et al. [13, 19] (see Fig. 1). The modified code successfully prevented the extensions of isolated deviation patch to the anterior section of the torso and around the armpits, and clearly separated the boundaries between the deviation patches in ST scans of patients with a double or triple scoliotic curves shown in Fig. 1. Moreover, we expect that the reliability of the method in repeating the analysis would increase by automating the patch isolation step and avoiding human intervention in the ST analysis process.

Accuracies of 65 and 60% were obtained in categorizing the severity of T-TL and L curves in the Validation cohort, respectively as show in Fig. 3. This level of accuracy was approximately the same as the accuracy obtained for the Training group, indicating repeatability of the classification model in the prediction of T-TL curves severity.

The distribution of MaxDev and RMS parameters of subjects in the Training group in Fig. 4 illustrated that the correlation of ST parameters with the curve severity in the T-TL region was better than in the L region, which is because of the fact that the soft tissue in the L area dampens the deformation of the vertebrae and might soften the effect of the curve in the surface of the torso, while for T-TL curves, the curvature of the vertebrae is transferred to the back surface of the torso through the rib cage and results in prominent deformation [16]. All ST scans with MaxDev less than 9.33 mm in Fig. 4, which were denoted by ◊ or ◆, had Cobb angle less than 15 degrees and were correctly classified using the original method developed by Komeili et al. [12].

The monitoring of T-TL and L curves progression were analyzed separately (results are not shown) and no difference in the sensitivity, specificity, and accuracy was obtained if T-TL and L curves were analyzed in one

group. Therefore, for the monitoring of scoliotic curve, T-TL and L curves were mixed and analyzed using only one classification tree which is likely more practical clinically (Fig. 6). The variation of ST parameters in this study was correlated with the progression of the Cobb angle measured in radiographs with a sensitivity of 67% for the Validation group in Fig. 6. However, some negative changes in ΔRMS and ΔMaxDev were obtained for patients with a positive ΔCA in Fig. 7. The proposed threshold of 9.33 mm for isolating the deviation patches in this study resulted in smaller accuracy and specificity in monitoring curve progression specifically for patients with mild and moderate curves in the baseline. Excluding areas with the deviation less than 9.33 mm from the deviation patches provided less information about the torso shape for monitoring the deformities over time. Therefore, any change in the areas with the deviation less than 9.33 mm over time was not included in the analysis, which led to the misclassification of multiple curves especially in the patients with moderate scoliotic curves, where relatively small portion of torso had deviations greater than 9.33 mm (see Fig. 7). Our results showed that curve progression monitoring appears to be 100% (4/4) accurate for patients with severe scoliotic curve in baseline who progressed in the follow-up scans (tabulated results are not shown). Therefore, monitoring mild and moderate scoliotic curves that present smaller asymmetry on the torso surface with respect to the severe curves, using the modified asymmetry analysis method in this study involves a higher risk of false positive. The case-by-case investigation of patients who were incorrectly identified in the Progression group (false positive) showed that 55% of the population had truly a larger Cobb angle in the follow-up radiographs compared to the baseline. However, the positive increase of Cobb angle was not significant enough to be considered as a progression, i.e., ΔCA in the range of 0–5 degrees. Although a follow-up radiograph is not necessary for this group of patients, considering the error in Cobb angle measurements and the small degree of progression in many of the participants might sufficiently justify taking a radiograph in the follow-up.

The overall sensitivities in identifying curve severity in this study were similar to the corresponding values in Komeili et al. [22], 95 and 94%, respectively (Fig. 5). The reduction in the overall accuracy (i.e. 82 to 65%) in identifying the severity of the curve using ST parameters in this study with respect to Komeili et al. [22] was caused by a larger false positive error rather than false negative error, i.e. classifying a considerable number of the deviation patches of patients with mild scoliotic curves in the moderate/severe group. One third of the misclassified mild curves had a Cobb angle in the range of 20–25 degrees, which is on the margin of the mild-moderate severity definition used in the scoliosis clinic. It should be noted that, there is a ±5° inter- and intra-observer error in the measurements of *Cobb angle* [23, 24], therefore there is a possibility that some of the misclassified mild curves with *Cobb angle* in the range of 20–25 degrees could have been diagnosed as moderate if the radiograph assessment had been repeated.

The overall sensitivity of 95% in Fig. 5 indicates a high ability to detect moderate/severe curves which are more susceptible to progress than mild curves and thus do require further attention. Taking full torso radiograph in the follow-up visits is the standard for all patients at the scoliosis clinics, hence, subjects whose classification was false positive would not get more radiographs than others without ST assessment, and we would still prevent radiograph exposure for some truly negative cases. Komeili et al. [15] reported a predicted 44% reduction in the radiograph acquisition if they combined the ST analysis with the radiograph assessment in the monitoring of curve progression. Because of the slightly lower accuracy observed in this study in screening for curve progression, we estimate a 5% lower reduction of the need for radiograph compared with the work of Komeili et al. [15]. Nevertheless, the asymmetry analysis improvements suggested in this study would result to a more conservative monitoring. Because of the higher sensitivity obtained (Fig. 5b) a lower number of patients would suffer from missing the opportunity of an early diagnosis of curve progression by using our improved ST analysis.

We had enough data for statistical analyses, however we have to acknowledge that only 39 patients in the Training group had curve progression, which may not represent the diversity of scoliotic curve types, such as single and double curves. Another limitation of our study is exclusion of trunk axial rotation in our predictions, which is an important piece of information for clinicians in prescribing patient specific braces. It may be possible to improve the accuracy of curve progression diagnosis if more ST parameters, such as curvature of back valley [25] and trunk rotation [26], were combined with the *RMS* and *MaxDev* parameters included in this study. The strong correlation between deviation patches and spinal curve location can also provide good information about the kyphosis and lordosis angles obtained from radiographs, which, however, may not be necessary if the proposed method is used only in scoliosis cases clinics. Our asymmetry analysis is compatible with the ST database of those clinics that do not use the same acquisition system in capturing the full torso geometry as we do. The markerless feature of the asymmetry analysis reduced the common limitations of ST methods, such as dependency of the method to specific local marker-based measurements, and data acquisition technique. Having the 3D geometry of the torso, in normal posture, is the only required condition for using this method. Our strategy in classifying curve severity and curve progression could also be followed in other ST classification systems, in which the cosmetic parameters of the torso are correlated to the scoliotic curve characteristics. Our conservative approach in minimizing the number of false progression and false moderate/severe in the classification system may result in a lower overall accuracy, however it would reduce the risk of missing a progressed or moderate/severe curve, which is the main concern in replacing radiographs with ST assessments in scoliosis clinics.

Conclusion

The modified thresholds used to define asymmetry patches successfully separated the deviation patches in the upper two-third (T-TL) section from the lower one-third part (Lumbar) section and eliminated the manual work, which was previously necessary for isolating the deviation patches in some patients. The modified thresholds used in this study, allow automation of the analysis and led to the same level of sensitivity in identifying the curve severity as in our previous work. Similarly, the modified analysis led to similar sensitivity for monitoring the progression of the scoliotic curve as our previous work. Despite the novel method being unfortunately associated with a higher risk of misclassification of cases with no progression, significant numbers of patients (approximately 39%) may be able to avoid radiographs confident that their curves did not progress.

Abbreviations
2D: Two Dimension; 3D: Three Dimension; ACC: Accuracy; AIS: Adolescent Idiopathic Scoliosis; L: Lumbar; MaxDev: Maximum deviation of the colour patch; RMS: Root Mean Square of distances between matched points; SE: Sensitivity; SP: Specificity; ST: Surface Topography; T-TL: Thoracic - Thoracolumbar; ΔCA: Change of *Cobb angle*; ΔMaxDev: Change in maximum deviation of the colour patch; ΔRMS: Change in root mean square of the colour patch deviation

Acknowledgements
Not applicable.

Funding
The authors gratefully acknowledge the financial support from the Scoliosis Research Society (SRS).

Authors' contributions
MG, AK, YL, ECP, SA have designed the study. MG analyzed and interpreted the patient data. All authors read and approved the final manuscript.

Authors' information
Maliheh Ghaneei was admitted as an M.Sc. student in the Department of Civil & Environmental Engineering, University of Alberta in 2016. Her current research interests include scoliosis, surface topography, and neural network.
Dr. Amin Komeili developed the original 3D asymmetry analysis of the torso in his PhD study. He published four journal papers with an emphasis on spine deformity and surface topography.

Dr. Yong Li, holding his Ph.D. degree in structural engineering and his M.A. degree in applied mathematics from UC San Diego, is active in research on probabilistic methods, statistical modeling & learning, reliability & risk analysis.

Dr. Eric Parent is Associate Professor of Physical Therapy, in the Faculty of Rehabilitation Science at University of Alberta. His physiotherapy and M.Sc. degrees were completed at Université Laval and his Ph.D. at University of Alberta.

Dr. Samer Adeeb finished his Ph.D. in Structural Engineering / Biomechanics and joined the Structures Group at the University of Alberta in 2007. His research is the study of the variation of the healthy anatomy of musculoskeletal components.

Competing interests

The authors declare that they have no competing interests.

Author details

[1]Department of Civil and Environmental Engineering, Donadeo-ICE, University of Alberta, 9203 116th St, Edmonton, AB T6G 1R1, Canada. [2]Faculty of Kinesiology, University of Calgary, Calgary, Canada. [3]Department of Physical Therapy, Faculty of Rehabilitation Medicine, University of Alberta, Edmonton, Canada.

References

1. Rogala EJ, Drummond DS, Gurr J. Scoliosis: incidence and natural history. A prospective epidemiological study. J Bone Joint Surg Am. 1978;60(2):173–6.
2. Roach JW, et al. Adolescent idiopathic scoliosis. Lancet. 2008;371(9623): 1527–37.
3. Cobb RJ. Outline for the study of scoliosis, Instructional Course Lectures. Am Acad Orthop Surg. 1948;5:261–75.
4. Thulbourne T, Gillespie R. The rib hump in idiopathic scoliosis. Measurement, analysis and response to treatment. J Bone Joint Surg (Br). 1976;58(1):64–71.
5. Ronckers CM, Doody MM, Lonstein JE, Stovall M, Land CE. Multiple diagnostic X-rays for spine deformities and risk of breast cancer. Cancer Epidemiol Biomark Prev. 2008;17(3):605–13.
6. Doody MM, Lonstein JE, Stovall M, Hacker DG, Luckyanov N, Land CE. Breast cancer mortality after diagnostic radiography: findings from the U.S. scoliosis cohort study. Spine (Phila Pa 1976). 2000;25(16):2052–63.
7. Hoffman DA, Lonstein JE, Morin MM, Visscher W, Harris BS 3rd, Boice JD Jr. Breast cancer in women with scoliosis exposed to multiple diagnostic x rays. J Natl Cancer Inst. 1989;81(17):1307–12.
8. Ronckers CM, Land CE, Miller JS, Stovall M, Lonstein JE, Doody MM. Cancer mortality among women frequently exposed to radiographic Examinations for Spinal Disorders. Radiat Res. 2010;174(1):83–90.
9. Nash CL, Gregg EC, Brown RH, Pillai K. Risks of exposure to X-rays in patients undergoing long-term treatment for scoliosis. J Bone Joint Surg. 1979;61(3):371–4.
10. Levy AR, Goldberg MS, Mayo NE, Hanley JA, Poitras B. Reducing the lifetime risk of cancer from spinal radiographs among people with adolescent idiopathic scoliosis. Spine (Phila Pa 1976). 1996;21(13):1540–7; discussion 1548.
11. Don S. Radiosensitivity of children: potential for overexposure in CR and DR and magnitude of doses in ordinary radiographic examinations. Pediatr Radiol. 2004;34 Suppl 3:S167–72; discussion S234–41.
12. Komeili A, Westover LM, Parent EC, Moreau M, El-Rich M, Adeeb S. Surface topography asymmetry maps categorizing external deformity in scoliosis. Spine J. 2014;14(6):973–983.e2.
13. Ajemba PO, Durdle NG, Raso VJ. Characterizing torso shape deformity in scoliosis using structured splines models. IEEE Trans Biomed Eng. 2009;56(6): 1652–62.
14. Lam GC, Hill DL, Le LH, Raso JV, Lou EH. Vertebral rotation measurement: a summary and comparison of common radiographic and CT methods. Scoliosis. 2008;3:16.
15. Komeili A, Westover L, Parent EC, El-Rich M, Adeeb S. Monitoring for idiopathic scoliosis curve progression using surface topography asymmetry analysis of the torso in adolescents. Spine J. 2015;15(4):743–51.
16. Giacomelli P. Apache Mahout Cookbook; 2013. p. 1–250.
17. Jaremko JL, et al. Estimation of spinal deformity in scoliosis from torso surface cross sections. Spine (Phila Pa 1976). 2001;26(14):1583–91.
18. Hill S, et al. Assessing asymmetry using reflection and rotoinversion in biomedical engineering applications. Proc Inst Mech Eng H. 2014;228(5): 523–9.
19. Zhou X-H, McClish DK, Obuchowski NA. Electronic Book Collection and Wiley InterScience (Online service). In: Statistical methods in diagnostic medicine. Hoboken: Wiley; 2011.
20. Hill DL, et al. Evaluation of a laser scanner for surface topography. Stud Health Technol Inform. 2002;88:90–4.
21. Soucacos PN, et al. Assessment of curve progression in idiopathic scoliosis. Eur Spine J. 1998;7(4):270–7.
22. Komeili A, Westover L, Parent EC, El-Rich M, Adeeb S. Correlation between a novel surface topography asymmetry analysis and radiographic data in scoliosis. Spine Deform. 2015;3(4):303–11.
23. Gross C, Gross M, Kuschner S. Error analysis of scoliosis curvature measurement. Bull Hosp Jt Dis Orthop Inst. 1983;43(2):171–7.
24. He J-W, et al. Accuracy and repeatability of a new method for measuring scoliosis curvature. Spine (Phila Pa 1976). 2009;34(9):E323–9.
25. Thériault J, Cheriet F, Guibault F. Automatic Detection of the Back Valley on Scoliotic Trunk Using Polygonal Surface Curvature. In: Image Analysis and Recognition. Berlin: Springer Berlin Heidelberg; 2008. p. 779–88.
26. Samuelsson L, Noren L. Trunk rotation in scoliosis. The influence of curve type and direction in 150 children. Acta Orthop Scand. 1997;68(3):273–6.

22

The head shaft angle is associated with hip displacement in children at GMFCS levels III-V - a population based study

L Finlayson[1], T Czuba[2], M S Gaston[3], G Hägglund[4*] (iD) and J E Robb[5]

Abstract

Background: An increased Head Shaft Angle (HSA) has been reported as a risk factor for hip displacement in children with cerebral palsy (CP) but opinions differ in the literature. The purpose of this study was to re-evaluate the relationship between HSA and hip displacement in a different population of children with CP.

Methods: The Cerebral Palsy Integrated Pathway Scotland surveillance programme includes 95% of all children with CP in Scotland. The pelvic radiographs from 640 children in GMFCS levels III-V were chosen. The most displaced hip was analysed and the radiographs used were those taken at the child's first registration in the database to avoid the potential effects of surveillance on subsequent hip centration. A logistic regression model was used with hip displacement (migration percentage [MP] ≥40%) as outcome and HSA, GMFCS, age and sex as covariates.

Results: The MP was ≥40% in 118 hips with a mean HSA of 164° (range 121–180°) and < 40% in 522 hips with a mean HSA of 160° (range 111–180°). The logistic regression analysis showed no significant influence of age and sex on MP in this population but a high GMFCS level was strongly associated with hip displacement. An increased HSA was also associated with hip displacement, a 10° difference in HSA for children adjusted for age, sex, and GMFCS gave an odds ratio of 1.26 for hip displacement equal or above 40% ($p = 0.009$) and hips with HSA above 164.5 degrees had an odds ratio of 1.96 compared with hips with HSA below 164.5 degrees ($p = 0.002$).

Conclusion: These findings confirm that HSA is associated with hip displacement in children in GMFCS levels III-V.

Keywords: Children, Cerebral palsy, Hip displacement, Head shaft angle

Background

For hip surveillance in cerebral palsy (CP) it is important to identify risk factors for hip displacement both for the treatment of the individual child and to optimise the monitoring programme. Young age and severe limitation of gross motor function as measured with the Gross Motor Function Classification System (GMFCS) are known risk factors.

The measurement of the head-shaft angle (HSA, Fig. 1) was popularised by Southwick [1] to measure the degree of slip in slipped upper femoral epiphysis. Foroohar et al. [2] evaluated the relationship between the femoral shaft and head in children with cerebral palsy (CP) and compared the HSA in children with CP with the HSA in

typically developing children. They also evaluated the HSA in children with CP who had significant hip displacement. They concluded that the HSA was greater in children with CP and more pronounced in those at risk for displacement and that the evaluation of HSA may be prudent in children with CP.

Lee et al. [3] analysed HSA, Migration Percentage (MP) and the neck-shaft angle (NSA) in 384 patients with CP. They found a higher correlation between NSA and MP than between HSA and MP and concluded that the NSA appeared to be more clinically relevant than the HSA in evaluating proximal femoral deformity in patients with CP. However, the material included children up to 17 years of age some of whom did not have a well demarcated growth plate, making HSA measurement less reliable. Subsequently, van der List et al. [4] reported from a retrospective study that the HSA decreased over

* Correspondence: gunnar.hagglund@med.lu.se
[4]Lund University Department of Clinical Sciences, Orthopedics, Lund, Sweden
Full list of author information is available at the end of the article

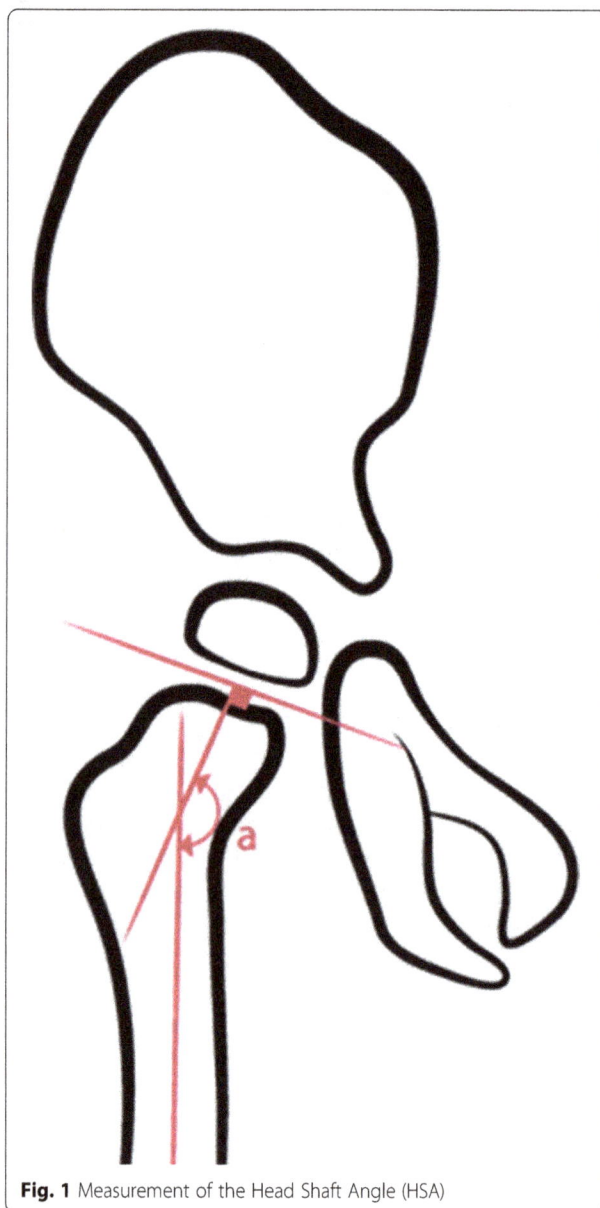

Fig. 1 Measurement of the Head Shaft Angle (HSA)

time in normal hips and children in GMFCS levels II-III but not in GMFCS levels IV-V, the two groups most at risk of developing hip subluxation. In the same year, van der List et al. [5] concluded from a retrospective cohort that, at age two years, the GMFCS and HSA were valuable predictors for hip displacement, but at the age of four years, only the MP should be used in the prediction of hip displacement. These studies seemed to confirm that the HSA was higher in GMFCS IV-V children at least up to the age of two years, but that the effect of age on the HSA as a predictor of hip displacement was less clear.

Hermanson et al. [6] reported on a total population of children with CP in a defined geographical area followed up for five years or until the development of a MP $\geq$ 40% of either hip within five years. The use of MP 40% as cut

off was chosen as hips with MP $\geq$ 40 have a high risk for further displacement, indicating the need for surgical intervention [7]. They concluded that a high HSA was a risk factor for hip displacement in children with CP. However, in 2016 Chougule et al. [[8] reported no statistically significant correlation between HSA and hip migration in children with CP aged 3–18 years in GMFCS levels III-V.

These seemingly contradictory reports on the relationship between the HSA, age and GMFCS as a risk factor for hip displacement prompted the present study from another defined population of children with CP. The Cerebral Palsy Integrated Pathway Scotland (CPIPS) surveillance programme includes 95% of all children with CP in Scotland. We have used radiographs from this total population to analyse the effect of HSA on hip displacement defined as MP $\geq$ 40%.

Methods

Radiological data from all children in GMFCS levels III-V was used in the analysis. Children receive a pelvic radiograph on first registration in the programme. This is taken in a standardised position which is used across Scotland [9]. Subsequent radiographs are taken according to a protocol based on age and GMFCS. In this study all radiographs taken at first registration into the programme of children in GMFCS levels III-V were used for analysis to avoid potential effects of surveillance on subsequent hip centration. Radiographs showing femoral osteotomy before inclusion in the programme were excluded. Hips were defined as displaced if the MP was $\geq$40%. The most displaced hip from each child was analysed. The HSA for all radiographs were measured by one observer (LF). The MP for the index radiograph had been previously been recorded in the database by clinicians responsible for the individual care of the children.

Two logistic regression models were used with hip displacement (MP $\geq$40%) as the outcome. In the first model the following covariates were used: HSA and age (both continuous), GMFCS (categorical, level III as reference), sex (categorical, female as reference). For the second model a ROC curve analysis between HSA and MP $\geq$40% was done. The ideal cut-off point was selected as the point that maximizes the product of specificity and sensitivity. HSA was dichotomised according to the ideal cutoff point and in the second model the HSA was analysed as a categorical covariate related to this cutoff value. The other covariates were similar to the first model.

The statistical analyses were performed using STATA 13 software.

Results

There were 640 children with a mean age of 8.2 years (range 0–19 years, 271 female and 369 male) fulfilling the inclusion criteria (Fig. 2). Their distribution by GMFCS

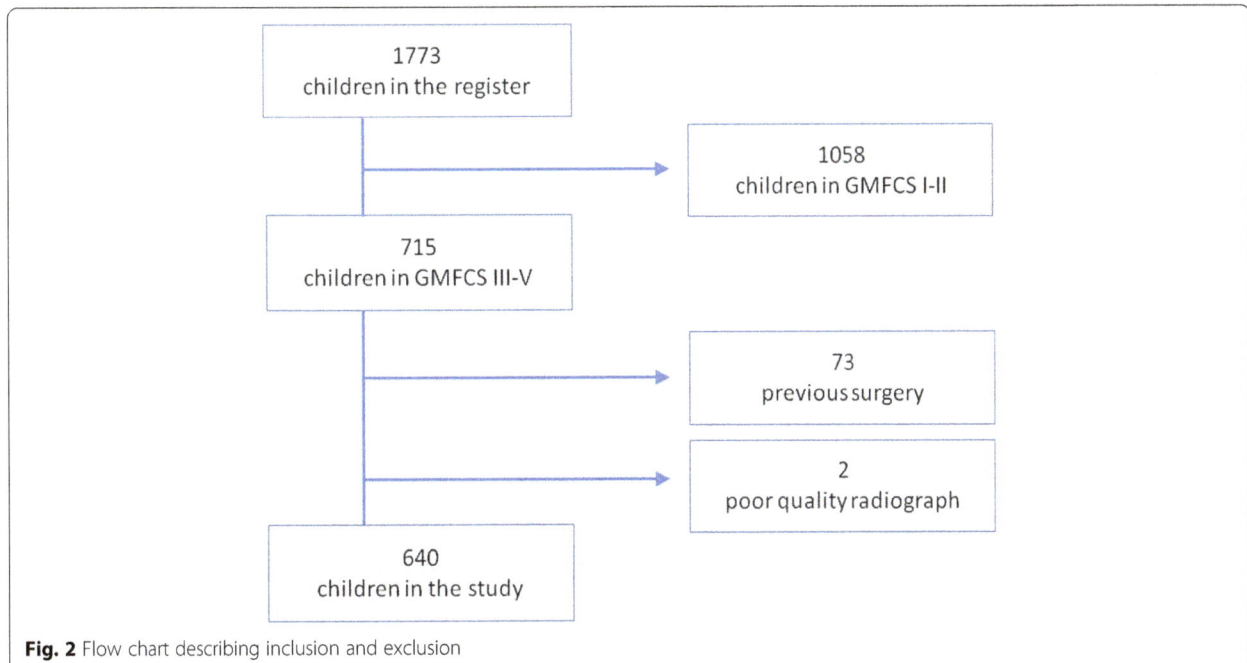

Fig. 2 Flow chart describing inclusion and exclusion

level was as follows: III - 160, IV - 184 and V - 296. One hundred and eighteen hips had a MP ≥40% in which the mean HSA was 164° (range 121–180°). Five hundred and twenty two hips with a MP < 40% had a mean HSA of 160° (range 111–180°). The first logistic regression analysis using HSA as a continuous variable showed no influence of age and sex had on MP but a high GMFCS level was strongly associated with hip displacement (Table 1). HSA was also statistically significantly associated with hip displacement. A 10° difference in HSA for patients adjusted for age, sex, and GMFCS gave an odds ratio of 1.26 for hip displacement to a MP $\geq$ 40% (p = 0.009) (Table 1). The ROC curve analysis between HSA and MP ≥40% showed that the ideal cutoff point was HSA =164,5 degrees. The second logistic regression analysis showed that HSA above 164.5 degrees had an odds ratio of 1.96 for MP ≥40% (Table 2).

Discussion

This study has confirmed Hermanson et al's [6] findings that a high HSA is a risk factor for hip displacement in children with CP. Both studies used defined populations of children with CP and thus probably avoided selection biases. The present study does not give prospective information on HSA changes over time, unlike Hermanson et al's study, because radiological data was taken from radiographs at the time of first registration of children into the surveillance programme. It does, however, provide information on the HSA without the potentially confounding influence of surveillance on hip centration.

The findings of the present study differ from those of Chougule et al. [8] who reported no statistically significant correlation between HSA and hip migration in children with CP aged 3–18 years in GMFCS levels III-V. There are some differences between the two studies which may explain the respective conclusions. Chougule et al. [8] used a linear regression model in their statistical analysis and randomised hips by laterality in the study design. There is a floor and ceiling effect for MP at 0% and 100% that may limit the usefulness of linear regression analysis which is not seen with logistic regression, where a binary outcome of hip 'displaced' or 'not displaced' was used and set at MP ≥ 40%. Randomisation

Table 1 Logistic regression estimates on the effect of HSA, GMFCS-level and age on MP using HAS as continuous variable

	Odds Ratio	95% CI		P
HSA[a]	1.26	1.06	1.50	0.009
GMFCS IV	2.86	1.39	5.90	0.004
GMFCS V	4.17	2.13	8.16	0.000
Age[b]	1.03	0.99	1.08	0.174
Sex[c]	0.94	0.62	1.42	0.763

[a]degrees, [b]years, [c]female as reference

Table 2 Logistic regression estimates on the effect of HSA, GMFCS-level and age on MP with HSA dichotomized

	Odds Ratio	95% CI		P
HSA[a]	1.96	1.29	3.00	0.002
GMFCS IV	2.78	1.35	5.74	0.006
GMFCS V	3.98	2.03	7.80	0.000
Age[b]	1.03	0.99	1.08	0.134
Sex[c]	0.94	0.62	1.42	0.755

[a]HSA < 164,5 degrees as reference [b]years, [c]female as reference

by laterality may also dilute a study population of hips at risk for displacement. Children in higher GMFCS levels may have pelvic obliquity and the abducted hip would most probably have a MP within normal limits and the opposite, adducted, hip an abnormal MP. For this reason we analysed the most displaced hip in each child. Van der List et al. [5] used both hips in their analyses and also did a logistic regression analysis for displacement with MP ≥40%.

The present study does have limitations. A single observer measured the HSA in all 640 hips. Training in the measurement was given and, reassuringly, Hermanson et al. [10] have reported excellent observer reliability for HSA. The present study is based on the radiographs of children at the time of registration into the CPIPS programme and effects of time or intervention on hip centration or HSA were not considered. The results are only valid for the age range and range of HSA-angle in the material.

Conclusion

This study, which was based on a total CP population, has confirmed that HSA is associated with hip displacement in children in GMFCS levels III-V.

Abbreviations
CI: Confidence Interval; CP: Cerebral palsy; GMFCS: Gross Motor Function Classification Scale; HSA: Head Shaft Angle; MP: Migration Percentage; ROC: Receiver operation characteristic

Acknowledgements
We gratefully acknowledge the contributions of all clinicians who have or continue to provide data on their patients for CPIPS.

Funding
No funding was obtained for this study.

Authors' contributions
JER, MG and GH conceived the research question, MG the data collection, LF the radiographic measurements, and TC the statistical analyses. JER was the major contributor in writing the manuscript to which all authors also contributed. All authors have read and approved the final manuscript.

Competing interests
The authors declare that they have no competing interests.

Author details
[1]University of Edinburgh, Edinburgh, Scotland. [2]Epidemiology and Register Center South, Lund, Sweden. [3]Department of Orthopaedic Surgery, Royal Hospital for Sick Children, Edinburgh, Scotland. [4]Lund University Department of Clinical Sciences, Orthopedics, Lund, Sweden. [5]School of Medicine, University of St Andrews, St. Andrews, Scotland.

References
1. Southwick WO. Osteotomy of the lesser trochanter for slipped capital femoral epiphysis. J Bone Joint Surg Am. 1967;49A:803–35.
2. Foroohar A, McCarthy JJ, JJ YD, Clarke S, Brey J. Head-shaft angle measurement in children with cerebral palsy. J Pediatr Orthop. 2009;29:248–50.
3. Lee KM, Kang JY, Chung CY, Kwon DG, Lee SH, Choi IH, Cho TJ, Yoo WJ, Park MS. Clinical relevance of valgus deformity of proximal femur in cerebral palsy. J Pediatr Orthop. 2010;30:720–5.
4. van der List JP, Witbreuk MM, Buizer AI, van der Sluijs JA. The head–shaft angle of the hip in early childhood. A comparison of reference values for children with cerebral palsy and normally developing hips. Bone Joint J. 2015a;97B:1291–5.
5. van der List JP, Witbreuk MM, Buizer AI,van der Sluijs JA. The prognostic value of the head-shaft angle on hip displacement in children with cerebral palsy. J Child Orthop 2015b; 9:129–135.
6. Hermanson M, Hägglund G, Riad J, Wagner P. Head-shaft angle is a risk factor for hip displacement in children with cerebral palsy. Acta Orthop. 2015;86:229–32.
7. Hägglund G, Lauge-Pedersen H, Persson M. Radiographic threshold values for hip screening in cerebral palsy. J Child Orthop. 2007;1:43–7.
8. Chougule S, Dabis J, Petrie A, Daly K, Gelfer Y. Is head–shaft angle a valuable continuous risk factor for hip migration in cerebral palsy? J Child Orthop. 2016;10:651–6.
9. Kinch K, Campbell DM, Maclean JG, Read HS, Barker SL, Robb JE, Gaston MS. How critical is patient positioning in radiographic assessment of the hip in cerebral palsy when measuring migration percentage? J Pediatr Orthop. 2015;35:756–61.
10. Hermanson M, Hägglund G, Riad J, Rodby-Bousquest E. Inter- and intrarater reliability of the head-shaft angle in children with cerebral palsy. J Child Orthop. 2017;11:256–62.

23

Bicycling participation in people with a lower limb amputation: a scoping review

Jutamanee Poonsiri[1,3]* (iD), Rienk Dekker[1], Pieter U. Dijkstra[1,2], Juha M. Hijmans[1] and Jan H. B. Geertzen[1]

Abstract

Background: To review literature on bicycling participation, as well as facilitators and barriers for bicycling in people with a lower limb amputation (LLA).

Methods: Peer-reviewed, primary, full text, studies about bicycling in people with a LLA from midfoot level to hemipelvectomy were searched in Pubmed, Embase, Cinahl, Cochrane library, and Sportdiscus. No language or publication date restrictions were applied. Included full-text studies were assessed for methodological quality using the Effective Public Health Practice Project tool. Data were extracted, synthesized and reported following Preferred Reporting Items for Systematic Review.

Results: In total, 3144 papers were identified and 14 studies were included. The methodological quality of 13 studies was weak and 1 was moderate. Bicycling participation ranged from 4 to 48%. A shorter time span after LLA and a distal amputation were associated with a higher bicycling participation rate particularly for transportation. In people with a transtibial amputation, a correct prosthetic foot or crank length can reduce pedalling asymmetry during high-intensity bicycling. People with limitations in knee range of motion or skin abrasion can use a hinged crank arm or a low profile prosthetic socket respectively.

Conclusion: People with a LLA bicycled for transportation, recreation, sport and physical activity. Adaptation of prosthetic socket, pylon and foot as well as bicycle crank can affect pedalling work and force, range of motion, and aerodynamic drag. Because the suggestions from this review were drawn from evidences mostly associated to competition, prosthetists should carefully adapt the existing knowledge to clients who are recreational bicyclists.

Keywords: Bicycling, Lower limb, Amputation, Prosthesis, Motivation

Background

In general bicycling has a number of physiological [1–4] and psychosocial benefits [5, 6]. Bicycling can, for instance, lower the risk of non-communicable diseases such as cardiovascular disease [1–3] and type 2 diabetes [7, 8]. Bicycling is thought to improve quality of life [9, 10]. People with a lower limb amputation (LLA) can also experience these benefits [9–11]. In addition, an increase in muscle strength of the intact and amputated limb as a result of regular bicycling [12] resulting in better walking [13, 14]. It is for the above mentioned reasons that enhancing the ability to perform physical activity (PA) such as bicycling for people with a LLA is important.

Bicycling is a low-impact activity as most of the body weight is supported by the bicycle's seat, and consequently relieving the load on the residual limb in people with a LLA. But bicycling requires more degrees of flexion at the hip, knee and ankle than walking [15, 16] which could be limited by designs and functions of prosthetic components. Some reviews have been performed to gain information on barriers and facilitators in PA or sports participation in the group of physically disabled persons and people with a LLA, but not focusing on bicycling [17, 18]. One review provided a way to adapt prostheses and bicycles for bicyclists with a transtibial amputation (TTA), however, no information for other

* Correspondence: j.poonsiri@umcg.nl
[1]Department of Rehabilitation Medicine, University of Groningen, University Medical Center Groningen, CB41, PO Box 30001, 9700 RB Groningen, The Netherlands
[3]Sirindhorn School of Prosthetics and Orthotics, Faculty of Medicine Siriraj Hospital, Mahidol University, Bangkok, Thailand
Full list of author information is available at the end of the article

levels of LLA nor were participation rates reported [19]. Another review on bicycling for different amputation levels of lower and upper limbs included studies without people with a LLA and included studies with people cycling on ergometers [20]. These inclusions limit clinical relevance of outcomes of that review [20].

Assessment of bicycling participation, and associated facilitators and barriers can identify the needs of people with a LLA. That insight can assist clinicians and researchers to design interventions that meet with the clients' goals and perspective and therefore may improve the participation in bicycling. Since bicycling has benefits, but information on participation in people with a LLA is lacking, the aim of this scoping review is to investigate and summarize bicycling participation rates in people with a LLA. The prevalence, frequency, duration and reasons for bicycling were identified. The second aim is to evaluate facilitators and barriers for bicycling in LLA.

Methods
Searches
Studies were searched in Pubmed, Embase, Cinahl, Cochrane library and Sportdiscus using a combination of Mesh terms and free texts. Part one of the search terms included MeSH terms and free texts relating to "amputee", "amputation" and "prosthesis" and part two included terms related to "bicycling" or "sport". Both parts were combined using "AND". The search strategies were initiated by information specialist (librarian) with extensive expertise in systematic review searching. No time and language restrictions were applied. Last search date was March 22, 2018. This review follows Preferred Reporting items for Systematic Reviews and Meta-Analyses (PRISMA) [21]. In line with PRISMA full electronic search strategies of five databases was presented (Additional file 1).

Participants
To be included, papers had to be about bicycling in people with a LLA either with or without a prosthesis, the minimum number of participants was one and the participants had to be human. At least one participant had to have a LLA from or proximal to midfoot level, but not above the hemipelvectomy level. Studies including multiple disabilities were only included when results for people with a LLA were reported separately. Papers were excluded if the participants use endoprostheses or implant devices.

Types of studies to be included
All types of study designs which are a peer reviewed primary research and published as a full-text paper were included. Reviews, books, notes, letters to editors, expert opinions, conference abstracts or proceedings were excluded.

Facilitators and barriers for bicycling
Factors influencing bicycling participation were classified into personal and environmental factors [22]. Any personal and environmental factors associated with bicycling were eligible. The personal and environmental factors associated with bicycling for all purposes were evaluated. The environmental factors make up physical, attitudinal and social environment in which people live such as prosthetic or assistive devices availability and access, infrastructure or policy [22]. The personal factors represent internal influences on functioning particular to the individual such as gender, motivation, self-efficacy, health status, or age [22]. Positive influences that help, motivate, or increase bicycling participation were considered facilitators. Negative influences that prevent, limit, or reduce bicycling were considered barriers.

Primary outcome(s)
1. Bicycling participation (prevalence, frequency, and duration) which must be performed by a person with a LLA on a bicycle, not being an ergometer.

Data extraction (selection and coding)
Two reviewers pilot tested assessments before each step of the review on papers not included in the review. Inter-rater agreement for titles and abstracts, and full text assessments were calculated using Cohen's kappa (k).

$$k = \frac{Po - Pe}{1 - Pe}$$

P_0 is the relative observed agreement between two reviewers, and P_e is the probability of chance agreement. K = 0 means there is no agreement, while K = 1 represents complete agreement between two reviewers. Low Cohen's kappa (k ≤0.40) represents poor agreement between reviewers. Reviewers, in this case, may interpret and understand selection criteria differently. Two reviewers (JP& JHBG) assessed the titles and abstracts independently. Papers were selected for full text assessment if there was a part of the title or abstract referring to people with a LLA and bicycling or PA, sport, exercise, or training. Papers were excluded if titles or abstracts mentioned a specified PA that was not bicycling such as running, jogging, or walking. Only papers that were excluded by both reviewers did not proceed to the full-text assessment (reviewers were JP& JMH). The reference lists of included studies and of relevant reviews were assessed similarly on title and abstract and full text. Disagreement between reviewers in the full-text assessment was discussed until consensus was reached. If no consensus could be reached, a third reviewer gave a binding verdict (RD). Data was extracted by 2 reviewers (JP&PD) using a data extraction form developed for this study (Additional file 2).

Risk of bias (quality) assessment

The quality of included studies was evaluated using the EPHPP (Effective Public Health Practice Project) tool. EPHPP tool was chosen due to the ability to assess the methodological quality of a range of study types regarding content validity and reliability [23–25]. Two reviewers (JP&RD) pilot tested the tool with excluded studies before assessing included studies. All studies were rated as strong, moderate or weak based on the rating of selection bias, study design, confounders, blinding, data collection method, and withdrawals and dropouts.

Strategy for data synthesis

Characteristics of included studies (study design, year of publication, study country), participant characteristics, amputation level, cause of amputation, outcome measure, findings related to factors associated with bicycling, percentage of participants riding the bicycle, and bicycling frequency and duration were reported according to PRISMA [21] and presented in the summary of findings table. Meta-analysis was not performed since the included studies were heterogeneous with regard to study populations, intervention, measure, and outcomes.

Results

Selected studies

After deduplication, 2904 titles and abstracts were screened of which 56 studies were included for the full-text screening (Cohen's kappa = 0.761). Fourteen studies met the inclusion criteria [26–39] (Cohen's kappa = 0.657) and were included for the quality assessment and data extraction (Fig. 1). One study was excluded because the study used mathematical model, so no participant in the study [40]. Seven articles were excluded because they were not primary research [41–47]. The other excluded studies were not about bicycling [48–75]. Full texts of 4 additional studies from the references of previous reviews and included studies were screened [26, 27, 76, 77]. Three of them passed to the full-text selection [26, 27, 76], two of which were about bicycling and therefore included for quality assessment and data extraction [26, 27].

Quantitative data relating to bicycling was not an inclusion criterion during titles and abstracts, and full text assessment. However, for data extraction, three studies were excluded due to the lack of quantitative data [78] and lack of separate reporting of information of people with a LLA [57, 79]. Sports popularity ranking was reported but not the number of people who took part in bicycling [78]. Participants of one study were grouped according to Para-cycling classification (C1-C5) which not only includes people with a LLA, but other types of impairments as well, such as hemiplegia, upper limb amputation, ataxia and spinal cord injury [79]. In addition, a study classified participants as physically challenged athletes including people with cerebral palsy, upper limb amputation, LLA and wheelchair users in which the people with a LLA could also be the wheelchair users [57]. Finally, a technical note about how to design a prosthetic shank was excluded due to a lack of quantitative data [80].

The study design and quality

In total, 7 cross-sectional [27, 32–37], 4 case reports [26, 30, 38, 39], 2 cross-over trials [28, 29], and a cohort study [31] were included, investigating 1 to 780 of people with a LLA (Table 1). The majority of studies recruited participants from one source which was laboratory [26, 28, 29, 38, 39] or clinic/center [27, 32, 33, 37]. One study analyzed results of 2 Paralympic Games, and 5 World Championships [31]. Eleven studies had weak study design [26, 27, 30, 32–39]. Moderate and strong design were given to a cohort [31] and 2 cross-over trials respectively [28, 29]. Twelve studies did not report how possible confounders were controlled for and did not report reliability and validity of outcome measures [26–29, 32–39]. Six studies that reported the percentage of participants at data collection more than 80% were rated strong regarding the EPHPP for drop-outs. Following the guidelines of the EPHPP [81], all studies except one had an overall rating of weak.

Bicycling participation - prevalence, frequency, duration

Information about bicycling participation and purposes were extracted from 7 surveys published between 1984 and 2014 and included 58–780 participants. The participants varied in age and were mostly male (62–98%) (Table 2). For transportation, 29 and 48% of people with a LLA bicycled in Slovenia and India, respectively [27, 33]. In the United States 12–48%% of people with a LLA bicycled for recreation or PA, in Slovenia this was 11%, and in the Netherlands 4–6% for sport [32, 34–37](Fig. 2 and Table 2). No reports of frequency and duration found from the included studies.

Bicycling facilitators and barriers

Table 2 presents factors associating to bicycling, bicycling purposes, and levels of amputation.

Transportation

Age, time since the LLA, and level of LLA were associated to bicycling participation [33]. People with

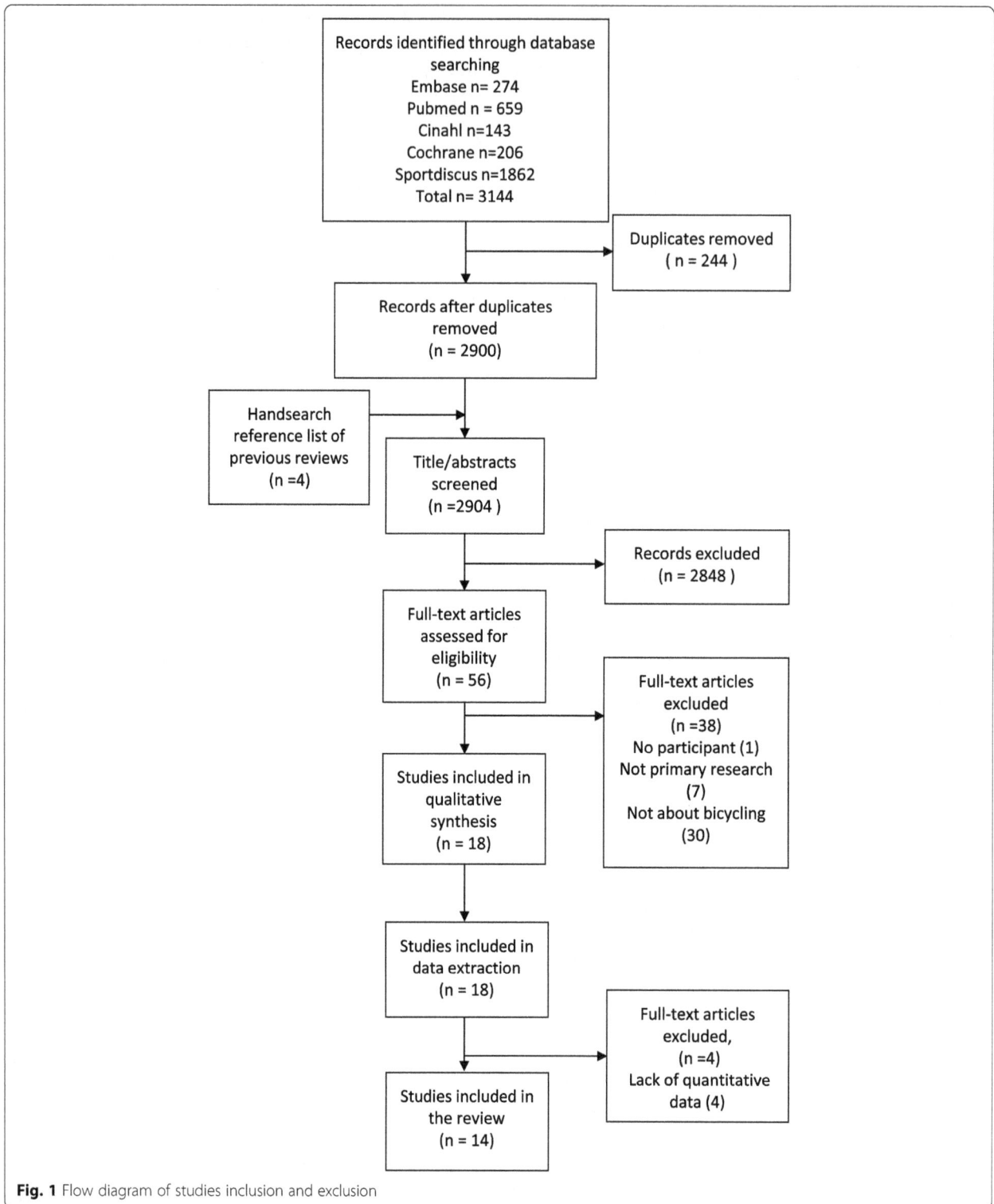

Fig. 1 Flow diagram of studies inclusion and exclusion

LLA who bicycled were younger than who stopped bicycling [33]. People with longer period after LLA stopped bicycling more than the people with shorter period after LLA [33]. People with a TTA traveled by bicycling more than people with a transfemoral amputation (TFA) [27, 33]. Half of Indian participants stopped traveling by bicycle after LLA while a few percent of participants never knew how to cycle [27].

Table 1 Quality of the included studies, based on the Effective Public Health Practice Project Tool

Ref	Selection Bias	Study Design	Confounders	Blinding	Data Collection	Drop-Outs	Global Rating
Narang et al. (1984) [27]	0	–	–	0	–	+	–
Burger et al. (1997) [32]	0	–	–	0	–	0	–
Burger et al. (1997) [33]	–	–	–	0	–	–	–
Mead(2005) [38]	–	-	–	0	–	+	–
Kars et al. (2009) [36]	–	–	–	0	–	–	–
Childers et al. (2011) [28]	–	+	–	0	–	+	–
Childers et al. (2011) [29]	–	+	–	0	–	+	–
Sprunger et al. (2012) [37]	–	–	–	0	–	–	–
Bragaru et al. (2013) [35]	–	–	–	0	–	–	–
Koutny et al. (2013) [26]	–	–	–	0	–	+	–
Littman et al. (2014) [34]	+	–	–	0	–	–	–
Scheepers (2015) [39]	–	–	–	0	–	+	–
Dyer and Woolley (2017) [30]	–	–	+	–	+	+	–
Dyer (2017) [31]	+	0	+	0	+	–	0
Totals							
weak(%)	10(71.4%)	11(79%)	12(86%)	12(86%)	12(86%)	6(43%)	13(93%)
moderate(%)	2(14.3%)	1(7%)	0	0	0	1(7%)	1(7%)
strong(%)	2(14.3%)	2(14%)	2(14%)	2(14%)	2(14%)	7(50%)	0

"Ref": reference, "+": strong, "0": moderate, "-": weak. The total at the bottom of Table 1 represents how weak, moderate and strong each criterion is

PA/ recreation/ sport

Having LLA and LLA level influenced bicycling for recreation. After LLA, people changed their recreational activities. Bicycling was the most popular activity before LLA, but the tenth after LLA [32]. The number of people with a TTA who bicycled was equal to TFA [34].

Competition

Three studies reported bicycling biomechanics in people with a TTA and the influence of adaptation of the prosthesis or the bicycle [26, 28, 29]. Pedaling work and force produced by the prosthetic and sound side were not the same, where the sound side contributed significantly more force [26, 29] and more work [28, 29] than the amputated side [26, 28, 29]. Pedaling asymmetry was also presented in able-bodied people, but to a smaller extent than in the people with a LLA [29]. When two prosthetic feet were compared, the aluminum or STIFF foot reduced work asymmetry more during high-intensity bicycling than the flexible carbon fiber dynamic response or FLEX-foot [29]. In low intensity, the FLEX and STIFF feet did not differ significantly in work asymmetry [29]. Furthermore, the ratio of forces orthogonal to the crank and the resultant force applied to the pedal which is called force effectiveness ratio were compared between the groups of able-bodied and people with a TTA. Pedaling force effectiveness ratio was not affected by the TTA or the applied prosthetic feet since the participants were able to

compensate and achieve the overall force effectiveness by using their sound side [28].

The length of a crank arm also influenced hip and knee kinematics [26]. Shortening the crank arm reduced asymmetry in hip and knee angles between both limbs, and moreover, reduced the higher muscles activity in the prosthetic side [26]. In individuals with limited knee range, a hinged crank arm enabled the person to bicycle using also the affected side. The crank arm was cut and reattached with the hinge at an appropriate level [38]. Design of socket was found to be associated with skin abrasion in high intensity bicycling. To prevent the abrasion, a conventional prosthesis socket made of a leather thigh cuff was replaced by a socket-less prosthesis [39]. The shape of the pylon was associated with aerodynamic drag, however, the measures performed during the tests did not show significant differences of the aero foil shaped pylon compared to the round shaped pylon [30, 31]. Analysis of data from C4 bicyclists competing in the Paralympic Games and World Championships revealed no advantages of use of prostheses, in relation to those participants who did not use prostheses [31].

Discussion

Health benefits from bicycling are apparent and bicycling serves as an alternative to other modes of transportation and exercise for LLA. After all, unlike running, skiing or golfing, recreational bicycling requires very little modifications to the people with a LLA to participate.

Table 2 Data summary of included studies

Authors (year)	Country	Study design	LLA No, Male	Age (mean ±SD/ range)	Amp Characteristics		Uni/Bilat	Results
					Cause	Level		
Bicycling participation								
**Burger et al. (1997) [32]	Slovenia	CS	228, 84%	53.3 ± 15.4	100%T	108TF, 114TT, 2KD, 4HD	NR	Recreation: • Before amputation: 38% bicycling • After amputation: 11% bicycling
Kars et al. (2009) [36]	Netherlands	CS	105, 66%	23–79	40% PVD, 31% T, 10% C, 19% other	27TF, 58TT, 1Hemipelvectomy, 5HD, 13KD, 1 AD	101/4	Sport: • 6% bicycling for sport • A minimal duration of half an hour of participation is required for sports
Sprunger et al. (2012) [37]	USA	CS	58 (100%VA)	48.3 ± 14.3	88% T, 12% PVD, DM, C, or infection	22 Gr1, 26 Gr2, 10 Gr3	48/10	Sport: • 45% bicycling (most popular)
Bragaru et al. (2013) [35]	Netherlands	CS	780, 62%	59.6 ± 14.8	27% PVD/DM, 73% non-PVD	261TF, 432TT, 87KD	736/44	Sports with a prosthesis: • Athletes are persons who joined sport at least 5 h a month • 4% of participants were athletes who cycle with a prosthesis
Littman et al. (2014) [34]	USA	CS	158, 98%, (100%VA)	65	36% T, 64%-NR	41TF, 62TT, 55PF	125/33	Physical activities: • 12% bicycling outdoors or on stationary bicycle (9%of PF, 12%of TT and 17% of TF)
Bicycling participation and facilitators and barriers for transportation								
Narang et al. (1984) [27]	India	CS	500, 95% (60% VA)	2–65#	82% T, 17% disease, 1% congenital	124TF, 308TT	432/68	• 48% used bicycle (60% of TT, 35%of TF and 18% of bilat) • 50% did not use bicycle (38%of TT, 63% of TF, 78% of bilat) • 2% never known how to cycle (2% of TT and TF and 4% of bilat)
**Burger et al. (1997) [33]	Slovenia	CS	223, 84%	54.4 ± 15.4	100% T	102TF, 115TT, 2KD, 4HD	203/20	• 29% used bicycle • 60%*** did not use bicycle (average 5.7 years older than those who use a bicycle) • 11% did not travel by bicycle both before and after amputation • TT amputees were more likely to bicycle than TF amputees
Bicycling facilitators and barriers in people with a TTA								
Childers et al. (2011) [28]*	USA	RCT	8, 75% (1Paralympic medalist) (control =9)	36.4 ± 10.4	7 T, 1 C	8 TT	8/0	Pedaling force effectiveness ratio was not significantly different between a STIFF foot and a FLEX foot
Childers et al. (2011) [29]*	USA	RCT	8, 75% (1Paralympic medalist) (control =9)	36.4 ± 10.4	NR	8 TT	8/0	Pedaling asymmetry in people with a TTA was significantly larger than in controls in low difficulty and time trial conditions (submaximal bicycling over a 6-min period). Work asymmetry was significantly greater than the force asymmetry in TT amputation group between both conditions. Work and

Table 2 Data summary of included studies (Continued)

Authors (year)	Country	Study design	LLA No, Male	Age (mean ±SD/ range)	Amp Characteristics Cause	Level	Uni/Bilat	Results
								force was provided more by the sound limb. Work asymmetry decreased when the STIFF foot was used during the time trial condition.
Koutny et al. (2013) [26]	Czech Republic	CR	1, 100% (athlete)	37	NR	1TT	1/0	After shortening of the bicycle's crank at the prosthetic limb, asymmetry of hip and knee kinematic reduced. Besides, muscle activity decreased during bicycling in seated position (vastus medialis, vastus lateralis, and gluteus maximus of both limbs) and climbing position (gluteus maximus of amputated limb). The sound side significantly produced more pedaling forces than the prosthetic side but this asymmetry was not influenced by the crank shortening.
Dyer and Woolley (2017) [30]	UK	CR	1, 100%	33	NR	1TT	1/0	An aero foil shaped pylon caused less, but not significant, aerodynamic drag than the round shaped pylon in both virtual elevation field and wind tunnel tests.
Dyer (2017) [31]	UK	Cohort	41,100%	NR	NR	41TT	41/0	The competitive bicyclists in C4 classification who used prosthesis were not faster when competing in 1 km time trial (world championships and Paralympic games) than the bicyclists without prosthesis.
Bicycling facilitators and barriers in Van Nes rotationplasty								
Mead (2005) [38]	Canada	CR	1, 100%	14	1 C	1 Van Nes rotationplasty	1/0	Limitation of knee flexion obstructed complete bicycling revolutions. By cutting a crank and adding a hinge in between two crank parts, the outer crank can swing down. The hinged-crank reduced amount of required knee flexion.
Scheepers et al. (2013) [39]	Netherlands	CR	1, 100%	18	1 C	1 Van Nes rotationplasty	1/0	The thigh cuff of a conventional prosthesis leads to perspiration, chaffing and skin abrasion in high-intensity bicycling. Replacing the thigh-cuff socket design and conventional prosthesis with the Socket-Less Rotationplasty Prosthesis for Cycling prevented abrasion.

"_" = weak; "0" = moderate; LLA = lower limb amputation; NO = number; SD = standard deviation; Amp = amputation; M = male; VA = veterans; Uni = unilateral; Bi = bilateral; CS = cross sectional; CR = case report; RCT = randomized control trial; PF = partial foot; TT = transtibial; TF = transfemoral; KD = knee disarticulation; HD = hip disarticulation; PVD = peripheral vascular disease; DM = diabetes; T = Trauma; C = Cancer; NR = not reported; Gr = group; Gr1 = TT and below; Gr2 = TF level and KD; Gr3 = above TF and all bilat; *,**,***have possibility of using the same group of participants in the studies of the same authors (Childers et al.** and Burger et al. ****); *** the percentage reported from this review (60%) is different from the original study (62%); #Age of participants at the time of a LLA–57% of participants aged between 21 and 30 years old at the time of survey

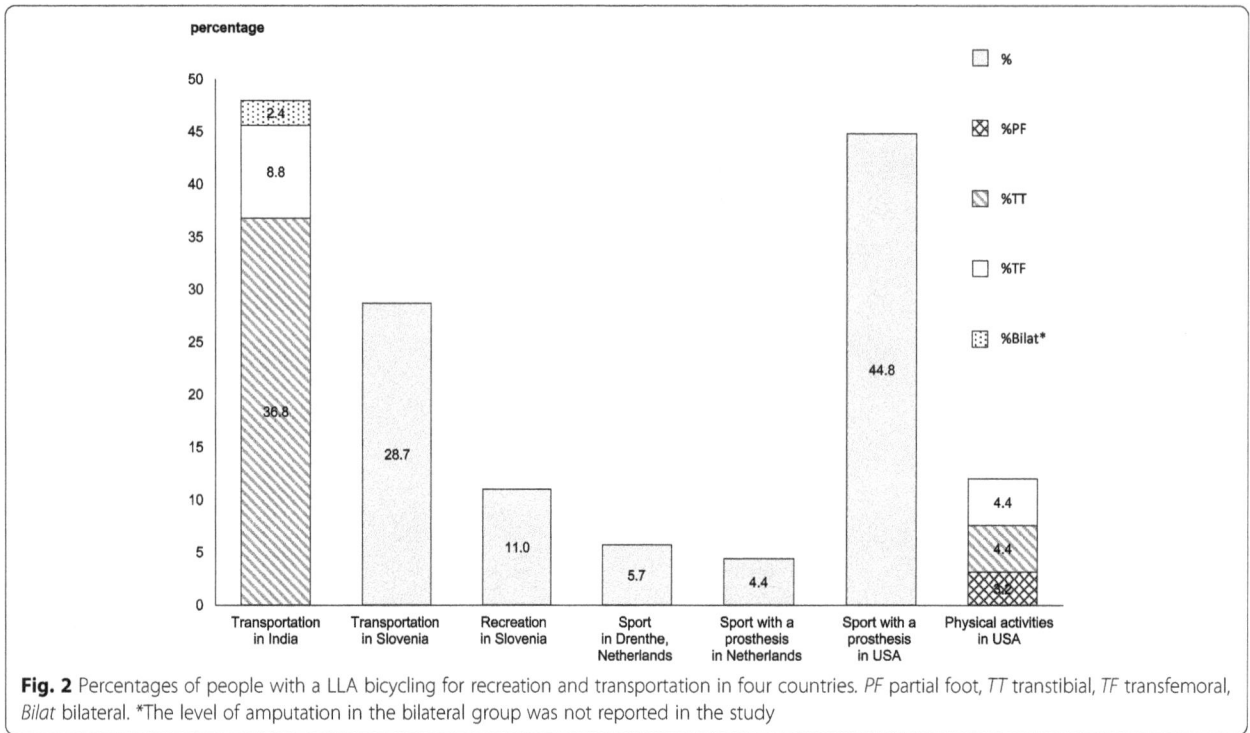

Fig. 2 Percentages of people with a LLA bicycling for recreation and transportation in four countries. *PF* partial foot, *TT* transtibial, *TF* transfemoral, *Bilat* bilateral. *The level of amputation in the bilateral group was not reported in the study

Bicycling should remain an integral component of rehabilitation and the return to recreation and vocation [82]. Bicycling participation ranged from 4 to 48%. Two studies done in the same country reported considerable differences within a country [34, 37]. People with a LLA bicycled for reasons of transportation, recreation, sport and physical activity [27, 32–37]. Data about frequency and duration of bicycling were not found from the included studies. Since most studies aimed to determine changes of lifestyle or activities after LLA, intensity, duration and frequency of PA were reported for the big picture of attended activities but not specifically for bicycling [34, 37].

In this study, we assumed that the studies are about bicycling outdoor if it was not specified in studies [32, 34–37]. There is one study that the term bicycling referred to both indoor and outdoor bicycling [34]. When participation rate was reported, two studies reported sport participation if a minimum duration of half an hour for each participation [36] or total of 5 hours participation a month [35] was met. Whereas, in 5 studies, duration was no concern as long as the people with a LLA reported riding the bicycle [27, 32–34, 37]. Consequently, the participation rates should be interpreted with caution. Definitions of bicycling participation should be reported in future studies.

The majority of participants in the included studies were males with a TTA or TFA. Males with a TTA were reported to participate in the bicycling the most. The overall gender distribution of people with a LLA is about 50% male and female [83]. Therefore, including considerably

more than 50% of male participants or veterans in studies [34, 37] may not represent the general population of people with a LLA. Although male, distal level of amputation and amputation due to trauma may associate to higher level of bicycling participation, the results of this review may not reflect the interest and purpose of bicycling of general populations with a LLA.

Bicycling was chosen as a form of transportation in Slovenia besides using cars and public transportations and was related to the level of independence [33]. A study from India investigated the functional capabilities of people after LLA and only included essential activities for daily living, vocational activities, and living arrangements in which bicycling was surveyed. It was demonstrated that bicycling was an important mode of transportation for civilians in India [27]. Both studies were done some decades ago; however, the recent studies did not show a difference in favor of other transportation modes in India especially in the group of low-income people [84, 85]. Socioeconomic status such as income or occupation may influence traveling by bicycling. A small number of participants could not ride the bicycle even before the amputation [27]. Knowledge or skill may facilitate bicycling participation. Two studies showed older age and longer time span after amputation [33] and level of LLA [27, 33] related to the reduce or stop traveling by bicycling. A change in lifestyle after the LLA was also reported in which bicycling became less popular after the LLA [29]. Disability, health, lack of energy and fatigue were personal barriers which were reported in a previous review of sports barriers and facilitators in adults with different types of physical disabilities [17]. It is possible that older people or a more proximal level of LLA may have more disabilities, health problems, less energy or more likely to be fatigue during bicycling. In contrast, for recreational bicycling, an equal number of veterans with a TFA and TTA was reported [34]. The relationship between amputation level and cause, these barriers and bicycling participation should be further studied.

Factors influencing competitive or high intensity bicycling were done in specific groups of bicyclists- TTA or Van Nes rotationplasty. Most studies investigated a small group of participants, mainly male, and having different bicycling experience [26, 28–30, 38, 39]. Only one study utilizing data of more than 8 participants ($N = 41$); however, the same participants were analyzed more than once [31].

For bicyclists with a TTA, the focus of research was towards asymmetry in force and work between sound and amputated side and ways to reduce this asymmetry for better performance [26, 28, 29]. Clinically, a STIFF foot reduced the pedaling work asymmetry in high-intensity or competitive bicycling [29] but not in recreational bicycling. In low-difficulty bicycling, no significant difference were found between the STIFF and the Flex foot suggesting a walking prosthetic foot may be adequate for recreational bicycling [29]. A pylon with an aerofoil shape caused less aerodynamic drag than the round shape [30]. On the one hand, a prosthetic foot and pylon influenced high intensity bicycling. On the other hand, while comparing between prosthetic and non-prosthetic bicyclists, there were no significant benefits reported from the prosthesis to the athletes [31]. Besides the kinetic asymmetry, there were hip and knee kinematic asymmetries which were reduced by shortening of the crank arm length on the amputated side [26]. The shortened crank arm also reduced the muscles activity on the amputated side [26]. Although the shortened crank arm improved the asymmetry in the person with a TTA in a case report [26], the same shortening may not give the same effects to other people with a TTA.

For a person with Van Nes rotationplasty, the socket design of walking prosthesis was a bicycling barrier because it caused skin abrasion [39]. Adding a hinge to the crank arm enabled a person with Van Nes rotationplasty with limited knee range of motion to bicycle [38]. Adaptation of the socket and crank arm might also facilitate bicycling in people with other types of LLA who have skin abrasions or limited knee ranges. The biomechanical effects from the prosthetic feet and crank arm shortening [26, 28, 29, 38] were also reported in a previous review of cycling with an amputation [20]. That review

focused on upper and lower limb amputee biomechanics, physiology, and assistive technology development and extracted data from expert opinions, reviews, and primary researches from 2004 to 2014 [20]. Articles without any participants and studies using ergometers were included [20], while the current review included only primary research of at least one human with LLA riding a normal bicycle from all publication years. Therefore, the objectives, methods and results of the previous review differ from the current review.

The personal factors for transportation by bicycling were age, time since LLA, and level of amputation. The prosthetic socket design can either be an environment facilitator or barrier for high-intensity bicycling. The STIFF foot and crank arm shortening were environmental facilitators for high-intensity bicycling. For people with a knee flexion limitation, the limitation was a personal barrier and the hinged crank arm was an environment facilitator. Other bicycling environment factors such as weather, cycling paths, physical and emotional support, individual and societal attitudes toward people with a LLA, public services, systems or policies were not reported.

Strengths and weaknesses

The search from 5 databases ensured that all medical and sports science articles could be included in this review. Eventually, only 14 studies were included showing this topic has not been explored very extensively.

Due to the small number of included studies with various focuses we were not fully able to answer the research questions of our study. Additionally the included studies had a high risk of bias. Though we focused more on the regular LLA, there were two case reports of Van Nes rotationplasty included in the review. It is understood that this special technique of LLA is very rare and the study designs were case reports, so the findings should be considered as low level evidence. Moreover, in the biomechanical studies in people with a TTA, the number of participants was also low and likely to be the same group of participants in the studies that have the same authors [28, 29]. Subsequently, the findings of this review may not reflect the general population of people with a LLA.

Conclusion

Multiple purposes of use of bicycles are exhibited in this study. After LLA, people stopped bicycle or changed leisure activity. Age, level of LLA, and time since LLA influenced bicycling participation. Although environmental factors were limited to prosthetic socket and pylon design, foot stiffness and bicycle's crank arm, arisen predominantly from small groups of bicyclists with a TTA and Van Nes rotationplasty, and mainly benefit to competition, some practical advices can be given. For instance, prosthetists may try to shorten the crank or use stiff foot if pedaling asymmetry is present. To supply prosthetists with sufficient additional knowledge in compiling an optimal prosthesis for bicycling, more research is necessary. Efforts towards studying facilitators and barriers for bicycling in a population with a LLA who are not athletes can benefit the general population with a LLA [9–14]. Further investigation of prosthetic and bicycle components in either competitive or recreational bicycling should include more participants, thus providing strong evidence for implementations by prosthetists or sport scientists.

Abbreviations
EPHPP: Effective Public Health Practice Project; LLA: Lower limb amputation; PA: Physical activity; PRISMA: Preferred Reporting Items for Systematic Reviews and Meta-Analyses; TFA: Transfemoral amputation; TTA: Transtibial amputation

Acknowledgements
We would like to thank the Medical Information Specialist, K.I. (Karin) Sijtsma for helping us to initiate and approve the search strategy.

Funding
Not applicable.

Authors' contributions
All authors contributed to conception and designed the review. JP& JHBG assessed the titles and abstracts. JP& JMH did the full-text assessment. JP and RD assessed the methodological quality of all studies. JP&PD extracted data. JP performed the searches on the databases. All authors were involved in data analysis, data interpretation, drafting and they all critically revised the manuscript. All authors have read and approved the manuscript.

Competing interests
The authors declare that they have no competing interests.

Author details
[1]Department of Rehabilitation Medicine, University of Groningen, University Medical Center Groningen, CB41, PO Box 30001, 9700 RB Groningen, The Netherlands. [2]Department of Oral and Maxillofacial Surgery, University of Groningen, University Medical Center Groningen, Groningen, The Netherlands. [3]Sirindhorn School of Prosthetics and Orthotics, Faculty of Medicine Siriraj Hospital, Mahidol University, Bangkok, Thailand.

References
1. Oja P, Titze S, Bauman A, de Geus B, Krenn P, Reger-Nash B, et al. Health benefits of cycling: a systematic review. Scand J Med Sci Sport. 2011;21:496–509.
2. Laverty AA, Mindell JS, Webb EA, Millett C. Active travel to work and cardiovascular risk factors in the United Kingdom. Am J Prev Med. 2013;45: 282–8.
3. Fox SM, Haskell WL. Physical activity and the prevention of coronary heart disese. Bull N Y Acad Med. 1968;44:950–9.
4. Oja P, Manttari A, Heinonen A, Kukkonen-Harjula K, Laukkanen R, Pasanen M, et al. Physiological effects of walking and cycling to work. Scand J Med Sci Sport. 1991;1:151–7.
5. Steptoe A, Butler N. Sports participation and emotional wellbeing in adolescents. Lancet. 1996;347:1789–92.
6. Eime RM, Young JA, Harvey JT, Charity MJ, Payne WR. A systematic review of the psychological and social benefits of participation in sport for children and adolescents: informing development of a conceptual model of health through sport. Int J Behav Nutr Phys Act. 2013;10:98.
7. Taddei C, Gnesotto R, Forni S, Bonaccorsi G, Vannucci A, Garofalo G. Cycling promotion and non-communicable disease prevention: health impact assessment and economic evaluation of cycling to work or school in Florence. PLoS One. 2015;10:e0125491.
8. Rasmussen MG, Grontved A, Blond K, Overvad K, Tjonneland A, Jensen MK, et al. Associations between recreational and commuter cycling, changes in cycling, and type 2 diabetes risk: a cohort study of Danish men and women. PLoS Med. 2016;13:e1002076.
9. Hutzter Y, Bar-Eli M. Psychological benefits of sports for disabled people: a review. Scand J Med Sci Sports. 1993;3:217–28.
10. Valliant PM, Bezzubyk I, Daley L, Asu ME. Psychological impact of sport on disabled athletes. Psychol Rep. 1985;56:923–9.
11. K a W, Hanson C, Levy CE. Effect of participation in physical activity on body image of amputees. Am J Phys Med Rehabil. 2002;81:194–201.
12. Nolan L. Lower limb strength in sports-active transtibial amputees. Prosthetics Orthot Int. 2009;33:230–41.
13. Renström P, LE Grimby G. Thigh muscle strength in below-knee amputees. Scand J Rehabil Med Suppl. 1983;9:–163, 73.
14. Isakov E, Burger H, Gregorič M, Marinček C. Isokinetic and isometric strength of the thigh muscles in below-knee amputees. Clin Biomech. 1996;11:233–5.
15. Ericson MO, Nisell R, Nemeth G. Joint motions of the lower limb during ergometer cycling. J Orthop Sports Phys Ther. 1988;9:273–8.
16. Timmer CAW. Cycling biomechanics: a literature review. J Orthop Sport Phys Ther. 1991;14:106–13.
17. Jaarsma EA, Dijkstra PU, Geertzen JHB, Dekker R. Barriers to and facilitators of sports participation for people with physical disabilities: a systematic review barriers to and facilitators of sports participation for people with physical disabilities: a systematic review. Scand J Med Sci Sports. 2014;24: 871–81.
18. Deans S, Burns D, McGarry A, Murray K, Mutrie N. Motivations and barriers to prosthesis users participation in physical activity, exercise and sport: a review of the literature. Prosthetics Orthot Int. 2012;36:260–9.
19. Bragaru M, Dekker R, Geertzen JHB. Sport prostheses and prosthetic adaptations for the upper and lower limb amputees: an overview of peer reviewed literature. Prosthetics Orthot Int. 2012;36:290–6.
20. Dyer B. Cycling with an amputation: a systematic review. Prosthetics Orthot Int. 2016;40:538–44.
21. Liberati A, Altman DG, Tetzlaff J, Mulrow C, Gøtzsche PC, Ioannidis JPA, et al. The PRISMA statement for reporting systematic reviews and meta-analyses of studies that evaluate health care interventions: explanation and elaboration. PLoS Med. 2009;6:1–28.
22. World Health Organization. International classification of functioning, disability and health: ICF. Geneva: World Health Organization; 2001.
23. Armijo-Olivo S, Stiles CR, Hagen NA, Biondo PD, Cummings GG. Assessment of study quality for systematic reviews: a comparison of the Cochrane collaboration risk of Bias tool and the effective public health practice project quality assessment tool: methodological research. J Eval Clin Pract. 2012;18:12–8.
24. Jackson N, Waters E. Criteria for the systematic review of health promotion and public health interventions. Health Promot Int. 2005;20:367–74.
25. Thomas BH, Ciliska D, Dobbins M, Micucci S. A process for systematically reviewing the literature: providing the research evidence for public health nursing interventions. Worldviews evidence-based Nurs. 2004;1:176–84.
26. Koutny D, Palousek D, Stoklasek P, Rosicky J, Tepla L, Prochazkova M, et al. The biomechanics of cycling with a Transtibial prosthesis: a case study of a professional cyclist. Int J Medical, Heal Biomed Bioeng Pharm Eng. 2013;7:812–7.
27. Narang IC, Mathur BP, Singh P, Jape VS. Functional capabilities of lower limb amputees. Prosthetics Orthot Int. 1984;8:43–51.
28. Childers WL, Gregor RJ. Effectiveness of force production in persons with unilateral transtibial amputation during cycling. Prosthetics Orthot Int. 2011; 35:373–8.
29. Childers WL, Kistenberg RS, Gregor RJ. Pedaling asymmetries in cyclists with unilateral transtibial amputation: effect of prosthetic foot stiffness. J Appl Biomech. 2011;27:314–21.
30. Dyer B, Disley BX. Validation of the virtual elevation field test method when assessing the aerodynamics of Para-cyclists with a uni-lateral trans-tibial amputation. Disabil Rehabil Assist Technol. 2018;13:107–11.
31. Dyer B. The impact of lower-limb prosthetic limb use in international C4 track Para-cycling. Disabil Rehabil Assist Technol. 2017;0:1–5.
32. Burger H, Marincek C. The life style of young persons after lower limb amputation caused by injury. Prosthetics Orthot Int. 1997;21:35–9.

33. Burger H, Marincek C, Isakov E. Mobility of persons after traumatic lower limb amputation. Disabil Rehabil. 1997;19:272–7.

34. Littman AJ, Boyko EJ, Thompson M Lou, Haselkorn JK, Sangeorzan BJ, Arterburn DE. Physical activity barriers and enablers in older veterans with lower-limb amputation. J Rehabil Res Dev 2014;51:895–906.

35. Bragaru M, Meulenbelt HEJ, Dijkstra PU, Geertzen JHB, Dekker R. Sports participation of Dutch lower limb amputees. Prosthetics Orthot Int. 2013;37:454–8.

36. Kars C, Hofman M, Geertzen JHB, Pepping G-J, Dekker R. Participation in sports by lower limb amputees in the province of Drenthe. The Netherlands Prosthet Orthot Int. 2009;33:356–67.

37. Sprunger NA, Laferrier JZ, Collins DM, Cooper RA. Utilization of prostheses and mobility-related assistive technology among service members and veterans from Vietnam and operation Iraqi freedom/operation enduring freedom. J Prosthetics Orthot. 2012;24:144–52.

38. Mead D. Development of a hinged crank arm to allow a subject with limited knee flexion to ride a bicycle. J Prosthetics Orthot. 2005;17:35–7.

39. Scheepers LG, Storcken JO, Rings F, Van horn Y, H a S. New socket-less prosthesis concept facilitating comfortable and abrasion-free cycling after van Nes rotationplasty. Prosthetics Orthot Int. 2014;39:161–5.

40. Childers WL, Gallagher TP, Duncan JC, Taylor DK. Modeling the effect of a prosthetic limb on 4-km pursuit performance. Int J Sports Physiol Perform. 2015;10:3–10.

41. Diaper N, Simpson LP. Supporting the GB Para-Cycling Team - A no compromise approach. Sport Exerc Sci. 2012:12.

42. Blum C, Ehrler S, Isner M-E. Assessment of therapeutic education in 135 lower limb amputees. Ann Phys Rehabil Med. 2016;59:e161.

43. Gailey R, Harsch P. Introduction to triathlon for the lower limb amputee triathlete. Prosthetics Orthot Int. 2009;33:242–55.

44. Haggstrom E, Hagberg K, Tranberg R. Implant loading during walking and riding a stationary bicycle with a bone-anchored transfemoral prosthesis - a pilot study using the iPec instrument. In: ISPO World Congress 2015 Abstract Book. Prosthetics Orthot Int. 2015;39(1_suppl):425.

45. Kegel B. Physical fitness: Sports and recreation for those with lower limb amputation or impairment. J Rehabil Res Dev Clin Suppl. 1985:1–125.

46. Rimaud D, Fernandez B, Chagnon P, Condemine A, Fayolle-Minon I, Calmels P. Vel'HandiRhone from leman to the sea: this cycling challenge was met by 15 disabled patients. Ann Phys Rehabil Med. 2012;55:e252.

47. Blokland I, Groot F, Houdijk H. Physical profile: An evidence- based exercise programme in rehabilitation. In: Abstracts of meeting DCRM November 2016. Clin Rehabil. 2017:835–41.

48. Childers WL, Kogler GF. Symmetrical kinematics does not imply symmetrical kinetics in people with transtibial amputation using cycling model. J Rehabil Res Dev. 2014;51:1243–54.

49. Childers WL, Perell-Gerson KL, Gregor RJ. Measurement of motion between the residual limb and the prosthetic socket during cycling. J Prosthetics Orthot. 2012;24:19–24.

50. Menaspà P, Rampinini E, Tonetti L, Bosio A. Physical fitness and performances of an amputee cycling world champion: a case study. Int J Sports Physiol Perform. 2012;7:290–4.

51. Mujika I, Orbañanos J, Salazar H. Physiology and training of a world-champion paratriathlete. Int J Sports Physiol Perform. 2015;10:927–30.

52. Muller EA, Hettinger T, Kuhm GG. Physiological studies of work in bicycling with an artificial leg. Z Orthop Ihre Grenzgeb. 1954;84:462–9.

53. Van Leeuwen HJ. Circulatory load in walking and cycling with upper leg prosthesis (Dutch). Ned Tijdschr voor Fysiother. 1976;86:2–3.

54. Wernke MM, Schroeder RM, Kelley CT, Denune JA, Colvin JM. SmartTemp prosthetic liner significantly reduces residual limb temperature and perspiration. J Prosthetics Orthot. 2015;27:134–9.

55. Boonstra AM, van Duin W, Eisma W. International forum. Silicone suction socket (3S) versus supracondylar PTB prosthesis with pelite liner: transtibial amputees' preferences. J Prosthetics Orthot. 1996;8:96–9.

56. Bragaru M, van Wilgen CP, Geertzen JHB, Ruijs SGJB, Dijkstra PU, Dekker R. Barriers and facilitators of participation in sports: a qualitative study on Dutch individuals with lower limb amputation. PLoS One. 2013;8: e59881.

57. Brueck CM. The role of topical lubrication in the prevention of skin friction in physically challenged athletes. J Sport Chiropr Rehabil. 2000;14:37–43.

58. Burgess EM, Hittenberger DA, Forsgren SM, Lindh DV. The Seattle prosthetic foot - a design for active sports: preliminary studies. Orthot Prosthetics. 1983;37:25–31.

59. Couture M, Caron CD, Desrosiers J. Leisure activities following a lower limb amputation. Disabil Rehabil. 2010;32:57–64.

60. Childers WL, Prilutsky BI, Gregor RJ. Motor adaptation to prosthetic cycling in people with trans-tibial amputation. J Biomech. 2014;47:2306–13.

61. Doukas WC, Hayda RA, Frisch HM, Andersen RC, Mazurek MT, Ficke JR, et al. The military extremity trauma amputation/limb salvage (METALS) study: outcomes of amputation versus limb salvage following major lower-extremity trauma. J Bone Joint Surg Am. 2013;95:138–45.

62. Ebrahimzadeh MH, Moradi A, Bozorgnia S, Hallaj-Moghaddam M. Evaluation of disabilities and activities of daily living of war-related bilateral lower extremity amputees. Prosthetics Orthot Int. 2016;40:51–7.

63. Gallagher P, O'Donovan M-A, Doyle A, Desmond D. Environmental barriers, activity limitations and participation restrictions experienced by people with major limb amputation. Prosthetics Orthot Int. 2011;35:278–84.

64. Gunawardena NS, de Alwis SR, Athauda T. Prosthetic outcome of unilateral lower limb amputee soldiers in two districts of Sri Lanka. J Prosthetics Orthot. 2004;16:123–9.

65. Karmarkar AM, Collins DM, Wichman T, Franklin A, Fitzgerald SG, Dicianno BE, et al. Prosthesis and wheelchair use in veterans with lower-limb amputation. J Rehabil Res Dev. 2009;46:567–76.

66. Kegel B, Webster JC, Burgess EM. Recreational activities of lower extremity amputees: a survey. Arch Phys Med Rehabil. 1980;61:258–64.

67. Sayed Ahmed B, Lamy M, Cameron D, Artero L, Ramdial S, Leineweber M, et al. Factors impacting participation in sports for children with limb absence: a qualitative study. Disabil Rehabil. 2018;40:1393–400.

68. Rinne MAH. Raaja-amputoitujen liikuntaharrastuksen motiivit ja rajoitukset. / Physical activity of limb amputees. Liik T. 1987;24:296–301.

69. Demets J, Weissland T, Metron D. Étude de faisabilité du pédalage unilatéral en réentraînement à l'effort chez le patient amputé de membre inférieur d'origine vasculaire : résultats préliminaires. / Feasibility of one-legged cycling exercise during rehabilitation training in lower limb a. Mov Sport Sci / Sci Mot. 2014:35–42.

70. Donachy JE, Brannon KD, Hughes LS, Seahorn J, Crutcher TT, Christian EL. Strength and endurance training of an individual with left upper and lower limb amputations. Disabil Rehabil. 2004;26:495–9.

71. Dyer B. The importance of aerodynamics for prosthetic limb design used by competitive cyclists with an amputation: an introduction. Prosthetics Orthot Int. 2015;39:232–7.

72. Eiser C, Cool P, Grimer RJ, Carter SR, Cotter IM, Ellis AJ, et al. Quality of life in children following treatment for a malignant primary bone tumour around the knee. Sarcoma. 1997;1:39–45.

73. Huonker M, Schmid A, Schmidt-Trucksass A, Grathwohl D, Keul J. Size and blood flow of central and peripheral arteries in highly trained able-bodied and disabled athletes. J Appl Physiol. 2003;95:685–91.

74. Kennedy AB, Trilk JL. A standardized, evidence-based massage therapy program for decentralized elite paracyclists: creating the model. Int J Ther Massage Bodyw Res Educ Pract. 2015;8:3–9.

75. Koopman ADM, Eken MM, van Bezeij T, Valent LJM, Houdijk H. Does clinical rehabilitation impose sufficient cardiorespiratory strain to improve aerobic fitness? J Rehabil Med. 2013;45:92–8.

76. Legro MW, Reiber GE, Czerniecki JM, Sangeorzan BJ. Recreational activities of lower-limb amputees with prostheses. J Rehabil Res Dev. 2010;38:319–25.

77. Yari P, Dijkstra PU, Geertzen JHB. Functional outcome of hip disarticulation and hemipelvectomy: a cross-sectional national descriptive study in the Netherlands. Clin Rehabil. 2008;22:1127–33.

78. Gailey RSJ. Recreational pursuits for elders with amputation. Top Geriatr Rehabil. 1992;8:39–58.

79. Wright RL. Positive pacing strategies are utilized by elite male and female Para-cyclists in short time trials in the velodrome. Front Physiol. 2015;6:425.

80. Dyer B, Woolley H. Development of a high-performance transtibial cycling-specific prosthesis for the London 2012 Paralympic games. Prosthetics Orthot Int. 2017;41:498–502.

81. Effective Public Health Practice Project. Quality Assessment Tool For Quantitative Studies. Effective Public Health Practice Project. https://merst.ca/ephpp/.

82. United Nations. Convention on the rights of persons with disabilities. Treaty Ser. 2006;2515:3 doi:UN Doc. A/61/611 (2006).

83. Unwin N. Epidemiology of lower extremity amputation in centres in Europe, North America and East Asia. Br J Surg. 2000;87:328–37.

24

Physical activity status by pain severity in patients with knee osteoarthritis: a nationwide study in Korea

Hye-Young Shim[1,2†], Mira Park[1†], Hee-June Kim[3], Hee-Soo Kyung[3] and Ji-Yeon Shin[4*]

Abstract

Backgrounds: Few reports have explored the extent to which physical activity is affected by pain severity in knee osteoarthritis (KOA) patients. We used national representative data to investigate the physical activity of KOA patients compared to the general population to determine what proportion of patients met physical activity recommendations and to explore how the proportion changes with pain severity.

Methods: We used data from the fifth Korean National Health and Nutrition Examination Survey (KNHANES V; 2010–2012). In total, 1279 participants aged ≥50 years who had radiographic KOA and who evaluated knee pain on a numerical rating scale were selected. KOA was assessed using the Kellgren–Lawrence system. The Korean short version of the International Physical Activity Questionnaire was used to measure physical activity status. We used the physical activity recommendations of the American College of Rheumatology Work Group Panel when evaluating the extent of activity in KOA patients.

Results: Only 18.6% of KOA patients met the osteoarthritis expert panel recommendations, lower than in the general population (23.2%; $p = 0.003$). The percentages that met the recommendations in the none to mild pain group, moderate pain group, and severe pain group were 23.4%, 17.6%, and 18.3%, respectively ($p = 0.341$). In terms of flexibility, a somewhat higher percentage of those with moderate pain engaged in physical activity compared to those with little or no pain (17.1% vs. 12.3%), but the difference was not significant ($p = 0.585$).

Conclusions: Regardless of pain severity, overall physical activity was suboptimal in Korean KOA patients. It is important to emphasize to osteoarthritis patients in clinical settings the need for physical activity, and a policy-based effort is required to facilitate appropriate exercise.

Keywords: Osteoarthritis, Knee, Physical activity, Exercises, Pain

Background

Knee osteoarthritis (KOA) is a degenerative joint disease that is common in the elderly; however, it also affects younger people [1]. KOA symptoms can limit physical activity and cause debilitating pain [1]. The World Health Organization (WHO) estimates that around 13–15% of adults aged over 55 years have KOA worldwide [2]. In Korea, because of the rapid aging of the population, it is expected that the burden of disease caused by osteoarthritis will increase, and care and management are thus becoming increasingly important [3]. If KOA symptoms lead to decreased mobility of the patients, then, patients can be more dependent on others and their quality of life can be compromised [4, 5]. The goal of KOA management is to improve quality of life and physical function, thereby, minimizing disability in daily life.

Considerable evidence suggests that physical activity can improve physical function [6, 7], reduce pain, and improve patient-reported disabilities [6, 7]. Currently, several different guidelines emphasize the importance of physical activity. The Osteoarthritis Research Society International (OARSI) document [8] recommends land- or water-based exercise and strength training as appropriate, and the

---

* Correspondence: nunmulgyupda@hanmail.net
†Hye-Young Shim and Mi-Ra Park contributed equally to this work.
⁴Department of Preventive Medicine, School of Medicine, Kyungpook National University, Daegu, Republic of Korea
Full list of author information is available at the end of the article

American Academy of Orthopedic Surgeons (AAOS) [9] recommends that patients with symptomatic KOA engage in self-management programs; perform strengthening, low-impact aerobic exercises; and engage in physical activity consistent with the national guidelines. The American College of Rheumatology Work Group Panel [10] proposed that KOA patients perform 30 min of moderate-intensity (50–70% maximal heart rate) exercise 3 days a week. In addition, the American Geriatrics Society Panel on Exercise and Osteoarthritis [11] recommended engaging in muscle-strengthening activity 2–3 days/week and in flexibility activity 3–5 days/week. In Korea, exercise guidelines [12] recommend low-impact aerobic exercise.

However, there have not been enough studies that examined whether KOA patients engage in appropriate physical activity, especially in East Asia, although several Western studies have reported that the physical activity rates were suboptimal [13]. Moreover, recent studies have shown that osteoarthritis patients are at a higher risk for cardiovascular disease and death because of insufficient physical activity [14]. Thus, from the perspectives of both public health and geriatrics it is important for patients with osteoarthritis to maintain an appropriate level of physical activity.

Pain is one of the major symptoms of osteoarthritis [15]. The extent of pain is associated with decreased physical activity [15]. However, few reports have explored the extent to which physical activity is affected by pain severity in KOA patients.

The populations of Korea and other East Asian countries are aging rapidly, and their body mass indices [16] and lifestyles [17] differ from those of Western populations. Therefore, more evidence with respect to physical activity status of KOA patients in East Asia is needed.

In this study, we aimed to 1) investigate the levels of physical activity among KOA patients compared to the general population, 2) determine the proportion of KOA patients who meet the physical activity recommendations, and 3) examine how the proportion changes with pain severity among KOA patients, by using data from a nationally representative Korean population.

Methods

Data sources

We used data from the fifth Korea National Health and Nutrition Examination Survey (KNHANES V; 2010–2012); KNHANES is an ongoing, multicomponent, nationally representative survey of the noninstitutionalized Korean population administered by the Korea Centers for Disease Control and Prevention (KCDC). The survey uses a multi-stage clustered probability design, creating sampling units from household registries that vary by sex, region, and age group. The KNHANES

V (2010–2012) survey evaluated a total of 576 primary sampling units and 11,520 households from approximately 200,000 geographically defined primary sampling units for the whole country over 3 years [18]. Each KNHANES assessment consists of a health interview, a health examination, and a nutrition survey. We extracted data from the health interview and health examination; we included sociodemographic factors, physical activity parameters, details of morbidities, and radiographic findings. The details of the survey methods and contents have been described elsewhere [18, 19]. The survey was approved by the institutional review board (IRB) of the KCDC in 2010–2012 (approval nos. 2010-02CON-21C, 2011-02CON-06-C, and 2012-01EXP-01-2C).

Radiographic examination of the knee and definition of KOA

In KNHANES 2010–2012, osteoarthritic radiological examinations were performed on those aged ≥50 years. Of the 25,534 individuals who participated, 9514 individuals age > 50 years were subjected to radiographic examination of the knee joints in mobile examination cars based in four different provinces. All examinations were performed by four trained radiologists using digital X-ray machines (SD3000 Synchro Stand; SYFM, Namyangju, South Korea). Bilateral anterior-posterior, lateral (30° flexion), and weight-bearing anterior-posterior plain radiographs of the knees were taken. Two radiologists performed individual radiographic evaluations referencing the Kellgren–Lawrence grading system (0 = normal, 1 = suspicious, 2 = mild osteoarthritis, 3 = moderate osteoarthritis, and 4 = severe osteoarthritis) [20]. We defined KOA of Kellgren–Lawrence grade ≥ 2 as radiographic KOA.

To ensure the reliability and validity of osteoarthritis examination, quality control was conducted through 1) professional surveyor education, 2) equipment quality control, and 3) quality control of the radiograph reading system.

Concerning surveyor education, a site survey management manual was developed and directed to the professional surveyors. Before the start of the osteoarthritis examination, the surveyors were educated about bone and joint digital radiography filming by using the manual. With respect to equipment quality control, an area was selected randomly each month among 192 survey districts and on-site visits were performed more than 20 times in a year. Regular inspection of measurement equipment was conducted once a year. Daily equipment inspection was conducted according to the inspection items designated by the professional inspector on the day of the survey, and any problem with the equipment was immediately reported and addressed with corrective actions. The quality of X-ray imaging by different radiographers was assessed using the newly developed "Knee

Joint Clinical Image Evaluation Form." The average score for bone and joint radiograph quality was 87.76 out of 100. Concerning the quality control of the radiograph reading system, data from the osteoarthritis examination using the reading system was uploaded to and downloaded from Webhard, and graded after double reading by two radiologists, using the Kellgren–Lawrence grading system. In 2010 and 2011, the radiographic digital images were graded by two radiologists. In 2012, one of the two radiologists read all images, and 5% of the images were read by another radiologist. If the grades differed by more than two points, those digital data were read by another radiologist. Inter-rater and intra-rater reliabilities were assessed annually. The measurement methods and quality control procedures are described in detail elsewhere [21, 22].

Pain inclusion criteria

Knee pain was assessed in those participants who complained of pain on > 30 days during the previous 3 months using the question "Please describe the average pain in the knee joint, regardless of the medication used? Please indicate this on a 0~10-point scale with higher scores representing greater pain severity." The numerical rating scale (NRS) answers were divided into three groups (0–3 points = none to mild pain, 4–6 points = moderate pain, ≥7 points = severe pain) [23].

Of the 9514 participants aged ≥50 years who underwent radiographic examinations, 3483 had radiographic KOA. Of these, 1279 who had NRS data were included as the final study subjects.

Physical activity

The KNHANES 2010–2012 physical activity questionnaire was based on the Korean short version of the International Physical Activity Questionnaire (IPAQ) [24]. This consists of six questions: the number of days on which vigorous physical activity was performed in the previous 7 days, and the usual duration of such activity; the number of days on which moderate physical activity was performed in the previous 7 days, and the usual duration of such activity; and the number of days on which the subject walked for at least 10 min at a time during the previous 7 days, and the usual duration of walking. The numbers of days on which muscle-strengthening and flexibility activities were performed during the previous 7 days was also noted.

Based on the short-form IPAQ responses, physical activity was divided into three categories [25]: inactive (Category 1), minimally active (Category 2), and health-enhancing physical activity (HEPA; Category 3). The inactive group (Category 1) reflected the lowest level of physical activity. Those who did not meet the criteria for Categories 2 or 3 were considered inactive. The minimally active group (Category 2) included those who engaged in a) ≥20 min of daily vigorous activity on ≥3 days, or b) ≥30 min of moderate-intensity activity or walking on ≥5 days, or c) any combination of walking and moderate- or vigorous-intensity activity on ≥5 days that summed to ≥600 MET-min/week. The HEPA group (Category 3) met either of the following criteria: a) vigorous-intensity activity at least 3 days summing to ≥1500 MET-min/week or b) any combination of walking and moderate- or vigorous-intensity activity that summed to ≥3000 MET-min/week. The methods for calculating activity are described in the IPAQ guidelines [25].

The American College of Rheumatology Work Group Panel has recommended physical activity or exercise at least 3 days a week (at 50–70% maximal heart rate) for KOA patients [10] (hereafter, the "OA expert panel recommendation"). We classified patients as meeting the recommendation or not meeting the recommendation. In addition, based on the recommendations of the American Geriatrics Society Panel on Exercise and Osteoarthritis [11], we categorized patients according to whether they met the recommendations in terms of muscle-strengthening and flexibility activity. The group that met the recommendation for muscle-strengthening activity engaged in such activity 2–3 days/week; those who did not meet the recommendation did so on ≤1 or ≥ 4 days/week. The group that met the recommendation for flexibility activity engaged in such activity 3–5 days/week; those who did not meet the recommendation did so on ≤2 or ≥ 6 days/week.

Other characteristics of the participants

Age (50–59, 60–69, and ≥ 70 years), monthly household income (in quartiles), education level (less than or equal to elementary school, middle school, high school, and college or higher), and marital status (with or without spouse [separated, bereaved, divorced]) were the sociodemographic factors evaluated. Income per adult equivalent was calculated as household income divided by the square root of the number of persons in the household. Depressive mood was explored using the question "Have you ever felt sad or desperate over the past year for 2 consecutive weeks or more?" The possible responses were "yes" or "no." Body mass index (BMI) was calculated as body weight divided by height squared (kg/m^2); participants with BMI ≥25.0 kg/m^2 were considered obese according to WHO criteria [26]. The number of comorbidities was the sum of diseases diagnosed by a doctor. Smoking status was categorized as smoker or nonsmoker. Alcohol consumption was categorized based on high-risk drinking (more than seven drinks at a time for males and five for females) and as never or low (< 1 episode/month of high-risk drinking), moderate (1–3 episodes/month), and excessive (≥4 episodes/month) drinking [27].

Statistical analysis

The chi-square test was used to compare the characteristics of KOA patients to those of the general population and also to analyze physical activity status by pain severity. Univariable and multivariable logistic regression was performed to identify factors affecting the inability to meet the recommendations of the osteoarthritis expert panel in terms of physical activity. Logistic regression yielded odds ratios (ORs) and 95% confidence intervals (CIs). A two-tailed p value < 0.05 was deemed statistically significant in all analyses. All analyses were performed using SAS ver. 9.4 (SAS Institute Inc., Cary, NC, USA).

Results

Table 1 compares the general characteristics and physical activity of KOA patients with those of the general population older than 50 years of age. Of the 1279 KOA patients, 221 (16.5%) were males and 1058 (83.5%) were females. The percentage of females was higher among KOA patients (83.5%) than in the general population (49.7%). The percentage of low-income KOA patients was twice that in the general population (53.1% vs. 25.4%, respectively). KOA patients also had less education and a more depressive mood than the general population. In terms of physical activity as classified by the IPAQ, more KOA patients were inactive (61.1%) than in the general population (53.3%; $p < 0.001$). Only 18.6% of KOA patients met the OA expert panel recommendations, lower than in the general population (23.2%; $p = 0.003$). The proportions of KOA patients who met recommendations for muscle-strengthening and flexibility activity were 4.3% and 15.8%, significantly lower than in the general population (14.6% and 26.2%, respectively; $p < 0.001$).

Table 2 shows physical activity status by pain severity among KOA patients. According to pain severity, 152 (11.9%), 434 (33.9%), and 693 (54.1%) patients had none to mild, moderate, and severe pain, respectively. Regardless of pain severity, overall physical activity was suboptimal. The level of physical activity did not differ significantly by pain severity. This was true for all types of physical activity, including IPAQ, muscle-strengthening, and flexibility activity. The proportions of minimally HEPA+ active patients by increasing pain severity were 47.4%, 38.5%, and 38.9%, respectively ($p = 0.142$). The proportions who met OA expert recommendations by increasing pain severity were 23.4%, 17.6%, and 18.3%, respectively ($p = 0.341$). Overall, the group with little or no pain engaged in slightly more physical activity than the group with severe pain, but the difference was not statistically significant. Those with moderate and severe pain exhibited little difference in physical activity. In terms of IPAQ, muscle-strengthening, and OA expert

panel–recommended activity, the group with severe pain engaged in somewhat more physical activity than the group with moderate pain, but the difference was not statistically significant. In terms of flexibility activity, the group with little or no pain engaged in less activity than the group with moderate pain (12.3% vs. 17.1%), but again the difference was not statistically significant ($p = 0.585$; Table 2).

We performed logistic regression analyses to identify factors affecting the inability of KOA patients to meet the OA expert recommendations. In univariable analyses, KOA patients aged 70 years or older were less likely to meet the recommendations (OR = 0.6, 95% CI = 0.38–0.96; Table 3) and patients with a spouse were more likely to meet the recommendations (OR = 1.6, 95% CI = 1.16–2.24; Table 3). Those who drank to excess were more likely to meet the recommendations (OR = 2.0, 95% CI = 1.17–3.52; Table 3). In multivariable analyses, however, the above three variables were no longer significant. Only > 3 comorbidities was associated with an inability to meet the recommendations (OR = 0.5, 95% CI = 0.27–0.94; Table 3).

Discussion

We measured the proportions of KOA patients who met physical activity recommendations and assessed physical activity status by pain severity. The percentage of KOA patients who met the physical activity guidelines of OA expert panel recommendation [10] was 18.6%, lower than in the general population. In addition, physical activity status did not differ significantly by pain level, being uniformly suboptimal.

Low levels of physical activity by osteoarthritis patients have been reported in previous studies [13, 23, 28, 29]. In a U.S.-based study [23], osteoarthritis patients were less likely than adults without arthritis to engage in recommended levels of physical activity as in our study. In the study, 32.3% of osteoarthritis patients met the OA expert panel recommendation, which was significantly lower than the proportion of 39.5% reported for the adults without arthritis [23]. One meta-analysis found that the proportion of osteoarthritis patients who met the recommendation of ≥150 min per week of moderate to vigorous physical activity (MVPA) in bouts of ≥10 min (the physical activity level recommended for general adults) was only 13% and that the proportion of those who met the recommendation of at least 10,000 steps per day (another popular physical activity recommendation) was 19% [13], which were suboptimal proportions, as our study showed.

Pain is reported to be one of the primary causes of reduced physical activity among osteoarthritis patients [30, 31], because pain can be experienced during the performance of an activity. Although the group with

Table 1 Comparison of the general characteristics and physical activity of knee osteoarthritis patients and the general population aged ≥50 years

	Knee osteoarthritis patients (≥50 years of age) (N = 1279)		General population (≥50 years of age) (N = 7917)		P-value
	n	Weighted %	n	Weighted %	
Sex					
Male	221	16.5%	3707	50.3%	< 0.001
Female	1058	83.5%	4210	49.7%	
Age					
50–59 years	154	15.1%	3226	52.3%	< 0.001
60–69 years	423	33.0%	2601	27.1%	
≥ 70 years	702	51.8%	2090	20.6%	
Monthly household income					
Low	677	53.1%	2189	25.4%	< 0.001
Moderate to low	290	23.5%	2053	26.2%	
Moderate to high	157	12.9%	1716	23.4%	
High	136	10.6%	1869	25.1%	
Education level					
≤ Elementary	1010	80.4%	3402	41.4%	< 0.001
Middle school	152	11.3%	1422	19.7%	
High school	92	6.8%	2033	26.5%	
≥ College	23	1.5%	1040	12.4%	
Marital status					
With spouse	504	42.5%	1427	17.8%	< 0.001
Without spouse	767	57.5%	6416	82.2%	
Depressive mood					
No	991	77.3%	6752	85.1%	< 0.001
Yes	279	22.7%	1128	14.9%	
Body mass index					
> 25 kg/m^2	500	43.7%	4258	61.5%	< 0.001
≤ 25 kg/m^2	620	56.3%	2582	38.5%	
Number of comorbidities					
0	360	28.7%	3141	42.6%	< 0.001
1	441	35.2%	2574	31.7%	
2	292	22.3%	1447	17.4%	
≥ 3	186	13.9%	755	8.3%	
Cigarette smoking					
Nonsmoker	1168	90.6%	6554	79.5%	< 0.001
Smoker	104	9.4%	1326	20.5%	
Alcohol consumption					
Never	700	54.1%	2957	34.2%	
Low	345	27.3%	2114	25.1%	< 0.001
Moderate	150	11.6%	1574	21.0%	
Excessive	77	7.0%	1232	19.7%	
IPAQ					
Inactive	752	61.1%	4200	53.3%	< 0.001
Minimally active	352	25.9%	2443	30.1%	

Table 1 Comparison of the general characteristics and physical activity of knee osteoarthritis patients and the general population aged ≥50 years *(Continued)*

	Knee osteoarthritis patients (≥50 years of age) (N = 1279)		General population (≥50 years of age) (N = 7917)		P-value
	n	Weighted %	n	Weighted %	
HEPA active	166	13.0%	1233	16.5%	
Muscle-strengthening activity (2–3 days/week)					
Not met	1219	95.7%	6793	85.4%	< 0.001
Met	60	4.3%	1124	14.6%	
Flexibility activity (3–5 days/week)					
Not met	1081	84.2%	5870	73.8%	< 0.001
Met	198	15.8%	2047	26.2%	
Osteoarthritis expert panel recommendation[a]					
Not met	1014	81.4%	6071	76.8%	0.003
Met	256	18.6%	1804	23.2%	

IPAQ International physical activity questionnaire, *HEPA* Health-enhancing physical activity
[a]Osteoarthritis expert panel recommendation: Performance of 30 min of moderate-intensity (50–70% maximal heart rate) physical activity or exercise at least 3 days a week

none to mild pain engaged in slightly more physical activity than did the other groups, we found no proportional decrease in physical activity by pain severity, regardless of the type of activity. Indeed, in terms of flexibility activity, the group with severe pain exercised more than the group with little or no pain. However, the proportions of patients who met the recommended physical activity guidelines were notably suboptimal, even in the group with little or no pain. In this group, the proportions satisfying the recommended physical activity, muscle-strengthening,

and flexibility activity recommendations were only 23.4%, 7.0%, and 12.3%, respectively. Although studies on the extent of physical activity according to pain severity in KOA patients are rare, White et al. [32] reported results similar to ours in that physical activity status was not statistically different according to pain level. Their study also showed that pain level did not significantly affect the attainment of the recommended physical activity levels [32]. The study was conducted by dividing male and female patients, and the percentages of men meeting the guidelines were

Table 2 Physical activity status by pain severity among knee osteoarthritis patients (N = 1279)

	Pain Severity						P-value
	None to mild (n = 152)		Moderate (n = 434)		Severe (n = 693)		
	n	Weighted %	n	Weighted %	n	Weighted %	
IPAQ[a]							
Inactive	80	52.6	244	61.6	428	61.1	0.142
Minimally active	47	31.1	130	27.9	175	25.9	
HEPA active	25	16.3	57	10.6	84	13.0	
Muscle-strengthening activity (2–3 days/week)[a]							
Not met	140	93.0	414	96.3	665	95.9	0.309
Met	12	7.0	20	3.7	28	4.1	
Flexibility activity (3–5 days/week)[a]							
Not met	133	87.7	355	82.9	593	84.3	0.585
Met	19	12.3	79	17.1	100	15.7	
Osteoarthritis expert panel recommendation[a,b]							
Not met	116	76.6	338	82.4	560	81.7	0.341
Met	35	23.4	93	17.6	128	18.3	

Pain severity was categorized using numerical rating scale: 0–3 = none to mild pain, 4–6 = moderate pain, and 7–10 = severe pain
IPAQ International physical activity questionnaire, *HEPA* Health-enhancing physical activity
[a]The totals do not equal 1279 because of missing data
[b]Osteoarthritis expert panel recommendation: Performance of 30 min of moderate-intensity (50–70% maximal heart rate) physical activity or exercise at least 3 days a week

Table 3 Factors associated with compliance with the exercise recommendations of experts on osteoarthritis[a]

| | Univariable analyses | | Multivariable analyses[b] | |
	OR	95% CI	OR	95% CI
Sex				
Male	reference	– –	reference	– –
Female	0.8	0.57 1.24	1.0	0.55 1.64
Age				
50–59 years	reference	– –	reference	– –
60–69 years	1.0	0.62 1.60	1.0	0.61 1.77
≥ 70 years	0.6	0.38 0.96	0.7	0.38 1.20
Monthly household income				
Low	reference	– –	reference	– –
Low to moderate	1.2	0.86 1.80	1.2	0.76 1.77
Moderate to high	0.8	0.47 1.35	0.6	0.34 1.14
High	1.3	0.80 2.11	1.1	0.61 1.90
Education level				
≤ Elementary school	reference	– –	reference	– –
Middle school	1.2	0.73 1.85	0.8	0.48 1.48
High school	1.3	0.76 2.30	1.2	0.64 2.33
≥ College	2.1	0.80 5.30	1.9	0.67 5.51
Marital status				
With spouse	reference	– –	reference	– –
Without spouse	1.6	1.16 2.24	1.3	0.90 2.00
Depressive mood				
No	reference		reference	
Yes	1.3	0.89 1.81	1.5	0.98 2.19
Body mass index				
> 25 kg/m²	reference	– –	reference	– –
≤ 25 kg/m²	1.1	0.79 1.54	1.0	0.71 1.46
Cigarette smoking				
Nonsmoker	reference	– –	reference	– –
Smoker	0.6	0.33 1.20	0.6	0.26 1.18
Alcohol consumption				
Never	reference	– –	reference	– –
Low	0.7	0.50 1.09	0.7	0.46 1.09
Moderate	1.6	1.05 2.53	1.3	0.78 2.27
Excessive	2.0	1.17 3.52	1.6	0.77 3.16
Knee pain severity				
None to mild	reference	– –	reference	– –
Moderate	1.0	0.63 1.69	0.9	0.53 1.59
Severe	0.8	0.51 1.34	0.8	0.48 1.39
Number of comorbidities				
0	reference	– –	reference	– –

Table 3 Factors associated with compliance with the exercise recommendations of experts on osteoarthritis[a] *(Continued)*

| | Univariable analyses | | Multivariable analyses[b] | |
	OR	95% CI	OR	95% CI
1	0.9	0.61 1.31	0.9	0.59 1.37
2	0.9	0.60 1.38	0.8	0.50 1.29
≥ 3	0.6	0.34 1.01	0.5	0.27 0.94

Pain severity was categorized using numerical rating scale: 0–3 = none to mild pain, 4–6 = moderate pain, and 7–10 = severe pain
OR Odds ratio, CI Confidence interval
[a]Performance of 30 min of moderate-intensity (50–70% maximal heart rate) physical activity or exercise at least 3 days a week
[b]The model included sex, age, monthly household income, education level, marital status, depressed mood, body mass index, cigarette smoking, alcohol consumption, knee pain severity, and number of comorbidities

10.9%, 8.8%, and 12.9% and those of women were 11.0%, 8.6%, and 6.7% in the no, mild, and moderate/severe pain groups, respectively, with no apparent statistically significant differences [32]. These findings suggest that pain is not a critical barrier to performing exercise in osteoarthritis patients.

We performed multivariable analyses to explore further whether factors other than pain were associated with KOA patients' (non)fulfilment of exercise recommendations. Previous studies found that physical activity was reduced in patients of older age [33, 34], on lower incomes [33], who were less educated [33], who were obese [35], and who received little social support [29]. In our study, we found that only the number of comorbidities was statistically significant. The more the comorbidities, the less the physical activity, as also reported by Dunlop et al. [33]. We found no significant factors other than poor health (i.e., three or more comorbidities), which suggests that there may be other factors not investigated in the survey besides the well-known individual factors that affect the physical activity status of osteoarthritis patients.

Together, our results suggest that barriers other than pain may cause KOA patients not to meet physical activity recommendations. Several possibilities are apparent. First, KOA patients may receive insufficient education in clinical settings. Currently, no treatment completely cures osteoarthritis [32]. When KOA patients visit clinics, the principal aim of conservative treatment is to minimize pain and limitations of joint function using pharmacological or nonpharmacological approaches. Of nonpharmacological treatments, appropriate physical activity is reportedly effective in maintaining joint mobility and improving muscle strength [36], and all major arthritis guidelines recommend moderate exercise [8–10]. However, in clinical settings, patients may be inadequately informed about how physical activity would assist them, types of exercise, and how often they should exercise. In fact, when we additionally assessed the experience of receiving education about arthritis management in osteoarthritis patients, more than 90% of all patients answered that they had not received any relevant education (Additional file 1: Table S1). Various institutional problems may be at play, including exercise education fees, too many patients per doctor, and a prohibitive payment system. Further research is needed to explore how to emphasize the importance of physical activity and the provision of appropriate guidelines.

Second, it is possible that although patients may wish to exercise, the absence of specific exercise guidelines (on kinds of exercise or the intensity and duration of exercise) renders engaging in activity difficult in the presence of pain. In fact, no specific activity guidelines are available for KOA patients with different grades of pain [8–11]. A systematic analysis of practice guidelines targeting osteoarthritis patients found that the guidelines varied by research group, institute, and professional society, as well as over time, and were based on lower-quality evidence [37]. The specific type of activity; the intensity, amount, and frequency of activity; the initial extent of joint exercise; how such exercise should be gradually increased; the duration of rest periods; and protective equipment by pain level all need to be included in the guideline.

Our study has certain limitations. First, this was a cross-sectional study, and we thus cannot address cause-and-effect questions. Second, information bias may have been at play; we used self-reported data to obtain information on physical activity and other variables. Third, and related to the second limitation, we did not use activity monitors such as accelerometers or heart-rate meters to measure physical activity. Rather, we used the self-administered IPAQ. Thus, the recorded physical activity levels may have been less accurate than those of studies that used activity monitors as surrogate markers of physical activity [38]. However, the IPAQ is a valid measurement tool, as reliable and valid as activity monitors in comparisons performed in about 12 countries, and is used in the U.S. National Health Interview Survey and various surveys conducted by the World Health Organization [24]. Fourth, as the study investigated Korean patients, caution should be taken when generalizing our results to other races with different lifestyles and anthropometric characteristics. Moreover, as our study population comprised > 80% women, caution is needed when generalizing our results to the entire KOA population.

Despite these limitations, our study is meaningful in that we investigated the physical activities of radiographically diagnosed osteoarthritis patients nationwide, calculated the proportions of such patients who met physical activity recommendations in terms of various types of activity, and explored physical activity status by severity of pain.

Conclusions

We found that only 18.6% of Korean KOA patients met the physical activity recommendations, which was significantly lower than the proportion of 23.3% reported for the general population. Regardless of pain severity, overall physical activity was suboptimal in KOA patients. The proportion of patients who met OA expert recommendations was 23.4%, 17.6%, and 18.3% in the none to mild, moderate, and severe pain groups, respectively. In the clinical setting, it is important to emphasize the need for physical activity to patients with osteoarthritis, and a policy-based effort is required to develop physical activity guidelines that reflect pain severity and facilitate the delivery of appropriate exercise.

Abbreviations
AAOS: American Academy of Orthopedic Surgeons; CI: Confidence interval; HEPA: Health-enhancing physical activity; IPAQ: International Physical Activity Questionnaire; KCDC: Korea Centers for Disease Control and Prevention; KNHANES: Korea National Health and Nutrition Examination Survey; KOA: Knee osteoarthritis; NRS: Numerical rating scale; OARSI: Osteoarthritis Research Society International; OR: Odds ratio; WHO: World Health Organization

Acknowledgements
Not applicable.

Funding
This work was supported by 1) Bio & Medical Technology Development Program of the National Research Foundation (NRF) funded by the Korean government, MSIP (No. 2016M3A9B694241) and 2) National Research Foundation of Korea (NRF) grant funded by the Korea government (MSIT) (NRF-2017R1C1B5018142).

Authors' contributions
JYS designed the project, performed the statistical analysis and interpretation of data, and revised critical point. HYS and MRP drafted the first version of the manuscript. HJK reviewed and revised the manuscript. HSK Contributed to the analysis and interpretation of data. All authors read and approved the final manuscript.

Competing interests
The authors declare that they have no competing interests.

Author details
[1]Department of Preventive Medicine, School of Medicine, Eulji University, Deajeon, Republic of Korea. [2]Department of Rehabilitation Medicine, Seoul National University Bundang Hospital, Seoul National University College of Medicine, Seongnam, Republic of Korea. [3]Department of Orthopaedic Surgery, School of Medicine, Kyungpook National University, Kyungpook National University Hospital, Daegu, Republic of Korea. [4]Department of Preventive Medicine, School of Medicine, Kyungpook National University, Daegu, Republic of Korea.

References
1. Breedveld F. Osteoarthritis—the impact of a serious disease. Rheumatology (Oxford). 2004;43(suppl_1):i4–8.
2. World Health Organization and Global Alliance for Musculoskeletal Heath: WHO World Report on Ageing and Health. 2015. http://bjdonline.org/who-strategy-and-action-plan-for-ageing-and-health-background-paper/. Accessed 3 Aug 2017.
3. Lee HS. Prevalence of osteoarthritis and related risk factors in the elderly: data from the fifth Korea National Health and nutrition examination survey (KNHANES V), 2010~ 2012. J Korean Diet Assoc. 2014;20(2):99–109.

4. Yang S, An J. Health status, health behavior and quality of life in the elderly with osteoarthritis. Nurs Sci. 2011;23(2):23–33.

5. Hartman CA, Manos TM, Winter C, Hartman DM, Li B, Smith JC. Effects of T'ai Chi training on function and quality of life indicators in older adults with osteoarthritis. J Am Geriatr Soc. 2000;48(12):1553–9.

6. Fransen M, McConnell S, Harmer AR, Van der Esch M, Simic M, Bennell KL. Exercise for osteoarthritis of the knee: a Cochrane systematic review. Br J Sports Med. 2015. https://doi.org/10.1136/bjsports-2015-095424.

7. Juhl C, Christensen R, Roos EM, Zhang W, Lund H. Impact of exercise type and dose on pain and disability in knee osteoarthritis: a systematic review and meta-regression analysis of randomized controlled trials. Arthritis Rheumatol. 2014;66(3):622–36.

8. McAlindon TE, Bannuru RR, Sullivan M, Arden N, Berenbaum F, Bierma-Zeinstra S, Hawker G, Henrotin Y, Hunter D, Kawaguchi H. OARSI guidelines for the non-surgical management of knee osteoarthritis. Osteoarthr Cartil. 2014;22(3):363–88.

9. Jevsevar DS, Brown GA, Jones DL, Matzkin EG, Manner PA, Mooar P, Schousboe JT, Stovitz S, Sanders JO, Bozic KJ. The American Academy of Orthopaedic surgeons evidence-based guideline on: treatment of osteoarthritis of the knee. J Bone Joint Surg. 2013;95(20):1885–6.

10. McGibbon CA. Work group recommendations: 2002 exercise and physical activity conference, St. Louis, Missouri. Arthritis Rheum. 2003;49(2):261–2.

11. Lundebjerg N. Exercise prescription for older adults with osteoarthritis pain: consensus practice recommendations. J Am Geriatr Soc. 2001;49(6):808–23.

12. Korean Knee Society Subcommittee on Osteoarthritis Guidelines. Guidelines for the treatment of osteoarthritis of the knee, Korean knee society subcommittee on osteoarthritis guidelines. J Korean Knee Soc. 2010;22(1):69–74.

13. Wallis J, Webster K, Levinger P, Taylor N. What proportion of people with hip and knee osteoarthritis meet physical activity guidelines? A systematic review and meta-analysis. Osteoarthr Cartil. 2013;21(11):1648–59.

14. Rahman MM, Kopec JA, Anis AH, Cibere J, Goldsmith CH. Risk of cardiovascular disease in patients with osteoarthritis: a prospective longitudinal study. Arthritis Care Res (Hoboken). 2013;65(12):1951–8.

15. Dekker J, Boot B, van der Woude LH, Bijlsma J. Pain and disability in osteoarthritis: a review of biobehavioral mechanisms. J Behav Med. 1992;15(2):189–214.

16. Yoon YS, Choi HS, Kim JK, Kim YI, Oh SW. Differences in the associations of anthropometric measures with insulin resistance and type 2 diabetes mellitus between Korean and US populations: comparisons of representative nationwide sample data. Obes Res Clin Pract. 2016;10(6):642–51.

17. Ha JK, Kim JG, Lee MC, Wang JH, Research Committee for Development of a Novel Knee Evaluation System of Korean Knee Society. What symptoms are more important for Korean patients in knee osteoarthritis? Development and validation of the Korean knee score. Knee Surg Relat Res. 2012;24(3):151–7.

18. Kweon S, Kim Y, Jang M-j, Kim Y, Kim K, Choi S, Chun C, Khang Y-H, Oh K. Data resource profile: the Korea national health and nutrition examination survey (KNHANES). Int J Epidemiol. 2014;43(1):69–77.

19. Kim Y. The Korea National Health and nutrition examination survey (KNHANES): current status and challenges. Epidemiol Health. 2014;36: e2014002.

20. Kellgren J, Lawrence J. Radiological assessment of osteo-arthrosis. Ann Rheum Dis. 1957;16(4):494–502.

21. Lee S, Kim SJ. Prevalence of knee osteoarthritis, risk factors, and quality of life: the fifth Korean National Health and nutrition examination survey. Int J Rheum Dis. 2015;20(7):809–17.

22. Korea Centers for Disease Control and Prevention. Korea National Health and nutrition examination survey V, the third year (2012): professional surveyor education and quality control for osteoarthritis examination. Seoul: Korea Centers for Disease Control and Prevention; 2012.

23. Shih M, Hootman JM, Kruger J, Helmick CG. Physical activity in men and women with arthritis: National Health Interview Survey, 2002. Am J Prev Med. 2006;30(5):385–93.

24. Oh JY, Yang YJ, Kim BS, Kang JH. Validity and reliability of Korean version of international physical activity questionnaire (IPAQ) short form. J Korean Acad Fam Med. 2007;28(7):532–41.

25. International Physical Activity Questionnaire Research Committee: Guidelines for data processing and analysis of the International Physical Activity Questionnaire (IPAQ)–short and long forms. 2005. http://www.ipaq.ki.se/. Accessed 30 Aug 2017.

26. Zheng W, McLerran DF, Rolland B, Zhang X, Inoue M, Matsuo K, He J, Gupta PC, Ramadas K, Tsugane S. Association between body-mass index and risk of death in more than 1 million Asians. N Engl J Med. 2011;364(8):719–29.

27. Kang K, Sung J, Kim CY. High risk groups in health behavior defined by clustering of smoking, alcohol, and exercise habits: National Health and nutrition examination survey. J Prev Med Public Health. 2010;43(1):73–81.

28. Dunlop DD, Song J, Semanik PA, Chang RW, Sharma L, Bathon JM, Eaton CB, Hochberg MC, Jackson RD, Kwoh CK. Objective physical activity measurement in the osteoarthritis initiative: are guidelines being met? Arthritis Rheum. 2011;63(11):3372–82.

29. Rosemann T, Kuehlein T, Laux G, Szecsenyi J. Factors associated with physical activity of patients with osteoarthritis of the lower limb. J Eval Clin Pract. 2008;14(2):288–93.

30. Somers TJ, Keefe FJ, Pells JJ, Dixon KE, Waters SJ, Riordan PA, Blumenthal JA, McKee DC, LaCaille L, Tucker JM. Pain catastrophizing and pain-related fear in osteoarthritis patients: relationships to pain and disability. J Pain Symptom Manag. 2009;37(5):863–72.

31. Steultjens M, Dekker J, Bijlsma J. Avoidance of activity and disability in patients with osteoarthritis of the knee: the mediating role of muscle strength. Arthritis Rheum. 2002;46(7):1784–8.

32. White DK, Tudor-Locke C, Felson DT, Gross KD, Niu J, Nevitt M, Lewis CE, Torner J, Neogi T. Do radiographic disease and pain account for why people with or at high risk of knee osteoarthritis do not meet physical activity guidelines? Arthritis Rheum. 2013;65(1):139–47.

33. Dunlop DD, Song J, Semanik PA, Sharma L, Chang RW. Physical activity levels and functional performance in the osteoarthritis initiative: a graded relationship. Arthritis Rheum. 2011;63(1):127–36.

34. De Groot I, Bussmann J, Stam H, Verhaar J. Actual everyday physical activity in patients with end-stage hip or knee osteoarthritis compared with healthy controls. Osteoarthr Cartil. 2008;16(4):436–42.

35. Farr JN, Going SB, Lohman TG, Rankin L, Kasle S, Cornett M, Cussler E. Physical activity levels in patients with early knee osteoarthritis measured by accelerometry. Arthritis Care Res (Hoboken). 2008;59(9):1229–36.

36. Vaishya R, Pariyo GB, Agarwal AK, Vijay V. Non-operative management of osteoarthritis of the knee joint. J Clin Orthop Trauma. 2016;7(3):170–6.

37. Feuerstein JD, Pelsis JR, Lloyd S, Cheifetz AS, Stone KR. Systematic analysis of the quality of the scientific evidence and conflicts of interest in osteoarthritis of the hip and knee practice guidelines. Semin Arthritis Rheum. 2016;45:379–85 Elsevier.

38. Veenhof C, Huisman P, Barten J, Takken T, Pisters M. Factors associated with physical activity in patients with osteoarthritis of the hip or knee: a systematic review. Osteoarthr Cartil. 2012;20(1):6–12.

25

A novel MRI- and CT-based scoring system to differentiate malignant from osteoporotic vertebral fractures in Chinese patients

Zi Li[1,2†], Ming Guan[1†], Dong Sun[3], Yong Xu[1], Feng Li[1] and Wei Xiong[1*] ⓘ

Abstract

Background: Various types of magnetic resonance imaging (MRI) and computed tomography (CT) findings are used to differentiate malignant vertebral fractures (MVFs) from osteoporotic vertebral fractures (OVFs). The distinguishing ability of any single finding is limited. This study developed a novel scoring system that integrates multiple MRI and CT signs for improved accuracy of differential diagnosis between MVFs and OVFs.

Methods: A total of 150 MVFs and 150 OVFs in thoracolumbar vertebrae were analyzed. MRI and CT images were obtained within 2 months of the probable time of fracture. The sensitivity and specificity of 15 MRI and CT image findings were evaluated. A stepwise discriminant analysis using these signs as variables was used to create a scoring system to differentiate MVFs from OVFs.

Results: All 15 image findings had strong specificity and moderate sensitivity. Seven MRI and three CT image findings were selected and assigned integral values in the final scoring system. A total score of 4 or greater points indicated MVF, whereas a total score of 3 or fewer points indicated OVF. The classification accuracy was 98.3% in the test set.

Conclusions: This novel scoring system using MRI and CT radiologic findings to differentiate MVFs from OVFs in Chinese patients was efficient with high accuracy and good applicability.

Keywords: Computed tomography, Discriminant analysis, Magnetic resonance imaging, Malignant vertebral fracture, Osteoporotic vertebral fracture

Background

Vertebral fractures caused by benign or malignant lesions are common among the elderly. Identifying the etiology of spinal fractures at an early stage is critical to determine the clinical course, treatment, and prognosis [1–4]. Common features of osteoporotic vertebral fracture (OVF) and malignant vertebral fracture (MVF), including age group, clinical symptoms, and history of inadequate trauma, make differential diagnosis challenging. Open biopsy is considered the benchmark to diagnose musculoskeletal lesions, with 98% accuracy [5]. Its clinical application has been limited due to increased morbidity and a significant risk of complications [6, 7]. Percutaneous biopsy, a less invasive option recommended as an alternative for open biopsy, has a wide range of reported accuracy rates from 16 to 92% and a complication rate between 0 and 10% [8].

Modern radiological imaging techniques, including magnetic resonance imaging (MRI) and computed tomography (CT), have good predictive value for differential diagnosis. Multiple-image findings are utilized to distinguish between MVFs and OVFs [1, 3, 4, 9, 10]. Single-image findings have limited distinguishing ability and are not considered sufficiently sensitive or specific, such as fluid sign and pedicle involvement [1, 11, 12]. Misdiagnosis or delayed diagnosis of MVF is not uncommon in clinical practice, potentially due in part to

* Correspondence: xcxgreatwellus@hotmail.com
†Zi Li and Ming Guan contributed equally to this work.
[1]Department of orthopedics, Tongji Hospital, Tongji Medical College, Huazhong University of Science and Technology, 1095#, Jiefang Ave, Wuhan, Hubei, China
Full list of author information is available at the end of the article

confusing MRI and CT image findings. Unnecessary biopsy and pathological examinations of OVF patients diminishes the medical treatment experience and increases the risk and cost to the patient.

Integrating characteristic image findings can improve the accuracy of differential diagnosis. Discriminant analysis is a generally accepted statistical method that combines multiple features to separate or characterize two or more classes of clinical issues [13–15]. Two earlier studies attempted to create a scoring system to distinguish MVFs from OVFs using discriminant analysis, but the etiology types for malignant cases [16] or the sample sizes were limited [17].

This study utilized a large sample of Chinese patients to generate a novel scoring system to differentiate MVFs from OVFs using MRI and CT image findings.

Methods

All OVF and MVF cases contained in the electronic records archives of the department of spine surgery for the period January 2013 to March 2018 were included in the study. Our institutional Ethics Review Board approved the study protocol. Informed and written concent was obtained from all patients. MRI images were obtained using two 3.0 T magnetic resonance scanners (Siemens Healthcare, Skyra, Germany; GE Healthcare, Discovery MR750, USA). Images of 5-mm thick contiguous or vertebral bodies and disc level CT sections were performed using a 16-detector CT scanner (GE Healthcare, LightSpeed 16, USA) and 1.25-3 mm thick reconstruction slices with no overlap were obtained for evaluation. The inclusion and exclusion criteria listed below were used to further refine selection of the sample.

Inclusion criteria

1. A definitive diagnosis was required for inclusion. Patients included in the group of MVF required an exact pathologic diagnosis for one vertebrae (positive percutaneous transpedicular biopsy or pathological specimen through spinal surgery). OVF diagnosis was verified by benign histologic pathology, or not aggravated or improving clinical symptoms with restoration of vertebral signal intensity on MRI observed for a period of at least 2 months [16].
2. Only thoracolumbar vertebral lesions were included.
3. An MRI or CT was obtained within 2 months of the probable day of fracture.

Exclusion criteria

1. Neurogenic tumor cases, such as schwannoma or neurofibroma.

2. MVF patients who had already received an operation, irradiation, or biopsy.
3. Concomitant cases of OVF and MVF.
4. Severe trauma cases, such as a traffic accident or high falling injury.

A total of 150 OVFs and 150 MVFs in 226 Chinese patients were selected. The 300 vertebral fracture images were reviewed by two orthopedic surgeons (Zi Li and Ming Guan each with 2 years of experience) and one musculoskeletal radiologist (Dong Sun with 2 years of experience). A total of 15 key findings (12 MRI and 3 CT) previously proposed in the literature was applied to image evaluation. Discrepancies were resolved by debate until consensus was achieved. The sensitivity and specificity of each finding was then calculated.

MRI finding
Pattern change of vertebrae signal intensity
A lesion is likely malignant when the observed geometric pattern of vertebral signal intensity is round (Fig. 1, F1) [2, 12, 18, 19]. A band-like appearance is often seen in OVF (Fig. 1, F2) [12, 19, 20]. A whole vertebrae diffused with abnormal signal indicates MVF (Fig. 1, F3); OVF is implied if a normal signal remains [11, 12, 19, 21].

Contour of the anterior or posterior wall border
OVF is implied when there is a sharp protrusion in the posterior superior border of the vertebral body (Fig. 1, F4); a smoothly blunt protrusion in the posterior border of the vertebral body is often seen in MVF (Fig. 1, F5) [20, 22]. An anterior vertebral convexity indicates a higher likelihood of MVF than OVF (Fig. 1, F6) [23].

Paravertebral solid mass
A paravertebral solid mass is more commonly detected in MVF than OVF (Fig. 1, F7). Spinal tumors are usually solid masses rather than cystic masses which are commonly detected in infectious cases, especially in the spinal tuberculosis [11, 18, 24].

Cleft formation ("fluid sign")
Fluid sign refers to a cleft configuration with a signal as low as that of water in T1WI and as high as that of water in T2WI (Fig. 1, F9) [2, 12, 19, 23, 24]. It supports a diagnosis of OVF rather than MVF.

Asymmetry of signal intensity change in axial image
The symmetry of the signal intensity change in vertebrae indicates OVF, whereas asymmetry of the signal intensity change indicates MVF (Fig. 1, F10) [18].

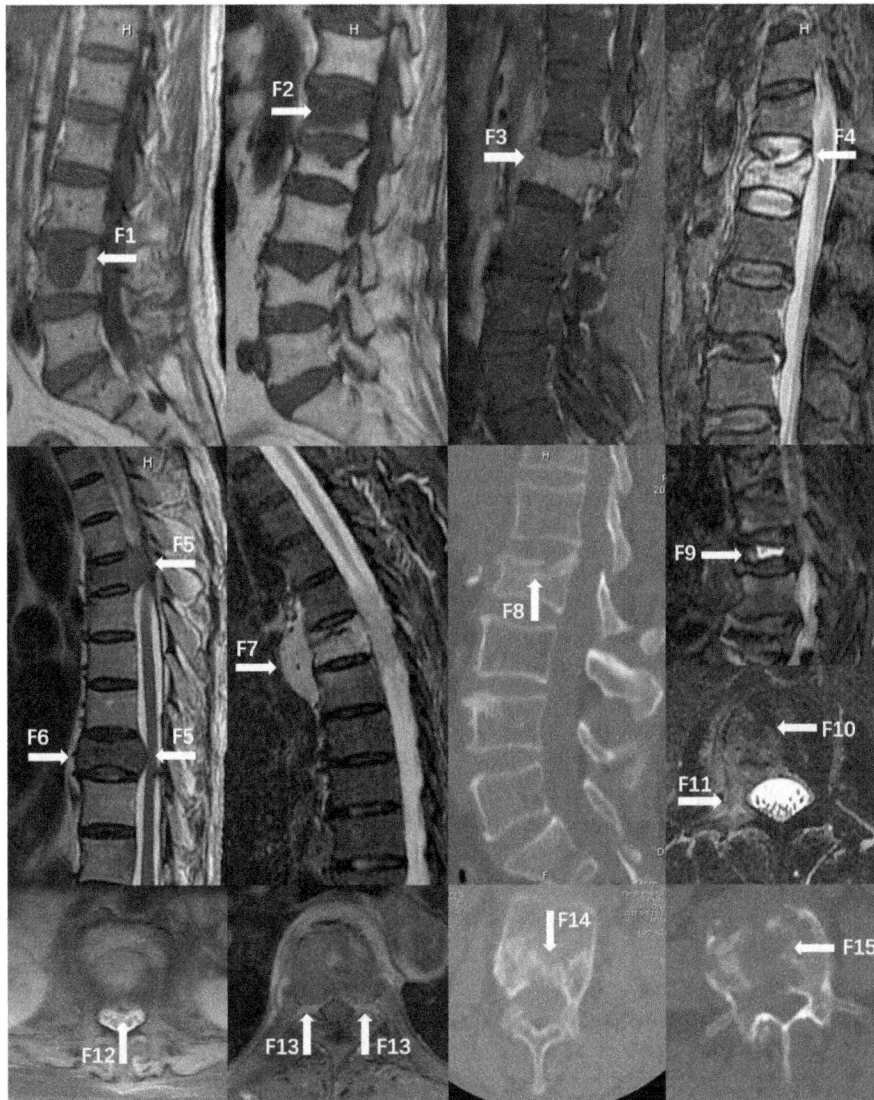

Fig. 1 Key radiological magnetic resonance imaging (MRI) and computed tomography (CT) findings. F1 indicates a round vertebral signal intensity change (metastasis of prostate cancer); F2 indicates a band-like vertebral signal intensity change (osteoporotic vertebral fracture [OVF]); F3 indicates a diffuse vertebral signal intensity change (metastasis of lung cancer); F4 indicates a superior sharp protrusion of the posterior wall border (OVF); F5 indicates a smoothly blunt protrusion of the posterior wall border (metastasis of bladder cancer); F6 indicates an anterior vertebral convexity (metastasis of bladder cancer); F7 indicates a paravertebral solid mass (lymphoma); F8 indicates a sclerotic band beneath the end plate (OVF); F9 indicates a cleft fluid sign (OVF); F10 indicates an asymmetry in signal intensity (metastasis of kidney cancer); F11 indicates a pedicle involvement (metastasis of kidney cancer); F12 indicates a single-peaked posterior wall protrusion (OVF); F13 indicates a double-peaked posterior wall protrusion (metastasis of prostate cancer); F14 indicates a vertebral fracture without osteolysis (OVF); F15 indicates an osteolytic destruction (metastasis of lung cancer)

Pedicle involvement
A signal intensity change encompassing half of the pedicle is judged as pedicle involvement and indicates MVF (Fig. 1, F11) [12, 19, 20].

Pattern of posterior wall protrusion in axial image
The normal pattern of posterior wall protrusion in OVF is single-peaked (Fig. 1, F12). The pattern of posterior wall protrusion in MVF is usually double-peaked (Fig. 1, F13) [18].

CT imaging finding
Sclerotic band beneath the end plate
The sclerotic band refers to a zone of trabeculae compaction and late reactive callus that has a high density in CT after osteoporotic fractures, usually accompanied by a deformed end plate (Fig. 1, F8) [19, 25].

Relationship between fracture and osteolysis

An apparent vertebral fracture line without osteolysis, with no tumor cells invading, is often seen in OVF (Fig. 1, F14). The osteolytic destruction of the vertebral cortex or body is observed in 97% of MVF cases (Fig. 1, F15) [18, 19, 25].

After image evaluation, a stepwise discriminant analysis was used to produce the scoring system. Discriminant analysis is a generalized statistical method that generates a suitable combination of features that separate or characterize two or more classes of objects [26]. Each image finding was considered a dummy variable, and multiple linear regression analysis was implemented with corresponding discriminant coefficients as scores, and constants as discriminant threshold. The stepwise method selects the "best" variables automatically in the analysis when comparing many variables. Starting with a situation that does not include any variables, the variable with the largest *F to Enter* value greater than the entry criteria (set by default as 3.84) is included in the analysis at each step. The variables with *F to Enter* values < 3.84 are left out of the analysis until no more are added. The error rate of discrimination is calculated by the leave-one-out cross validation method: any sample is regarded as a test case and the remaining samples are regarded as a training set, detecting on the cycle until all samples have become test cases once. A novel scoring formula was obtained, with corresponding coefficients of selected predictors as scores and the discriminant threshold as a constant. All data were statistically analyzed using IBM SPSS version 19. Single parameters were analyzed using chi-square tests. A value of $p < 0.05$ was considered statistically significant.

Results

The MVF group had a younger mean age and lower proportion of females than the OVF group. The most common metastasis and primary neoplasms were lung cancer (35 cases) and multiple myeloma (21 cases), respectively. The clinical characteristics of the included cases are presented in Table 1. The calculated sensitivity and specificity of the 15 image findings included in the analysis are presented in Table 2.

Discriminant analysis

The 15 image findings listed in Table 2 were set as independent variables. A variable present in one vertebra was set as 1; if it was not present, the value was set as 0. Stepwise discriminant analysis was then performed. A total of ten selected findings with the corresponding coefficients and the constant in the result are presented in Table 3; the remaining five findings were excluded because of low tolerance. The classification accuracy of the stepwise discriminant analysis was 98.3%, Wilks' λ was 0.158 ($p < 0.001$), and the

Table 1 Clinical characteristics

Characteristics	MVF	OVF
n (vertebrae)	150	150
n (patients)	106	126
Gender (Male/Female)	74/32	34/92
Age (years), Mean ± SD (range)	55.5 ± 11.9 (23–75)	66.3 ± 7.6 (51–82)
Spinal level		
Thoracic, n (%)	70 (46.7%)	69 (46.0%)
Lumbar, n (%)	80 (53.3%)	81 (54.0%)
n (tumor type)		N/A
Lung	35	
Multiple myeloma	21	
Prostate	13	
Bladder	11	
Liver	9	
Kidney	8	
Lymphoma	7	
Breast	4	
Leukemia	4	
Osteosarcoma	3	
PNET	3	
Chondrosarcoma	2	
Other	30	

MVF metastatic vertebral fracture, *OVF* osteoporotic vertebral fracture, *PNET* peripheral neuroectodermal tumor, *N/A* not applicable

discriminant accuracy of the cross-validation (leave-one-out method) was 97.7%.

Decimal scores are not practical in clinical settings. To enhance practicability, we divided the constant and coefficients term by two and the results were rounded into integral numbers. Finally, a simplified scoring system was created (Table 4). A total score ≥ 4 indicates MVF, whereas a total score ≤ 3 points indicates OVF. The classification accuracy of the simplified scoring system was 98.3%, equal to the original discriminant analysis. Only three OVF and two MVF cases were incorrectly classified by the simplified scoring system.

Discussion

A stepwise discriminant analysis was used to create a novel simple scoring system to differentiate MVF from OVF using MRI and CT image findings, with a discriminant accuracy of 98.3%.

Relatively low sensitivity and high specificity were calculated for image findings. The distinguishing ability of any single radiological finding was limited. The rational application of discriminant analysis to integrate different image findings was a statistically valid and logical method to maximize the diagnostic accuracy rate. A total of 15 significant image findings were

Table 2 Sensitivity and specificity of key MRI and CT findings

Radiological Findings	Implication	Sensitivity (%)	Specificity (%)	p-value
MRI findings				
Pattern change of vertebrae signal intensity				
Round	MVF	43	99	< 0.001
Band like	OVF	58	97	< 0.001
Diffuse	MVF	79	91	< 0.001
Shape of posterior wall protrusion				
Superior sharp	OVF	43	87	< 0.001
Smoothly blunt	MVF	57	96	< 0.001
Anterior vertebral convexity	MVF	23	97	< 0.001
Paravertebral solid mass	MVF	63	99	< 0.001
Fluid sign	OVF	29	99	< 0.001
Asymmetry of signal intensity change	MVF	80	87	< 0.001
Pedicle involvement	MVF	86	79	< 0.001
Shape of posterior wall protrusion				
Single peaked	OVF	26	88	< 0.05
Double peaked	MVF	35	97	< 0.001
CT findings				
Sclerotic band beneath the end plate	OVF	65	99	< 0.001
Fracture without osteolysis	OVF	59	99	< 0.001
Osteolytic destruction	MVF	63	98	< 0.001

CT computed tomography, *MRI* magnetic resonance imaging, *MVF* malignant vertebral fracture, *OVF* osteoporotic vertebral fracture

Table 3 Result of the discriminant analysis

Radiological Findings	Discriminant coefficient
MRI findings	
Pattern change of vertebrae signal intensity	
Round	3.794
Band like	−1.730
Diffuse	4.238
Smoothly blunt border protrusion of the posterior wall	1.909
Paravertebral solid mass	4.250
Asymmetry of signal intensity change	4.559
Pedicle involvement	4.330
CT findings	
Sclerotic band beneath the end plate	−3.467
Fracture without osteolysis	−3.786
Osteolytic destruction	3.051
Discriminant threshold	7.272

CT computed tomography, *MRI* magnetic resonance imaging, *MVF* malignant vertebral fracture, *OVF* osteoporotic vertebral fracture

included as variables in the study based on previous research. Analysis of the input variable contribution to the output eliminated five findings, and the rational model was established. Only two previous studies have attempted to develop scoring systems to differentiate benign and malignant vertebral fractures using discriminant analysis [16, 17]. The score scale of the study from Yuzawa et al. was also based on MRI and CT signs, but had a limited sample size (100 cases), and radiologic findings yielded relatively low accuracy rates [17]. This study included four involved findings (pedicle involvement, paravertebral solid mass, fracture without osteolysis, and osteolytic destruction) not included in previous scoring systems.

The discriminant accuracy based on MRI or CT findings alone were 96.0 and 89.7%, respectively. These are slightly lower than the MRI findings accuracy of 96.6% reported by So Koto et al., who concluded that using MRI findings alone provides satisfactory accuracy for differential diagnosis [16]. Including findings, image judging criteria, sample size, and ethnicity may account for the different

accuracy rates. To improve accuracy, this study included CT image findings in the analysis. CT is the most suitable imaging technique to identify calcification, ossification, extent of lesion, and cortical outline with high spatial resolution [24]. The affordability and speed of CT scanning have made it a general imaging service in China. Supplementing MRI findings with CT are indispensable for differential diagnosis.

The sclerotic band beneath the end plate was an important finding in the scoring system. A faint band of sclerosis beneath the end plate refers to a zone of trabeculae compaction and late reactive callus, which has high density in CT after osteoporotic fracture and may be present for 8 to 10 weeks post-fracture [19]. Reactive sclerotic change was observed with 77.8% sensitivity and 90.0% specificity, indicating that sclerotic change on CT images was a statistically significant finding indicating benign lesion [25]. The discriminant accuracy decreased to 97.3% without the sclerotic band beneath the end plate, verifying the importance of the finding.

A total of 300 cases were included in this study, larger than any other sample in the literature. The tumor etiology was primarily primary and metastatic tumors. Pathological examination is considered the benchmark for tumor diagnosis, and all patients of MVF included in this study had exact pathologic diagnoses of one vertebrae (positive percutaneous transpedicular biopsy or pathological specimen through spinal surgery). In the study from Kato et al., metastatic tumor cases were diagnosed either by pathologic diagnosis or malignancy radiographic changes, which are less rigorous than the criteria used in this study [16].

Table 4 Modified scoring system for diagnosis of malignant vertebral fractures (MVFs)

Radiological Findings	Implication	Score
MRI findings		
Pattern change of vertebrae signal intensity		
Round	MVF	2
Band-like	OVF	−1
Diffuse	MVF	2
Smoothly blunt border protrusion of the posterior wall	MVF	1
Paravertebral solid mass	MVF	2
Asymmetry of signal intensity change	MVF	2
Pedicle involvement	MVF	2
CT findings		
Sclerotic band beneath the end plate	OVF	−2
Fracture without osteolysis	OVF	−2
Osteolytic destruction	MVF	2
Total score: OVF ≤ 3 and MVF ≥ 4		

CT computed tomography, *MRI* magnetic resonance imaging, *MVF* malignant vertebral fracture, *OVF* osteoporotic vertebral fracture

Combining 15 MRI and CT findings based on the available literature, and selecting 10 variables for the scoring system, yielded a system with discriminant accuracy higher than that achieved in previous studies.

There are several limitations to this study. Firstly, although CT findings can improve the discriminant accuracy for differentiating MVFs from OVFs, the hazards of radiation ionization would not be ignored. Secondly, there were many multiple malignant vertebral fractures in the available cases. Single vertebral involvement is the best operation indication for *en bloc* resection in malignant vertebral fractures [27]. One of the original objectives for this study was to contribute to the surgical decision for single vertebral pathologic fractures. Due to the limited sample size, vertebrae were used as the sample unit for assessment rather than patients. A multi-center approach to compile more cases of single pathological vertebral fracture can be used address this issue in the future. Additionally, clinical information including symptoms and tumor markers can assist clinicians with diagnoses and may be added to a future scoring system.

Conclusion
A novel scoring system based on MRI and CT image findings in Chinese patients was effective and convenient for differentiating MVFs from OVFs. A future multi-center validation is required to confirm the accuracy and practicability of the scoring system.

Abbreviations
CT: Computed tomography; MRI: Magnetic resonance imaging; MVF: Malignant vertebral fracture; OVF: Osteoporotic vertebral fracture

Acknowledgements
We thank all the patients involved in the study.

Funding
This work is supported by National Natural Science Foundation of China (No. 81571816).

Authors' contributions
ZL: study design, analyzing the data and writing the paper. MG: study design, interpreting the data and writing the paper. DS: analyzing the data. YX: critical revision. FL: critical revision. WX: study design and critical revision. All authors read and approved the final manuscript.

Competing interests
The authors declare that they have no competing interests.

Author details
[1]Department of orthopedics, Tongji Hospital, Tongji Medical College, Huazhong University of Science and Technology, 1095#, Jiefang Ave, Wuhan, Hubei, China. [2]Department of orthopedics, Taikang Tongji Hospital, Wuhan, Hubei, China. [3]Radiology department, Tongji Hospital, Tongji Medical College, Huazhong University of Science and Technology, 1095#, Jiefang Ave, Wuhan, Hubei, China.

References
1. Takigawa T, Tanaka M, Sugimoto Y, Tetsunaga T, Nishida K, Ozaki T. Discrimination between malignant and benign vertebral fractures using magnetic resonance imaging. Asian Spine J. 2017;11(3):478–83.
2. Thawait SK, Marcus MA, Morrison WB, Klufas RA, Eng J, Carrino JA. Research synthesis: what is the diagnostic performance of magnetic resonance imaging to discriminate benign from malignant vertebral compression fractures? Systematic review and meta-analysis. Spine. 2012;37(12):E736–44.
3. Cuenod CA, Laredo JD, Chevret S, Hamze B, Naouri JF, Chapaux X, Bondeville JM, Tubiana JM. Acute vertebral collapse due to osteoporosis or malignancy: appearance on unenhanced and gadolinium-enhanced MR images. Radiology. 1996;199(2):541–9.
4. Jung HS, Jee WH, McCauley TR, Ha KY, Choi KH. Discrimination of metastatic from acute osteoporotic compression spinal fractures with MR imaging. Radiographics. 2003;23(1):179–87.
5. Dupuy DE, Rosenberg AE, Punyaratabandhu T, Tan MH, Mankin HJ. Accuracy of CT-guided needle biopsy of musculoskeletal neoplasms. AJR Am J Roentgenol. 1998;171(3):759–62.
6. Rehm J, Veith S, Akbar M, Kauczor HU, Weber MA. CT-guided percutaneous spine biopsy in suspected infection or malignancy: a study of 214 patients. RoFo. 2016;188(12):1156–62.
7. Rimondi E, Staals EL, Errani C, Bianchi G, Casadei R, Alberghini M, Malaguti MC, Rossi G, Durante S, Mercuri M. Percutaneous CT-guided biopsy of the spine: results of 430 biopsies. Eur Spine J. 2008;17(7):975–81.
8. Metzger CS, Johnson DW, Donaldson WF 3rd. Percutaneous biopsy in the anterior thoracic spine. Spine. 1993;18(3):374–8.
9. Schwaiger BJ, Gersing AS, Baum T, Krestan CR, Kirschke JS. Distinguishing benign and malignant vertebral fractures using CT and MRI. Semin Musculoskelet Radiol. 2016;20(4):345–52.
10. Yuan Y, Zhang Y, Lang N, Li J, Yuan H. Differentiating malignant vertebral tumours from non-malignancies with CT spectral imaging: a preliminary study. Eur Radiol. 2015;25(10):2945–50.
11. Frighetto-Pereira L, Rangayyan RM, Metzner GA, de Azevedo-Marques PM, Nogueira-Barbosa MH. Shape, texture and statistical features for classification of benign and malignant vertebral compression fractures in magnetic resonance images. Comput Biol Med. 2016;73:147–56.
12. Abdel-Wanis ME, Solyman MT, Hasan NM. Sensitivity, specificity and accuracy of magnetic resonance imaging for differentiating vertebral compression fractures caused by malignancy, osteoporosis, and infections. J Orthop Surg. 2011;19(2):145–50.
13. Van Toen C, Street J, Oxland TR, Cripton PA. Cervical spine injuries and flexibilities following axial impact with lateral eccentricity. Eur Spine J. 2015;24(1):136–47.

14. Dolphens M, Cagnie B, Coorevits P, Vleeming A, Palmans T, Danneels L. Posture class prediction of pre-peak height velocity subjects according to gross body segment orientations using linear discriminant analysis. Eur Spine J. 2014;23(3):530–5.

15. Lin SP, Mandell MS, Chang Y, Chen PT, Tsou MY, Chan KH, Ting CK. Discriminant analysis for anaesthetic decision-making: an intelligent recognition system for epidural needle insertion. Br J Anaesth. 2012;108(2):302–7.

16. Kato S, Hozumi T, Yamakawa K, Saito M, Goto T, Kondo T. META: an MRI-based scoring system differentiating metastatic from osteoporotic vertebral fractures. Spine J. 2015;15(7):1563–70.

17. Yuzawa Y, Ebara S, Kamimura M, Tateiwa Y, Kinoshita T, Itoh H, Takahashi J, Karakida O, Sheena Y, Takaoka K. Magnetic resonance and computed tomography-based scoring system for the differential diagnosis of vertebral fractures caused by osteoporosis and malignant tumors. J Orthopaed Sci. 2005;10(4):345–52.

18. Cicala D, Briganti F, Casale L, Rossi C, Cagini L, Cesarano E, Brunese L, Giganti M. Atraumatic vertebral compression fractures: differential diagnosis between benign osteoporotic and malignant fractures by MRI. Musculoskelet Surg. 2013;97(Suppl 2):S169–79.

19. Kazawa N. T2WI MRI and MRI-MDCT correlations of the osteoporotic vertebral compressive fractures. Eur J Radiol. 2012;81(7):1630–6.

20. Cho WI, Chang UK. Comparison of MR imaging and FDG-PET/CT in the differential diagnosis of benign and malignant vertebral compression fractures. J Neurosurg Spine. 2011;14(2):177–83.

21. Barragan-Campos HM, Jimenez-Zarazua O, Mondragon JD. Diagnosis and treatment options of spinal metastases. Rev Invest Clin. 2015;67(3):140–57.

22. Ruivo C, Hopper MA. Spinal chondrosarcoma arising from a solitary lumbar osteochondroma. JBR-BTR. 2014;97(1):21–4.

23. Pongpornsup S, Wajanawichakorn P, Danchaivijitr N. Benign versus malignant compression fracture: a diagnostic accuracy of magnetic resonance imaging. J Med Assoc Thai. 2009;92(1):64–72.

24. Torres C, Hammond I. Computed tomography and magnetic resonance imaging in the differentiation of osteoporotic fractures from neoplastic metastatic fractures. J Clin Densitom. 2016;19(1):63–9.

25. Kim YS, Han IH, Lee IS, Lee JS, Choi BK. Imaging findings of solitary spinal bony lesions and the differential diagnosis of benign and malignant lesions. J Korean Neurosurg Soc. 2012;52(2):126–32.

26. McLachlan GJ. Discriminant analysis. Wiley Interdiscipl Rev: Comput Stat. 2012;4(5):421–31.

27. Hsieh PC, Li KW, Sciubba DM, Suk I, Wolinsky JP, Gokaslan ZL. Posterior-only approach for total en bloc spondylectomy for malignant primary spinal neoplasms: anatomic considerations and operative nuances. Neurosurgery. 2009;65(6 Suppl):173–81 discussion 181.

Can anthropometric, body composition, and bone variables be considered risk factors for musculoskeletal injuries in Brazilian military students?

Mauro A. S. Melloni*[ORCID], Josiel De Almeida Ávila, Mauro Alexandre Páscoa, Camila Justino De Oliveira Barbeta, Vagner Xavier Cirolini, Ezequiel M. Gonçalves and Gil Guerra-Júnior

Abstract

Background: Musculoskeletal injuries are the main cause of premature discharge from military service and can sometimes lead to permanent disabilities. Some intrinsic risk factors are well discussed in the literature. However, the relation between body composition variables and the risk for musculoskeletal injury is not well known or recognized.

Methods: This prospective study evaluated 205 Brazilian military students. At the beginning of military service, health status and sports experience prior to military service were registered. Anthropometric variables were evaluated, and bone and body composition variables were measured using dual-energy X-ray absorptiometry. The occurrence of musculoskeletal injuries throughout the year was registered at the military physiotherapy service. At the end of 1 year of follow-up, risk factors were analysed by comparing the variables between the injured and non-injured students.

Results: No difference in previous health status was found between injured and non-injured groups, whereas sports experience prior to military service was identified as a protective factor (Odds Ratio (OR) 0.323; 95% CI: 0.108–0.968; $p = 0.044$). Anthropometric, bone, and body composition variables could not be identified as risk factors for musculoskeletal injuries in Brazilian military students.

Conclusion: Anthropometric, bone, and body composition variables could not be considered risk factors for musculoskeletal injuries in Brazilian military students.

Keywords: Military, cumulative trauma disorders, body composition, risk factors

Background

Being healthy and physically fit is required in the military profession. Thus, some aspects of military physical training programs are important to ensure development of the physical and fitness skills required in the military profession. However, they can also lead to musculoskeletal injury (MI) and disabilities, which in turn result in premature discharge from military service [1, 2]. In this respect, a systematic review [2] showed a cumulative incidence ranging from 8 to 51% for MI related to military physical training, whereas a prospective study reported that almost 70% of participants followed up for 6 months presented with at least one type of MI, [3] concluding that MI is an important public health problem for the military.

The literature on general military health usually recognizes that overload injuries are more prevalent than traumatic injuries in the military population [4]. Furthermore, MI is highlighted as the main cause of premature discharge from military service [5] and the main reason for seeking medical care during the service [1]. Consequently, premature discharge from military service and the need for medical care owing to MI can result in

* Correspondence: mauromelloni@gmail.com
Departamento de Pediatria, Universidade Estadual de Campinas-Unicamp, Tessália Vieira de Camargo, 126, Cidade Universitária Zeferino Vaz, Campinas, SP Zip code: 13083-887, Brazil

financial and physical fitness losses and psychological changes, mainly in countries where military service is compulsory [5].

Many variables are reported as risk factors for MI related to military physical training. In general, these variables are usually classified as extrinsic (e.g. long weekly running distance, absence of sports experience prior to military service, smoking habit, and history of MI prior to military service) [5, 6] or intrinsic (e.g. low physical fitness, low educational level, large abdominal girth, high body mass index [BMI], and low body mass) [3–5].

Previous military studies have sought to identify anthropometric characteristics as risk factors for MI related to physical training. Those studies observed that BMI [3–5, 7] and waist circumference [3] were potential risk factors for MI. Thus, as the literature has selected anthropometric variables as risk factors, we hypothesized that a more specific body composition assessment can provide information regarding the predictive value of body components as risk factors for injuries in militaries.

In this regard, a Greek study that measured body fat percentage using bioelectrical impedance analysis confirmed the hypothesis by observing that adiposity expressed as body fat percentage can predict the risk for MI in militaries [8]. However, a glance at the literature exposes the current gap on this topic, because there are few studies that have investigated body composition variables as risk factors for MI. For example, to our knowledge no recent studies have measured fat-free mass, bone mineral content (BMC), and bone mineral density (BMD) to investigate the risk factors for MI in militaries. In this respect, dual-energy X-ray absorptiometry (DXA) is a well-adopted method to evaluate body composition in different populations, including children and adolescents, [9–11] individuals with different diseases [12] athletes, [13, 14] and also militaries, [15] mainly because it is considered non-invasive and fast and involves low radiation exposure [16–18]. Furthermore, another advantage of this method is that it can evaluate total or segmental (right and left sides of the upper and lower limbs and trunk) fat mass, BMC, and lean soft tissue as separate compartments with good accuracy and reliability [16–18], which can provide information regarding imbalances among different body tissues and segments. These imbalances can supposedly represent an additional risk for MI, as observed by a study on rugby athletes [19]. In that study, lower BMD, lower fat-free mass, higher fat mass, and higher body mass were considered risk factors for bone injuries [19]. Furthermore, considering that comparative tests have identified imbalances in limb performance as risk factors for MI [20, 21], we believe that it is important to

investigate if there are relationships between body composition imbalance in terms of limbs and the risk of injury. To our knowledge, this has not been investigated, especially using DXA. On the other hand, despite several advantages and the accuracy of DXA, its high cost and the need to visit specific research centres for evaluation may explain why few studies have adopted this method for investigating the risk factors for MI.

Thus, considering the fact that there are many studies focusing on the investigation of anthropometric variables as risk factors for MI in different populations, no studies have used DXA in militaries for the investigation of body composition as a risk factor for MI, this study aimed to verify the prevalence of MI in military students and to investigate the effect of total and segmental body composition assessed by DXA on the risk for MI in military students at the end of 1 year of military service.

Methods

This was a prospective study with a follow-up period of 9 months (from March to November 2013). The participants were military students from Escola Preparatória de Cadetes do Exército located in Campinas, São Paulo, Brazil. This school is responsible for the first year of study of cadets in the Brazilian army and annually receives 500 students approved in a public contest under a boarding school regime. The first 205 male students who agreed to participate in this study were included in a convenience sample. The inclusion criteria were recent inclusion in the army during the study period and the absence of any physical complaint or MI at the baseline evaluation at the beginning of military service. The study was approved by the ethics committee of the faculty of medical science of the Unicamp (n° 511.4610).

Baseline measurements

Participants underwent health status and body composition evaluation at the beginning of service in March 2013. Prior evaluation was performed at the Laboratory of Growth and Development in the Pediatric Investigation Center, University of Campinas, Campinas, São Paulo, Brazil. Participants were required to fill out a questionnaire that assessed demographic data and other potential risk factors such as history of chronic disease and MI prior to military service and physical activity experience.

Body mass was measured using a balance-beam scale (Filizola™) with a precision of 100 g that was graduated from 0 to 150 kg. Height was measured using a stadiometer (Holtain Ltd.™) with a precision of 1 cm. BMI was calculated using the formula weight/height^2.

Body composition and bone variables

Body composition and bone variables were measured using DXA (model iDXA, GE Healthcare Lunar, Madison, WI, USA). Fat mass (kg) and relative fat mass (%), BMC (kg), fat-free mass (kg), and BMD (g/cm^2) were estimated. In order to maximize the investigation on risk factors, we analysed the data for total and segmental (right and left sides of the lower and upper limbs and trunk) body composition and bone variables.

Training routine and injury registration

After baseline evaluation, participants started the military physical training program proposed and coordinated by the military school. This program comprised five weekly training sessions that each lasted for 1 h and 30 min. After some training sessions, according to their sporting abilities, some participants were selected to form school sports teams that would represent the military school in Brazilian military competitions. Consequently, a specific training period during the year was planned for some students according to the sports modality that they were recruited for. Sports training and military physical training were conducted at the same period. In case of health complaints, participants sought military school medical service. MI was diagnosed by a military physician and was defined as a musculoskeletal complaint that led to at least one instance of withdrawal from training or competition. In this case, the participant was referred to a military physiotherapy service, and the researcher proceeded with the injury registration. Injuries were classified according to aetiology as traumatic (a known trauma in a specific moment) or overload (non-traumatic mechanisms). At the end of the study period, we proceeded with the investigation on risk factors for general, traumatic, and overload injuries and lower and upper limb injuries (Fig. 1).

Statistical analysis

Data were analysed using SPSS version 16. Kolmogorov–Smirnov test was used to verify the normality of data. Independent-samples Student's t-test was used to compare the injured and non-injured militaries. To verify the association between MI and sample characteristics (sports team participation during the study, history of chronic disease or MI prior to military service, and sports experience prior to military service), chi-square test or Fisher's exact test was used. Logistic regression analysis was used to investigate the risk factors for MI, traumatic or overload injuries, and upper or lower limb injuries. The computation of odds ratios was included. The significance level was set at 5%.

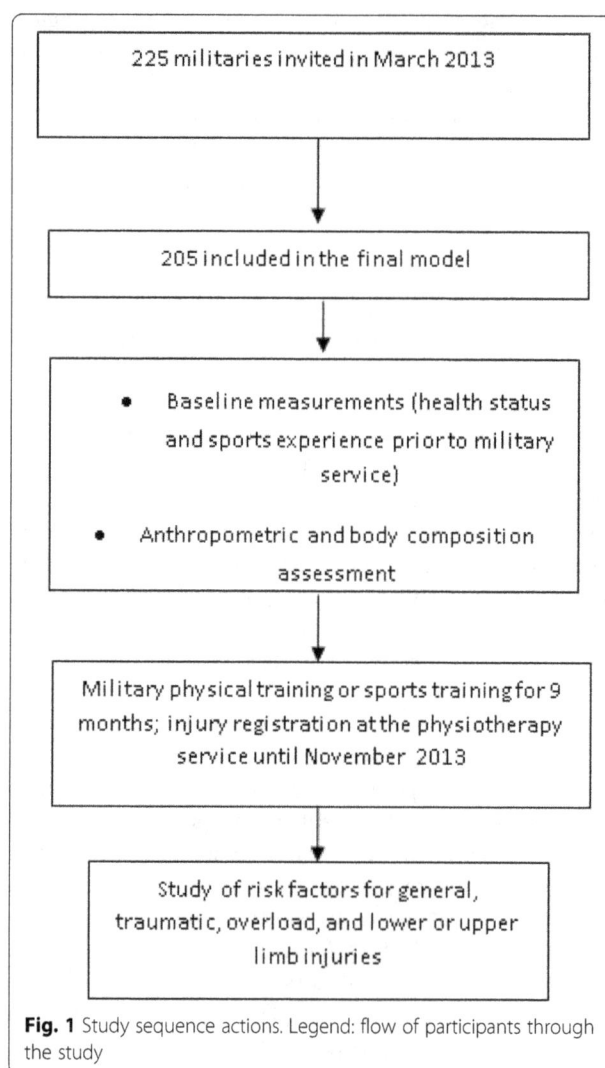

Fig. 1 Study sequence actions. Legend: flow of participants through the study

Results

During follow-up, 66 injuries were registered in 56 participants (27.3% of the sample), with 41 overload injuries (62.1%) and 25 traumatic injuries (37.8%). The most prevalent injuries observed were ankle sprain (16.6%) and medial tibial stress syndrome (15.1%). Most injuries occurred in the lower limbs (69.7%), followed by the upper limbs (25.7%) and spine (4.5%). The demographic and descriptive data of the total sample and comparison of anthropometric and body composition variables between the injured and non-injured groups are presented in Table 1. No differences between the injured and non-injured groups were found.

Similarly, no differences in sports team participation during the study (Chi-Square 0,010; $p = 0.92$), history of chronic disease (Fischer exact $p = 0.913$) or MI (Chi-Square = 2593; $p = 0.107$) prior to military service, and sports experience prior to military service (Fisher

Table 1 Demographic data of the total sample and comparison of anthropometric and body composition variables between the injured and non-injured groups

Variables	Total $n = 205$				Non-injured $n = 149$		Injured $n = 56$		P
	Mean	SD	Min	Max	Mean	SD	Mean	SD	
Age (years)	19.6	1.4	16.7	23.9	19.5	1.5	19.8	1.4	0.168
Height (cm)	176.2	6.4	160.3	192.4	175.8	6.4	177.3	6.1	0.111
Body mass (kg)	71.3	8.1	53.8	95.5	71.3	8.5	71.2	7.0	0.889
BMI (kg/m²)	22.9	2.1	17.62	28.8	23.1	2.1	22.6	2.0	0.187
FM (kg)	12.5	3.4	5.7	22.3	12.5	3.4	12.4	3.6	0.914
%FM	17.2	3.7	9.7	26.1	17.2	3.5	17.2	4.1	0.979
FFM (kg)	56.3	5.9	41.3	75.4	56.3	6.2	56.1	5.3	0.856
BMC (kg)	3.0	0.4	2.2	4.2	3.0	0.4	3.0	0.4	0.916
BMD (g/cm²)	1.229	0.095	0.989	1.561	1.230	0.093	1.227	0.101	0.874

Abbreviations: *SD* standard deviation, *BMI* body mass index, *FM* fat mass, *%FM* relative fat mass, *FFM* fat-free mass, *BMC* bone mineral content, *BMD* bone mineral density

exact $p = 0.51$) were found between the injured and non-injured groups.

Table 2 shows the results of logistic regression analysis to investigate the included variables as risk factors for MI.

Anthropometric variables were not found to be risk factors for MI (height OR = 1.040, 95% CI = 0.991–1.093, $p = 0.112$; body mass OR = 0.997, 95% CI = 0.960–1.036, $p = 0.888$; BMI OR = 0.903, 95% CI = 0.776–1.051, $p = 0.187$). An absence of sports team participation during follow-up and an absence of history of chronic disease or MI prior to military service were not found to be protective factors for MI. In contrast, sports experience prior to military service was found to be a protective factor for MI (OR = 0.32; 95% CI 0.108–0.968; $p = 0.04$). Logistic regression analysis for categorical variables are shown in Table 2.

The results of logistic regression analysis to investigate body composition variables as potential risk factors for general, traumatic, and overload injuries are presented in Table 3. None of the studied variables were found to be risk factors.

Finally, Table 4 presents the logistic regression results comparing body composition variables between the

Table 2 Logistic regression analysis of risk factors with respect to general sample characteristics for categorical variables

Variables	B	SE	OR	95% CI OR	P
Non-athlete[a]	0.078	0.312	1.081	0.587–1.994	0.802
No disease[b]	0.041	0.613	1.042	0.313–3.465	0.947
No previous injury[c]	0.553	0.316	1.739	0.935–3.233	0.080
Sports practice[d]	−1.129	0.559	0.323	0.108–0.968	0.044

Abbreviations: *B* beta coefficient of logistic regression, *SE* standard error, *OR* odds ratio, *95% CI* 95% confidence interval, *BMI* body mass index
[a]non-athlete during the follow-up
[b]no history of chronic disease prior to the service
[c]no history MI prior to the service
[d]sports experience prior to military service

non-injured group and the group with injury in the lower limbs and between the non-injured group and the group with injury in the upper limbs. Body composition variables were not found to be risk factors.

Discussion

Our prospective study with a follow-up period of 9 months investigated the prevalence of MI in Brazilian military students. We also sought to identify the risk factors for MI, overload and traumatic injuries, and upper and lower limb injuries. Of the participants, 27.3% presented with at least one type of MI, and overload injuries were the most prevalent (62.1%), with most injuries occurring in the lower limbs (69.7%). However, none of the studied body composition variables were found to be risk factors for MI, overload and traumatic injuries, or injuries in the lower or upper limbs. Finally, sports experience prior to military service was identified as a protective factor for MI.

The prevalence rate of almost 30% for MI in our study population reflects that MI is an important public health problem that deserves attention from military health-care providers, which has already been described by several studies. For example, an Iranian military study with a follow-up period of 1 year observed that MI accounted for 96% of health problems occurrence in one year of follow-up [1]. Moreover, a Finnish study demonstrated that 10% of a military sample was prematurely discharged from military service for medical reasons, mainly MI, and that premature discharge from military service was a potential risk factor for psychological problems, primarily in countries where military service is compulsory [22]. The findings of previous studies in the literature highlight the need for preventive strategies based on scientific knowledge about risk factors, considering the physical demands imposed on militaries in service that increase their risk for injury. Although we

Table 3 Logistic regression analysis to investigate body composition variables as risk factors for general, traumatic, and overload injuries

Variables	OR	General (total) (95% CI OR)	P	OR	Traumatic (95% CI OR)	P	OR	Overload (95% CI OR)	P
FM%	1.00	(0.92–1.09)	0.97	1.09	(0.97–1.23)	0.13	0.95	(0.84–1.07)	0.84
FM (kg)	1.00	(0.91–1.09)	0.91	1.06	(0.94–1.20)	0.30	0.95	(0.84–1.08)	0.50
BMC (kg)	1.04	(0.47–2.34)	0.91	1.21	(0.41–3.53)	0.71	0.88	(0.28–2.80)	0.84
FFM (kg)	1.00	(0.95–1.05)	0.85	0.97	(0.90–1.04)	0.46	1.01	(0.94–1.09)	0.63
BMD (g/cm^2)	0.77	(0.03–19.2)	0.87	1.91	(0.02–154.6)	0.77	0.24	(0.00–22.3)	0.54
FM, upper limbs (g)	1.00	(1.00–1.00)	0.81	1.00	(1.00–1.00)	0.52	1.00	(0.99–1.00)	0.63
FM, lower limbs (g)	1.00	(1.00–1.00)	0.86	1.00	(1.00–1.00)	0.30	1.00	(1.00–1.00)	0.31
FM, trunk (g)	1.00	(1.00–1.00)	0.98	1.00	(1.00–1.00)	0.33	1.00	(1.00–1.00)	0.72
FFM, upper limbs (g)	1.00	(1.00–1.00)	0.85	1.00	(1.00–1.00)	0.85	1.00	(1.00–1.00)	0.52
FFM, lower limbs (g)	1.00	(1.00–1.00)	0.75	1.00	(1.00–1.00)	0.50	1.00	(1.00–1.00)	0.77
FFM, trunk (g)	1.00	(1.00–1.00)	0.90	1.00	(1.00–1.00)	0.37	1.00	(1.00–1.00)	0.52
BMC, upper limbs (g)	1.00	(0.99–1.01)	0.94	0.99	(0.99–1.00)	0.87	1.00	(1.00–1.00)	0.87
BMC, lower limbs (g)	1.00	(1.00–1.00)	0.85	1.00	(1.00–1.00)	0.64	1.00	(1.00–1.00)	0.79
BMC, trunk (g)	1.00	(1.00–1.00)	0.82	1.00	(1.00–1.00)	0.75	1.00	(1.00–1.00)	0.88

Abbreviations: OR odds ratio, *95% CI* 95% confidence interval, *%FM* relative fat mass, *FM* fat mass, *BMC* bone mineral content, *FFM* fat-free mass, *BMD* bone mineral density, *NS* non-significant

Table 4 Logistic regression comparing the non-injured group and groups with lower or upper limb injury

Non-injured group vs. group with lower limb injury	B	SE	P	OR	(95% CI OR) Lower	Upper
Bone mass, left lower limb	−0.002	0.002	0.468	0.998	0.994	1.003
Bone mass, right lower limb	−0.002	0.002	0.403	0.998	0.993	1.003
Difference between the lower limbs	−0.005	0.011	0.673	0.995	0.975	1.017
Fat mass, left lower limb	0.000	0.000	0.641	1.000	0.999	1.000
Fat mass, right lower limb	0.000	0.000	0.599	1.000	0.999	1.000
Difference between the lower limbs	−0.001	0.002	0.701	0.999	0.996	1.003
Lean mass, left lower limb	0.000	0.000	0.394	1.000	1.000	1.000
Lean mass, right lower limb	0.000	0.000	0.390	1.000	1.000	1.000
Difference between the lower limbs	0.000	0.001	0.946	1.000	0.999	1.001
Non-injured group vs. group with upper limb injury	**B**	**SE**	**P**	**OR**	**Lower**	**Upper**
Bone mass, left upper limb	0.005	0.009	0.607	1.005	0.987	1.023
Bone mass, right upper limb	0.005	0.009	0.576	1.005	0.988	1.023
Difference between the upper limbs	0.008	0.033	0.801	1.008	0.944	1.077
Fat mass, left upper limb	−0.001	0.002	0.708	0.999	0.996	1.003
Fat mass, right upper limb	−0.001	0.002	0.602	0.999	0.995	1.003
Difference between the upper limbs	−0.002	0.005	0.723	0.998	0.990	1.007
Lean mass, left upper limb	0.000	0.001	0.985	1.000	0.999	1.001
Lean mass, right upper limb	0.000	0.001	0.991	1.000	0.999	1.001
Difference between the upper limbs	0.000	0.002	0.979	1.000	0.996	1.004

Abbreviations: B beta coefficient of logistic regression, *SE* standard error, *OR* odds ratio, *95% CI* 95% confidence interval

do not have epidemiologic data on other health problems in our study population, the incidence of MI in our study and previous epidemiologic studies in the literature can evidently justify the search for risk factors for MI.

With respect to the anatomical body parts affected, similar to our study, many studies have found a higher prevalence of injuries in the lower limbs. A Finnish study indicated a prevalence rate of 67% for lower limb injury in four cohorts followed up for 6 months [4], whereas another Finnish study reported a prevalence rate of 48% for lower limb injury in 944 conscripts who were followed up [3]. These results are consistent with those of our study, which showed that 69.7% of the injuries occurred in the lower limbs.

An interesting finding of our study is that sports experience prior to military service was a protective factor for MI, which is consistent with that of another military study [4]. According to Taanila et al. [4], previous experience of physical activity can produce overload on musculoskeletal structures prior to military service. In this case, we believe that previous physical activity programs can improve fitness and maturation of the musculoskeletal system. This could supposedly prepare participants for new training routines in the service, as the physical demands on them are lower than their less active counterparts. Such an idea was already previously proposed in the literature [23]. Moreover, this becomes evident in the study by Knapik et al. (2006) in which military low-fit recruits who participated in a pre-conditioning physical program before basic combat training tended to have a lower risk of injury during military service than low-fit recruits who did not participate in a pre-conditioning program [24].

This is particularly important for our study population, which was composed of students who supposedly had to spend part of their time studying for intelligence tests prior to military service. It is important to mention that, different from recruits, the military service as student in Escola Preparatória de Cadetes do Exército is not compulsory, and that before been considered approved to the service, participants underwent to a selection process composed by physical, health and intelligence test to be eligible.

However, it is important to mention that our main objective was to verify if anthropometric and body composition variables could be considered risk factors for MI. Despite our previous hypothesis, we could not identify any studied variables that could be considered risk factors for MI or overload or traumatic injuries. In this respect, no consensus on the relationship between body composition and anthropometric variables and the risk for MI exists in the literature.

Our hypothesis that anthropometric and body composition variables could be risk factors for MI was based on various previous studies. For example, in the military and athletic populations, higher BMI [3, 25], larger abdominal girth [3], and both low [26] and high body mass [27] were identified as risk factors for MI. Moreover, a high BMI was identified as a risk factor for MI in the lower limbs [28] and increased height was identified as a risk factor for MI [29]. Taking all these findings from previous studies into consideration, we formulated the hypothesis that body composition variables could also be risk factors for MI in our study population.

In contrast, although a small body of literature provides information on anthropometric variables as risk factors for MI, many studies that had the same objective refuted this hypothesis. For example, Rauh et al. observed that body mass, height, and BMI were not associated with incidence and risk of stress fractures or overload injuries in female recruits from the American Navy [30]. Moreover, some studies on athletes were not able to identify anthropometric variables as risk factors. For example, body mass was not considered a risk factor for MI in rugby athletes [31], and body mass, height, BMI, and body fat percentage measured by skinfold thickness were not identified as risk factors for MI in football athletes [32]. Consequently, the variability and inconsistency in results to date affect whether researchers can identify anthropometric variables as risk factors for MI.

Moreover, some studies sought to identify anthropometric variables as risk factors for specific injuries in militaries. Rauh et al. did not identify body mass, height, or BMI as a predictive factor for stress fractures [30] and Mahieu et al. did not also consider these variables as risk factors for calcaneus tendinopathy [33]. Further, Moen et al. did not identify body mass, height, BMI, maximal calf girth, and lean calf girth (maximal calf girth less calf skinfold) as risk factors for medial tibial stress syndrome [34].

Some hypotheses may potentially explain why our study, unlike other studies on militaries [3, 25] did not find a relation between anthropometric and body composition variables and the risk for MI. Our study population comprised students who were recently approved in a selection process prior to military service, which consisted of an intelligence test, followed by health examination and physical fitness tests. The characteristics of our study population may have reduced the variability in body composition variables in the students who were the sample population because of the physical fitness requirements to be approved in the selection process, which likely made our study population quite homogenous compared to the recruit population followed up in other studies. A study identified higher BMI as a risk factor for MI in American male recruits [35]. However, the mean BMI of the population in the previous study was 24.3 kg/m^2, whereas the mean BMI of our study population was 22.9 kg/m^2. Moreover, the standard deviation for BMI was 4.85 and 2.1 in the previous study and our study, respectively. It is also important to mention that no minimal physical fitness requirements for the recruits at the beginning of compulsory military service usually exist in Brazil; in contrast, the students in our study voluntarily participated in the military selection process, which had physical requirements for approval.

With respect to tools used to evaluate anthropometric and body composition variables in the previous studies, most investigations had measured anthropometric variables using simple and unspecific tools, and studies often failed to evaluate body composition variables or distinguish lean mass, fat mass, or bone variables. No military studies apparently used DXA to measure body composition variables to identify risk factors for MI in militaries. All anthropometric variables evaluated by the different aforementioned studies to date included body mass, height, BMI, abdominal girth, body fat percentage measured by skinfold thickness, maximal calf girth, and lean calf girth. In this regard, some disadvantages of DXA may explain why there are few studies, even with athletes, with the same objective as our study, that have investigated similar variables by using DXA: it is expensive, often not accessible to study centres, and is not portable.

A careful literature search revealed that a few studies indeed have used DXA with the same objective as the present study [36, 37] and suggests that many other body composition variables should be further investigated. In this respect, we found three studies that followed up athletes. Interestingly, of these three studies, only one identified body composition variables as risk factors. In this study, lower BMD, lower lean mass, lower bone (tibial) mass, higher fat mass, and higher body mass were associated with bone injuries [19]. The other two studies were not able to identify risk factors for stress fractures in cross-country athletes [36], and vertebral fractures in rugby athletes [37].

DXA continues to be considered the gold standard for evaluating BMD, being a non-invasive method that involves low radiation exposure, and demonstrates good accuracy with respect to total or segmental body composition evaluation [38].

However, aside from the advantages of the method, the fact that we could not find studies that used DXA to identify risk factors for MI in the militaries clearly indicates the current need for more studies adopting DXA with the same objective, preferably with a large sample of injured participants.

The small sample of injured participants can be considered a limitation of the present study, considering that there are previous studies with larger samples of significantly injured participants [3, 4], which gives them a higher statistical power for observing risk factors.

Furthermore, it would be interesting to register the severity of injuries as training days lost per injury, which would permit statistical analyses in groups categorized by severity. Finally, the cross-sectional design of body composition evaluation did not permit us to identify how body composition changed during military training. Thus, a no one-time point future study would be interesting.

However, considering the several strong points of this study and its results, and the evident variability of results found in the literature to date, this indicates the need for the identification of other intrinsic and extrinsic variables as risk factors. Our findings cannot confirm the relation between anthropometric and body composition variables and the risk for MI during military service.

Conclusion

MI is an important public health problem that causes premature discharge from military service; 30% of our study population presented with MI. Lower limb injuries were the most prevalent, mainly ankle sprain and medial tibial stress syndrome. Overload injuries were more prevalent than traumatic injuries. It was not possible to establish the relationship between anthropometric or body composition variables and risk for MI during military service in this population with the current sample size. However, future studies with data collected over multiple time-points or with more individuals may identify patterns of injury risk.

Abbreviations
BMC: Bone mineral content; BMD: Bone mineral density; BMI: Body mass index; DXA: Dual-energy X-ray absorptiometry; MI: Musculoskeletal injuries

Acknowledgments
The present study was developed at Escola Preparatória de Cadetes do Exército. We appreciate the excelent cooperation of the personnel of that military school over the course of the study and also thank EsPCEx commandant.

Authors' contributions
MASM, JAA, MAP, CJOB, VXC, EMG and GGJ contributed to all data analysis, interpretation and data acquisition. All authors made intellectual contribution to the study and reviewed the article. All authors read and approved the final manuscript.

Competing interests
The authors declare that they have no competing interests.

References
1. Mehri NS, Sadeghian M, Tayyebi A, et al. Epidemiology of physical injuries resulted from military training course. Iran J Military Med. 2010;12(2):89–92.
2. Kaufman KR, Brodine S, Shaffer R. Military training-related injuries. Surveillance, research, and prevention. Am J PrevMed. 2000;18(3S):54–63.
3. Taanila H, Suni J, Pihlajamaki H, et al. Aetiology and risk factors of musculoskeletal disorders in physically active conscripts: a follow-up study in the Finnish Defence Forces. BMC MusculoskeletDisord. 2010;11:146.
4. Taanila H, Suni JH, Kannus P, Pihlajamaki H, Ruohola JP, Viskari J, Parkkari J. Risk factors of acute and overuse musculoskeletal injuries among young conscripts: a population-based cohort study. BMC Musculoskelet Disord. 2015;16:104.
5. Taanila H, Hemminki AJM, Suni JH, Pihlajamaki H, Parkkari J. Low physical fitness is a strong predictor of health problems among young men: a follow-up study of 1411 male conscripts. BMC Musculoskelet Disord. 2011; 11:590.
6. Grier T, Canham-Chervak M, McNulty V, Jones BH. Extreme conditioning programs and injury risk in a US army brigade combat team. US ArmyMedDep J. 2013;36–47.
7. Kuikka PI, Pihlajamaki HK, Mattila VM. Knee injuries related to sports in young adult males during military service – Incidence and risk factors. Scand J Med Sci Sports. 2013;23:281–7.
8. Havenetidis K, Paxinos T. Risk factors for musculoskeletal injuries among Greek Army Officers Cadets undergoing basic combat training. Mil Med. 2011;176(10):1111–6.
9. Pietrobelli A, Andreoli A, Cervelli V, Carbonelli MG, Peroni DG, De Lorenzo A. Predicting fat-free mass in children using bioimpedance analysis. ActaDiabetol. 2003;40(Suppl. 1):S212–S15.
10. Nielsen BM, Dencker M, Ward L, Linden C, Thorsson O, Karlsson MK, et al. Prediction of fat-free body mass among 9- to 11-year-old Swedish children. Diabetes. ObesMetab. 2007;9:521–39.
11. Kriemler S, Puder J, Zahner L, Roth R, Meyer U, Bedogni G. Estimation of percentage body fat in 6- to 13-year-old children by skinfold thickness, body mass index and waist circumference. Br J Nutr. 2010;104:1565–72.
12. Albanese CV, Diessel E, Genant HK. Clinical applications of body composition measurements using DXA. J ClinDensitom. 2003;6:75–85.
13. Stewart AD, Hannan WJ. Prediction of fat and fat-free mass in male athletes using dual X-ray absorptiometry as the reference method. J Sports Sci. 2000;18(4):263–74.
14. Santos DA, Dawson JA, Matias CN, Rocha PM, Minderico CS, Allison DB, Sardinha LB, Silva AM. Reference values for body composition and anthropometric measurements in athletes. PLoS One. 2014;9(5):e97846. https://doi.org/10.1371/journal.pone.0097846. eCollection 2014.
15. Langer RD, Borges JH, Pascoa MA, Cirolini VX, Guerra-Júnior G, Gonçalves EM. Validity of Bioelectrical Impedance Analysis to Estimation Fat-Free Mass in the Army Cadets. Nutrients. 2016;8(3):121.
16. Mazess RB, Barden HS, Bisek JP, Hanson J. Dualenergy X-ray absorptiometry for total-body and regional bonemineral and soft-tissue composition. Am J ClinNutr. 1990;51:1106–12.
17. Svendsen OL, Haarbo J, Hassager C, Christiansen C. Accuracy of measurements of body composition by dual energy X-ray absorptiometry in vivo. Am J Clin Nutr. 1993;57:605–8.
18. Mattsson S, Thomas BJ. Development of methods for body composition studies. Phys Med Biol. 2006;51:203–28.
19. Georgeson EC, Weeks BK, McLellan C, Beck BR. Seasonal change in bone, muscle and fat in professional rugby league players and its relationship to injury: a cohort study. BMJ Open. 2012;2:e001400.

20. Silva A, Zanca G, Alves ES, Lemos VA, Gávea SA, Winckler C, Mattiello SM, Peterson R, Vital R, Tufik S, De Mello MT. Isokinetic assessment and musculoskeletal complaints in Paralympic athletes. Am J Phys Med Rehabil. 2015;0:1–7.
21. Freckleton G, Cook J, Pizzari T. The predictive validity of a single leg bridge test for hamstring injuries in Australian Rules Football Players. Br J Sports Med. 2014;48:713–7.
22. Taanila H, Hemminki AJM, Suni JH, Pihlajamaki H, Parkkari J. Low Physical Fitness is a strong predictor of health problems among young men: a follow-up study of 1411 male conscripts. BMC Public Health. 2011;11:590.
23. Jones BH, Thacker SB, Gilchrist J, Kimsey JRCD, Sosin DM. Prevention of lower extremity stress fractures in athletes and soldiers: a systematic review. Epidemiol Rev. 2002;24(2):228–47.
24. Knapik JJ, Darakjy S, Hauret KG, Canada S, Scott MAJS, Reger W, Marin R, Jones BH. Increasing the physical fitness of low-fit recruits before basic combat training: an evaluation of fitness, injuries, and training outcomes. Mil Med. 2006;171(1):45–54.
25. Grier T, Canham-Chervak M, McNulty V, Jones BH. Extreme conditioning programs and injury risk in a US Army Brigade Combate Team. Army Med Depart J. 2013:36–47.
26. Gastin PB, Meyer D, Huntsman E, Cook J. Increase in injury risk with low body mass and aerobic-running fitness in elite Australian football. Int J Sports Physiol Perform. 2015;10:458–63.
27. Gabbett TJ, Ullah S, Finch CF. Identifying risk factors for contact injury in professional rugby league players – Application of a frailty model for recurrent injury. J Sci Med Sport. 2012;15:496–504.
28. Nilstad A, Anderson TE, Bahr R, Holme I, Steffen K. Risk factors for lower extremity injuries in elite female soccer players. Am J Sports Med. 2014;42(4):940–8.
29. Faude O, Junge A, Kindermann W, Dvorak J. Risk factors for injuries in elite female soccer players. Br J Sports Med. 2006;40:785–90.
30. Rauh MJ, Macera CA, Trone DW, Shaffer RA, Brodine SK. Epidemiology of stress fracture and lower-extremity overuse injury in female recruits. Med Sci Sports Exerc. 2006;38(9):1571–7.
31. Fuller CW, Caswell SE, Zimbwa T. Do mismatches between teams affect the risk of injury in the rugby world cup? J Sci Med Sport. 2010;13:36–8.
32. Haxhiu B, Murtezani A, Zahiti B, Shalaj I, Sllamniku S. Risk factors for injuries in professional football players. Folia Med. 2015;57(2):138–43.
33. Mahieu NN, Witvrouw E, Stevens V, Van Tiggelen D, Roget P. Intrinsic risk factores for the development of Achilles tendon overuse injury: a prospective study. Am J Sports Med. 2006;34(2):226–36.
34. Moen MH, Bongers T, Bakker EW, Zimmermann WO, Weir A, Tol JL, Backx FJG. Risk factors and prognostic indicators for medial tibial stress syndrome. Scand J Med Sci Sports. 2012;22(1):34–9.
35. Jones BH, Bovee MW, Harris JM III, Cowan DN. Intrinsic risk factors for exercise related injuries among male and female army trainees. Am J Sports Med. 1993;21(5):705–10.
36. Roelofs EJ, Smith-Ryan AE, Melvin MN, Wingfield HL, Trexler ET, Walker N. Muscle size, quality, and body composition: characteristics of division I cross-country runners. J Strength Cond Res. 2015;29(2):290–6.
37. Hind K, Birrell F, Beck B. Prevalent morphometric vertebral fractures in professional male rugby players. PLoS One. 2014;9(5):e97427.
38. Lee SY, Gallagher D. Assessment methods in human body composition. CurrOpinClinNutrMetab Care. 2008;11(5):566–72.

27

Identifying individuals with chronic pain after knee replacement: a population-cohort, cluster-analysis of Oxford knee scores in 128,145 patients from the English National Health Service

Rafael Pinedo-Villanueva[1,2*] (iD), Sara Khalid[1], Vikki Wylde[3,5], Rachael Gooberman-Hill[3,5], Anushka Soni[1,4] and Andrew Judge[1,3,5]

Abstract

Background: Approximately one in five patients undergoing knee replacement surgery experience chronic pain after their operation, which can negatively impact on their quality of life. In order to develop and evaluate interventions to improve the management of chronic post-surgical pain, we aimed to derive a cut-off point in the Oxford Knee Score pain subscale to identify patients with chronic pain following knee replacement, and to characterise these patients using self-reported outcomes.

Methods: Data from the English Patient-Reported Outcome Measures (PROMs) programme were used. This comprised patient-reported data from 128,145 patients who underwent primary knee replacement surgery in England between 2012 and 2015. Cluster analysis was applied to derive a cut-off point on the pain subscale of the Oxford Knee Score.

Results: A high-pain group was identified, described by a maximum of 14 points in the Oxford Knee Score pain subscale six months after surgery. The high-pain group, comprising 15% of the sample, was characterised by severe and frequent problems in all pain dimensions, particularly in pain severity, night pain and limping, as well as in all dimensions of health-related quality of life.

Conclusions: Patients with Oxford Knee Score pain subscale scores of 14 or less at six months after knee replacement can be considered to be in chronic pain that is likely to negatively affect their quality of life. This derived cut-off can be used for patient selection in research settings to design and assess interventions that support patients in their management of chronic post-surgical pain.

Keywords: Chronic pain, Knee replacement, Cluster-analysis, Oxford knee score, Observational study, NHS England

Background

Pain and functional limitations due to knee osteoarthritis (OA) is a leading health concern and a major global contributor to years lived with disability [1]. For people living with advanced stages of the disease, knee replacement (KR) can be performed to provide pain relief, restore function, and improve quality of life. However, chronic pain after KR is common: approximately 20% of patients report moderate or severe pain at between 3 months and 5 years after surgery [2].

With approximately 700,000 KR performed per year in the US [3] and 108,000 performed during 2016 in England, Wales, Northern Ireland and the Isle of Man [4], large numbers of people are living with chronic pain after KR. These patients experience high levels of pain-related distress [5] and reduced ability to participate

* Correspondence: rafael.pinedo@ndorms.ox.ac.uk
[1]Nuffield Department of Orthopaedics, Rheumatology and Musculoskeletal Sciences, University of Oxford, Botnar Research Centre, Windmill Road, Headington, Oxford OX3 7LD, UK
[2]MRC Lifecourse Epidemiology Unit, University of Southampton, Southampton, UK
Full list of author information is available at the end of the article

in work, family life and valued social activities, which may contribute to social isolation [6].

Often patients do not seek care for chronic pain [7]. The ability to characterise and identify people with chronic pain following KR is a necessary first step to developing, evaluating, and implementing interventions which aim to improve the management of this condition. Although cut-off points on a visual analogue scale have been suggested to distinguish between mild, moderate and severe general pain [8], no standard cut-off points are available for patients following a KR. Identifying individuals with chronic pain early during their post-operative recovery will facilitate the delivery of timely and targeted interventions to improve pain outcomes. This requires a robust and standardised method for identifying people in chronic pain following KR that can be used across a range of research settings.

The aim of this study was to identify a cut-off point on the pain subscale of the commonly-used Oxford Knee Score (OKS) that can be used to identify patients with high levels of pain 6 months after KR.

Methods
Study design
Data were obtained from the patient-level, anonymized English NHS Patient-Reported Outcome Measures (PROMs) programme available from the NHS Digital website [9]. All patients undergoing KR through the English NHS, or on behalf of it, are eligible to be included in the programme. Two questionnaires are sent to participants before and after surgery by the PROMs programme, a disease-specific and a generic quality of life measure: the OKS [10] and the EQ-5D [11]. For this analysis, data were extracted for UK financial years 2012 through 2015.

Participants
Patients undergoing primary KR, with complete post-operative OKS were included in the present study. There were no restrictions on age or sex. The dataset did not include the indication for or type of surgery performed, hence records were included regardless of the underlying condition or type of KR. As the unit of analysis was KRs and records were fully anonymised, it was not possible to determine if patients had their contralateral knee replaced within the same period of analysis. It was therefore possible for patients to be included twice in the dataset.

Data and outcome measure
The OKS is a 12-item score which measures knee pain, stiffness, and functional disability within the previous 4 weeks [10]. Responses are scored using a 0–4 Likert scale. Item scores are summed to calculate a total score ranging from 0 (worst possible score) to 48 (best possible score). The PROMS programme collects post-operative data 6 months after surgery. Chronic post-surgical pain is widely accepted to be pain of at least three to 6 months duration that develops or increases in intensity after a surgical procedure and significantly affects health-related quality of life [12, 13]. This is applicable to KR, as most pain relief is obtained in the first three to 6 months [14, 15] and continuing pain at 6 months after surgery is a cause of dissatisfaction [16].

Previous work has identified pain- and function-related subscales within the OKS [17], with further details given in Additional file 1. A raw OKS pain subscale (OKS-PS) summary score can be calculated by summing the responses of its seven items, hence ranging from 0 (most pain) to 28 (least pain). Although the OKS, and particularly the pain subscale, could be considered an unidimensional measure of highly-correlated items, each item captures a different dimension of pain. Some pain items are highly intertwined with function, reflected by the inclusion of two items in both the pain and function components [17]. Our analysis allowed for each item to independently contribute to the generation of pain severity clusters.

Statistical methods
To identify the high-pain group, hierarchical clustering was used to group patients into clusters based on the similarity of their OKS-PS item scores. Hierarchical clustering is commonly used, easily interpretable and has been applied in several previous studies on knee pain in order to identify pain profiles, and broader subgroups which are then examined for correlation with pain [18–21]. Cluster analysis splits a set of participants into groups or clusters, so that participants within the same cluster are most similar, and any two clusters are as distinct as possible from one another. Agglomerative hierarchical clustering follows a sequence whereby clusters are repetitively merged until a pre-specified number of clusters is achieved, or all participants have been merged into one single cluster. We conducted agglomerative clustering with all patients beginning as individual clusters, which were then successively merged into all possible numbers of clusters, starting at two (the natural minimum) up to 28 clusters (the maximum, where each cluster would correspond to each possible value of the OKS-PS). This constituted the essence of our data-driven approach, considering all possibilities allowed by the data instead of setting discretionary limits on the number of clusters to be identified. We assumed that it is not known, a-priori, if subgroups of KR patients exist based on their levels of pain and, if so, how

many there are. By applying a data-driven approach, we allowed the model to answer these questions based on the features of our population.

For each set of clusters (2 to 28), the distribution of the OKS-PS corresponding to the highest-pain cluster, i.e. that reporting the lowest values, was examined. This was used to derive a cut-off point, defined as the highest value taken by the highest-pain cluster on the OKS-PS. Changes in the cut-off point as the number of clusters varied are reported. Further details on the methodology have been published previously [22].

Uncertainty around the cut-off point was measured undertaking a secondary analysis which repeated the hierarchical clustering on 100 random re-orderings of the sample, and by additionally applying k-means clustering, another commonly used method which adds an additional level of variability as cluster initialisation is randomly assigned in every iteration. To assess the choice of the cut-off point, sensitivity and specificity were calculated considering 'true cases' those patients included in the highest–pain cluster from the primary analysis at the lowest number of clusters (k) at which the cut-off was identified. These measures are useful because the analysis produced clusters based on answers to seven different items, hence clusters were likely to report overlapping overall OKS-PS scores. This secondary analysis was also conducted as an internal validation by exploring an alternative approach to generating cut-off points using the same data, although differently ordered.

Based on the cut-off point identified in the primary analysis, patients were placed into either a 'high-pain' or a 'low-pain' group, and scores reported for the overall OKS, OKS subscales, OKS-PS items, EQ-5D Visual Analogue Scale (VAS), and the EQ-5D summary score comprising mobility, self-care, usual activities, pain/discomfort, and anxiety/depression. EQ-5D dimensions are scored using a 1–3 Likert scale [11] and a summary index calculated by applying UK general population preference weights [23]. The summary score is anchored at 0 signifying 'death' and 1 'perfect health', negative values being possible and interpreted as health states worse than death. Answers to two questions about the results and impact of the surgery are also reported by group. Analyses were performed using Matlab R2015 and Stata.

Results

During the study period, 128,145 records from primary KR patients were reported in the PROMs dataset with returned post-operative questionnaires. Of these, 2081 (1.6%) records were excluded as they were missing ≥1 answers for the OKS-PS items. Therefore, 126,064 records were used for analysis, of which 54% were from females and 73% from patients aged 60–79 years. Table 1 shows participants' demographic characteristics.

Identification of a cut-off point

Figure 1 shows the distribution of different-size clusters over the OKS-PS summary score from the primary analysis. When the clustering algorithm derives $k = 2$ clusters, the OKS-PS distributions for the two clusters have a large overlap. As the number of derived clusters increases, the degree of overlap in their corresponding OKS-PS distributions reduces and both the mode and the upper limit shift. Figure 2 illustrates this shift in the resulting cut-off point, in particular how it decreases as the number of clusters increases from $k = 2$ to $k = 4$. However, for $k \geq 4$, the cut-off point remains constant at OKS-PS = 14, implying that the OKS-PS score range of 0–14 characterises the high-pain cluster whether the sample is split into four or more clusters. Using OKS-PS ≤ 14 to identify participants in chronic pain led to a sensitivity of 100% and specificity of 89%.

The cut-off points obtained through secondary analysis were different to that obtained through the primary analysis. As Fig. 2 shows, running 100 random re-orderings and applying hierarchical clustering led to a mean cut-off point at k = 4 clusters of OKS-PS = 18.5 (SD = 2.6), whilst when k-means was applied the mean cut-off was OKS-PS = 14.7 (SD = 0.9). The Figure also illustrates that these cut-off points are not constant with increasing numbers of clusters. At OKS-PS = 18.5, sensitivity and specificity were 100% and 74%, whereas at OKS-PS = 14.7 they were 100% and 89%, respectively.

Characterisation of the high-pain group

Using the OKS-PS cut-off of 14, a total of 18,522 out of 126,064 (14.7%) patients with KR were found to be in the high-pain group. Table 2 shows the demographics and outcome scores for the high- and low-pain groups.

Age and sex were largely similar between both groups, with the exception of a larger proportion of 50–59 year olds and lower proportion of 70–79 year olds in the high-pain compared to the lower-pain group. Pre-operatively, patients in the high-pain group reported worse pain, function and health-related quality of life. Post-operatively, outcomes were also poorer for the high-pain group. A higher percentage of the high-pain group judged the outcome of their operation as 'fair' or 'poor', and perceived little or no improvement in their symptoms from their pre-operative status. Figure 3 shows how the high-pain group consistently reported greater pain, in average, in all OKS-PS items. The greatest differences were reported in pain severity, limping and night pain. The overall improvement of the standardised OKS-PS (scale of 0–100) was 46 for the lower-pain group and 10 for the high-pain group. Outcomes in

Table 1 Cohort description

Observations: n	126,064
Gender: n (%)	
Female	68,114 (54%)
Male	49,306 (39%)
Not specified	106 (0%)
Missing	8538 (7%)
Age band: n (%)	
40–49 years of age	258 (0%)
50–59 years of age	11,380 (9%)
60–69 years of age	43,583 (35%)
70–79 years of age	48,073 (38%)
80–89 years of age	14,226 (11%)
90+ years of age	6 (0%)
Missing	8538 (7%)
Pre-op OKS score[1]	
Mean (SD)	19.0 (8)
Median (IQR)	19 (11)
Missing	1473 (1%)
Pre-op EQ-5D index[2]	
Mean (SD)	0.414(0.31)
Median (IQR)	0.587 (0.603)
Missing	7077 (6%)
Pre-op EQ-5D VAS[3] "Your own health state today"	
Mean (SD)	68.2(20)
Median (IQR)	70 (25)
Missing	13,110 (10%)
"How would you describe the results of your operation?" n (%)	
Excellent	31,827 (25%)
Very good	44,472 (35%)
Good	30,670 (24%)
Fair or Poor	18,355 (15%)
Missing	740 (1%)
"Overall, how are your problems now, compared to before your operation?" n (%)	
Much better	92,164 (73%)
A little better	20,276 (16%)
About the same	5775 (5%)
A little or much worse	7388 (6%)
Missing	461 (0%)
Post-op OKS score[a]	
Mean (SD)	35.2 (10)
Median (IQR)	37 (14)
Missing	46 (0%)

Table 1 Cohort description (Continued)

Observations: n	126,064
Post-op EQ-5D index[b]	
Mean (SD)	0.734(0.25)
Median(IQR)	0.760 (0.344)
Missing	6084 (5%)
Post-op EQ-5D VAS[c] "Your own health state today"	
Mean (SD)	73.8 (20)
Median (IQR)	80 (25)
Missing	6746 (5%)

[a]captures knee pain and function, scored from 0 to 48 where 0 indicates most and 48 least pain and functional limitations
[b]a health-related quality of life measure where 0 represents death and 1 refers to perfect health
[c]a Visual Analogue Scale ranging from 0 to 100, where 0 represents the worst and 100 the best imaginable health state

function were even worse for the high-pain group, with a mean improvement of 2 points compared to 27 for the lower-pain group. Post-operative health-related quality of life was also worse in the high-pain group, with lower scores by approximately the same magnitude across all five dimensions. As shown in Fig. 4, however, the median of the EQ-5D summary score for the high-pain group saw a larger improvement after surgery than the lower-pain group, but the middle half of the high-pain group remained essentially within the same range of scores reported pre-operatively. Notably, 17% of the high-pain group reported post-operative EQ-5D summary scores lower than zero, compared to less than 1% for the lower-pain group.

Discussion

Using data from a large cohort of patients in England, we have developed a standardised and robust method to identify people with chronic pain following primary KR. Clusters of patients were produced according to their responses to pain-related questions in the OKS. A specific group with the lowest OKS-PS, indicating high pain, was identified. Characterisation of this group showed an association with poor health-related quality of life. A cut-off was derived such that a patient with an OKS-PS score ≤ 14 6 months after KR could be considered to be in chronic pain which is likely to have a negative impact on health-related quality of life.

Our secondary analysis using hierarchical clustering and based on repetitive sampling with different ordering showed that the cut-off could be higher than 14. Differences between the primary and secondary analysis were due to the random data reordering in the latter and the high probability of ties during the clustering process. Ties are highly likely when the clustering variables are discrete and can only take a few values, such as in this

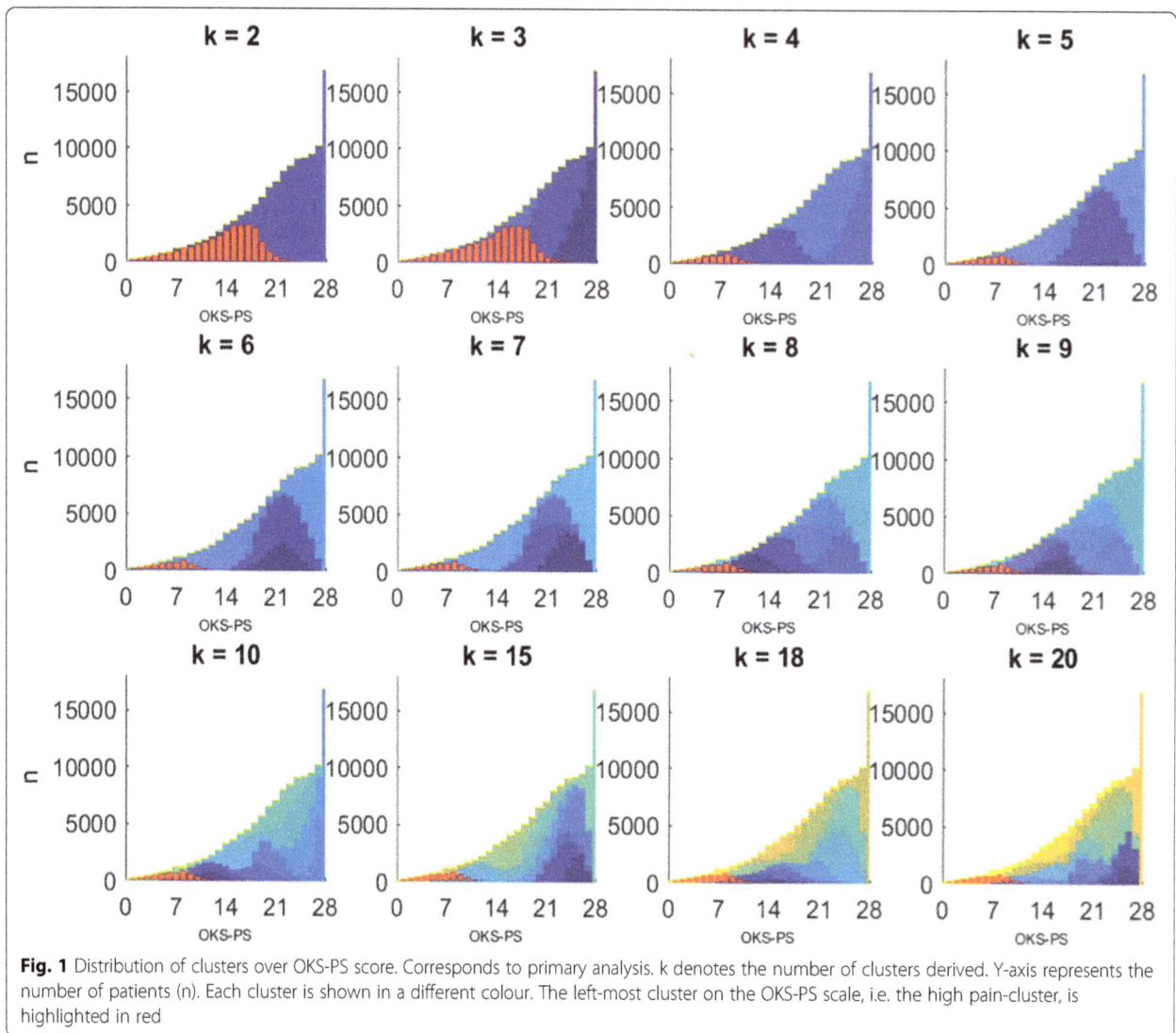

Fig. 1 Distribution of clusters over OKS-PS score. Corresponds to primary analysis. k denotes the number of clusters derived. Y-axis represents the number of patients (n). Each cluster is shown in a different colour. The left-most cluster on the OKS-PS scale, i.e. the high pain-cluster, is highlighted in red

case the OKS items which can only take the values 0 to 4. Each iteration of the clustering analysis produced different clusters as it faced ties in a different order every time, with this variation increased by the fact that the k-means method starts the clustering from random points every time. By conducting both analyses, we are able to provide a reference point for the cut-off value as well as a measure of its variability when the data and cluster initialisation are allowed to change randomly.

This cut-off point corresponds to the highest value in the OKS-PS for a participant in the high-pain group when four groups or clusters had been identified. This number of clusters is consistent with the number identified by previous studies also using cluster analysis. Egsgaard et al. identified four knee pain profiles based on biochemical and pain biomarkers, physical impairments, and psychological factors [20], whilst Frey-Law identified five distinct pain sensitivity profiles [21].

Identifying patients with chronic pain after KR revealed marked differences between the high- and lower- pain groups not only 6 months after the operation but also pre-operatively and with regards to patients' assessment of their outcomes. Expectedly, all measures of post-operative pain and health-related quality of life were worse for patients in the chronic-pain group. They reported significantly worse scores than their counterparts in all items of the OKS-PS items as well as in all health-related quality of life dimensions. Patients with chronic pain were characterised by high pain intensity and frequency, with severity, night pain, and limping as the most serious problems. Regarding health-related quality of life, those in chronic pain reported least problems in self-care and anxiety/depression but were still notably worse than the low pain-group in all dimensions of health-related quality of life. After the operation, one

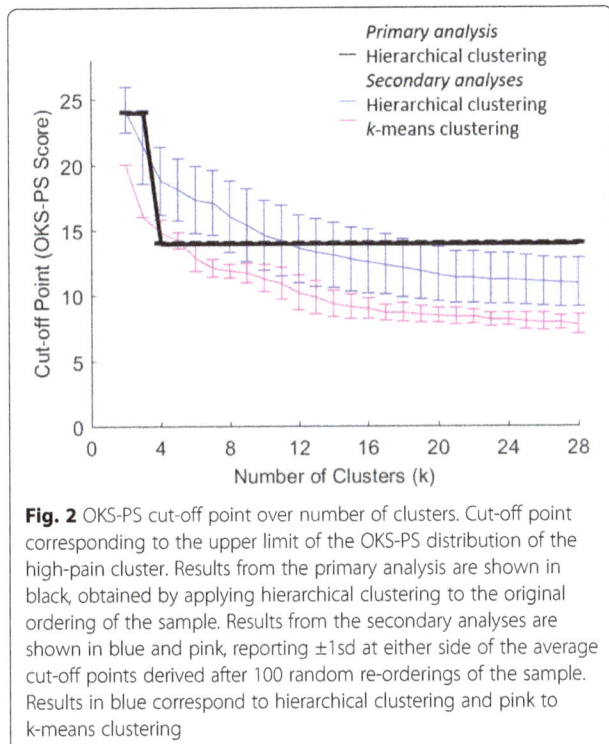

Fig. 2 OKS-PS cut-off point over number of clusters. Cut-off point corresponding to the upper limit of the OKS-PS distribution of the high-pain cluster. Results from the primary analysis are shown in black, obtained by applying hierarchical clustering to the original ordering of the sample. Results from the secondary analyses are shown in blue and pink, reporting ±1sd at either side of the average cut-off points derived after 100 random re-orderings of the sample. Results in blue correspond to hierarchical clustering and pink to k-means clustering

in six individuals with chronic pain reported scores considered to be worse than death.

There were some difficulties in applying the cut-off on the OKS-PS to identify patients in the highest-pain cluster. Specificity of 89% revealed that some of those scoring ≤14 in their OKS-PS were not in this highest-pain cluster but in others with likely similar characteristics. The heterogeneity of outcomes after surgery for the group scoring ≤14 reflects this. Despite function remaining essentially unchanged, 32% of patients reporting their problems being worse after surgery and 60% perceiving their operation either "fair" or "poor", in average their pain improved and 48% indicated that their problems had also improved after surgery. Therefore, this high-pain group did much worse than their counterparts, but many of them reported some improvement after surgery.

This problem could potentially be attenuated if several cut-off points based on various patient characteristics were identified. Such an approach has been used previously to identify thresholds for satisfaction after joint replacement, stratified by subgroups of baseline or change scores [24]. The authors found slight variation in the thresholds, although there was also great overlap between them. However, the groups were arbitrarily defined. We employed an data-driven approach, free from researcher intervention in the definition of groups or the number of clusters. There is no evidence to suggest that multiple cut-off points, for arbitrarily defined patient

Table 2 Cohort description by pain group

	Low pain (OKS-PS > 14)	High pain (OKS-PS ≤ 14)
Observations: n (%)	107,542 (85.3%)	18,522 (14.7%)
Gender: n (%)		
Female	57,771 (54%)	10,343 (56%)
Male	42,683 (40%)	6623 (36%)
Not specified	98 (0%)	8 (0%)
Missing	*6990 (7%)*	*1548 (8%)*
Age band: n (%)		
40–49 years of age	167 (0%)	91 (0%)
50–59 years of age	8668 (8%)	2712 (15%)
60–69 years of age	37,112 (35%)	6471 (35%)
70–79 years of age	42,070 (39%)	6003 (32%)
80–89 years of age	12,529 (12%)	1697 (9%)
90+ years of age	6 (0%)	0 (0%)
Missing	*6990 (7%)*	*1548 (8%)*
Pre-op OKS score[1]		
Mean (SD)	19.8 (8)	14.4 (8)
Median (IQR)	20 (11)	14 (10)
Missing	*1229 (1%)*	*244 (1%)*
Standardised pre-op OKS-Pain score [2]		
Mean (SD)	36.5 (16)	25.6 (15)
Median (IQR)	35.7 (21.42)	25.0 (21.42)
Missing	*1227 (1%)*	*243 (1%)*
Standardised pre-op OKS-Function score [3]		
Mean (SD)	48.0 (18)	36.4 (17)
Median (IQR)	45 (25)	35 (20)
Missing	*1185 (1%)*	*240 (1%)*
Pre-op EQ-5D index[4]		
Mean (SD)	0.442 (0.30)	0.249 (0.32)
Median (IQR)	0.620 (0.532)	0.159 (0.603)
Missing	*5887 (5%)*	*1990 (11%)*
Pre-op EQ-5D VAS[5] "Your own health state today"		
Mean (SD)	69.6 (19)	59.8 (22)
Median (IQR)	74 (25)	60 (35)
Missing	*10,807 (10%)*	*2304 (12%)*
"How would you describe the results of your operation?" n (%)		
Excellent	31,212 (29%)	615 (3%)
Very good	42,716 (40%)	1756 (9%)
Good	25,755 (24%)	4915 (27%)
Fair	6740 (6%)	7273 (39%)
Poor	602 (1%)	3740 (20%)
Missing	*517 (0%)*	*223 (1%)*
"Overall, how are your problems now, compared to before your operation?" n (%)		
Much better	89,210 (83%)	2954 (16%)

Table 2 Cohort description by pain group *(Continued)*

	Low pain (OKS-PS > 14)	High pain (OKS-PS ≤ 14)
A little better	14,271 (13%)	6005 (32%)
About the same	2286 (2%)	3489 (19%)
A little worse	1237 (1%)	3227 (18%)
Much worse	227 (0%)	2647 (14%)
Missing	*331 (0%)*	*150 (1%)*
Post-op OKS score[a]		
Mean (SD)	38.2 (7)	17.8 (6)
Median (IQR)	39 (11)	19 (8)
Missing	*44 (0%)*	*2 (0%)*
Standardised post-op OKS-Pain score[b]		
Mean (SD)	82.4 (14)	36.0 (12)
Median (IQR)	85.7 (25.0)	39.3 (17.9)
Missing	*0 (0%)*	*0 (0%)*
Standardised post-op OKS-Function score[c]		
Mean (SD)	75.4 (8)	38.8 (8)
Median (IQR)	80 (25)	40 (20)
Missing	*44 (0%)*	*2 (0%)*
Post-op EQ-5D index[d]		
Mean (SD)	0.792 (0.19)	0.395 (0.30)
Median (IQR)	0.796 (0.309)	0.516 (0.532)
Missing	*4934 (5%)*	*1150 (6%)*
Post-op EQ-5D VAS[e] "Your own health state today"		
Mean (SD)	76.9 (16)	55.1 (20)
Median (IQR)	80 (20)	55 (30)
Missing	*5413 (5%)*	*1333 (7%)*

[a]captures knee pain and function, scored from 0 to 48 where 0 indicates most and 48 least pain and functional limitations
[b]OKS Pain subscale as captured by seven questions, scored 0–100 where 0 indicates most and 100 least pain
[c]OKS Function subscale as captured by five questions, scored 0–100 where 0 indicates most and 100 least functional limitations
[d]a health-related quality of life measure where 0 represents death and 1 refers to perfect health
[e]a Visual Analogue Scale ranging from 0 to 100, where 0 represents the worst and 100 the best imaginable health state

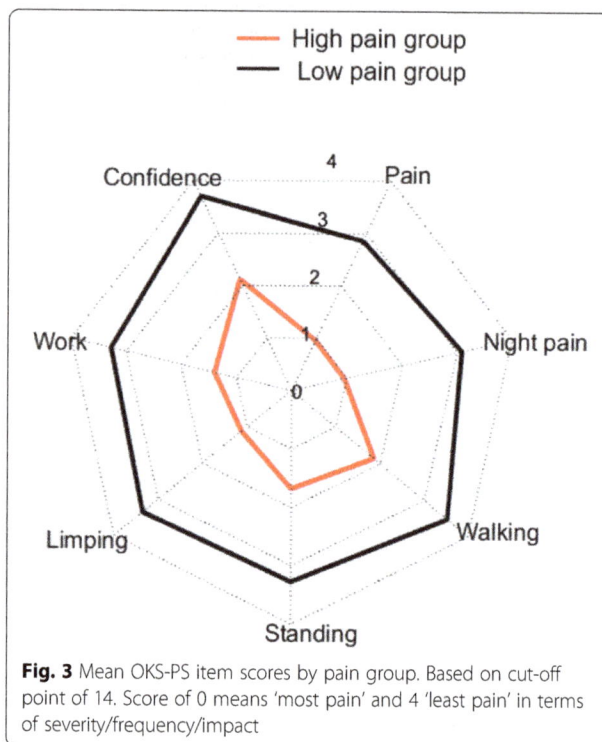

Fig. 3 Mean OKS-PS item scores by pain group. Based on cut-off point of 14. Score of 0 means 'most pain' and 4 'least pain' in terms of severity/frequency/impact

subgroups, would lead to more efficient classifications, but they would add a level of bias and make their potential application in clinical practice more complex.

Conducting a complete-case analysis was one limitation of this study. Results may therefore be affected as patients who did not complete all items of the OKS-PS may be different to those who did. However, only 1.6% of all patients in the dataset were excluded for incomplete data, thereby making any such bias unlikely. Large population cohorts such as the one used here also often suffer from loss to follow-up. In our study, however, only two patients who completed a pre-operative form did not complete the follow-up questionnaire, suggesting the data are representative of the English population.

Hierarchical cluster analysis has been used in a number of OA patient studies [18–21]. All of these studies used visual inspection of the dendogram (clustering diagram) in samples of 64 to 346 patients to identify the optimal number of clusters. Visual inspection is only practical in studies with small sample sizes. In this study, we applied data-driven clustering methods to a sample of over 120,000 KR patients and examined the highest OKS-PS value taken by the high-pain cluster without any discretionary framework imposed on the analysis. This is the first time, to our knowledge, that hierarchical clustering has been applied to large, real-world evidence data to identify groups based on their levels of chronic post-surgical pain.

The lack of a gold standard or other reference point for chronic pain following KR did not allow for a formal external validation of our method using a split sample of our data. However, our secondary analysis served as an internal validation as it evaluated the method by adding a second clustering approach whilst generating random orderings of the data. Our primary result of 14 fell within the ranges of values obtained from either method for all numbers of clusters between four and 19. In order to assess the generalisability of the cut-off point we identified as a screening tool for people with chronic pain following KR, a validation study using an external cohort is recommended.

Using the cut-off point of 14 in the OKS-PS identified in the primary analysis, 15% of primary KR patients in

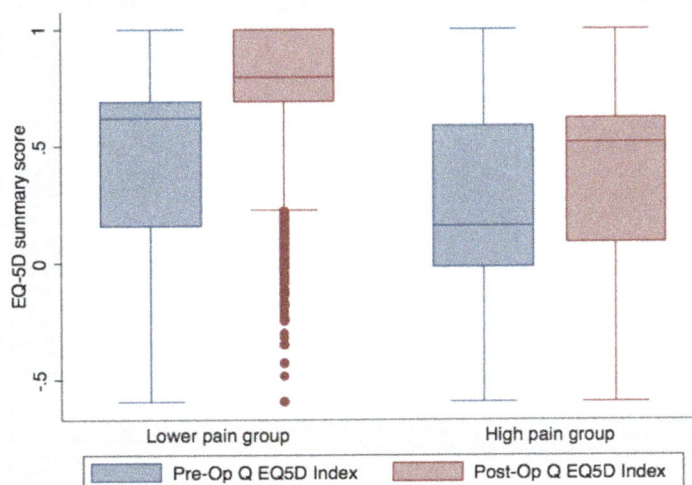

Fig. 4 Pre- and post-operative EQ-5D summary score by pain groups

England between 2012 and 2015 had chronic pain 6 months after their operation. This result is consistent with previous findings: a systematic review [2] found that 10–34% of patients reported moderate to severe chronic pain after KR. In one of the UK studies included in the review, 15% of TKR patients had severe to extreme pain three to 4 years after KR [25].

Conclusion

This study developed a cut-off score on a commonly used PROM to provide researchers with a standardised and validated approach to the identification of patients with chronic pain after TKR. We used a population-based observational cohort to identify a cut-off point in the Oxford Knee Score pain subscale of 14 at 6 months after KR which can be useful to select patients with chronic pain. Our secondary analyses indicated that the cut-off can be higher than 14. This cut-off point will facilitate the inclusion of a targeted group in clinical trials to help investigate pain characteristics, biological mechanism and evaluate interventions designed to improve support and management for people with KR who experience chronic pain. Given the growing number of KR operations being performed and the negative association found between chronic post-surgical pain and health-related quality of life, targeted interventions are likely to benefit many people. Identifying these individuals using a simple and commonly used questionnaire such as the OKS will also allow for the conduct of future qualitative studies to assess how the profile described here matches individuals' experiences, outcomes and expectations in other settings before broader uptake in clinical practice is considered.

Abbreviations

EQ-5D: Euro-Quol 5-dimension health-related quality of life questionnaire; KR: Knee replacement; NHS: National Health Service in England; NIHR: National Institute for Health Research; OA: Osteoarthritis; OKS: Oxford Knee Score; OKS-PS: Oxford Knee Score pain subscale; PROMs: Patient-Reported Outcome Measures; VAS: Visual Analogue Scale

Acknowledgements

We are thankful to all NHS patients whose anonymised records were used in this study as without their reported outcomes this research would not have been possible.

Funding

This article presents independent research funded by the National Institute for Health Research (NIHR) under its Programme Grants for Applied Research programme (RP-PG-0613-20001). This study was also supported by the NIHR Biomedical Research Centre at the University Hospitals Bristol NHS Foundation Trust and the University of Bristol. The views expressed in this publication are those of the authors and not necessarily those of the NHS, the National Institute for Health Research or the Department of Health. The funder had no involvement in the study design, data collection, analysis or interpretation, in the writing of the manuscript or the decision to submit for publication.

Authors' contributions

RPV, SK, VW, RGH, AS, and AJ all made substantial contributions to conception and design of the study. SK undertook the statistical analysis. RPV and SK drafted the manuscript with VW, RGH, AS and AJ revising it for important intellectual content. All authors read and approved the final manuscript.

Competing interests

All authors have completed the ICMJE uniform disclosure form. RGH and VW are members of the journal's editorial board, but as all other authors they have no other financial or personal relationships with other people or organisations that could inappropriately bias this work. AJ declares financial activities with Anthera Pharmaceuticals (through the Data Safety and Monitoring Board), the UK Renal Registry, Freshfields Brukhaus Deringer, and Roche, all outside the submitted work. RPV declares financial activities with Freshfields Brukhaus Deringer and Mereo Biopharma, both outside the submitted work as well.

Author details
[1]Nuffield Department of Orthopaedics, Rheumatology and Musculoskeletal Sciences, University of Oxford, Botnar Research Centre, Windmill Road, Headington, Oxford OX3 7LD, UK. [2]MRC Lifecourse Epidemiology Unit, University of Southampton, Southampton, UK. [3]Musculoskeletal Research Unit, Translational Health Sciences, Bristol Medical School, University of Bristol, Learning and Research Building, Level 1, Southmead Hospital, Bristol BS10 5NB, UK. [4]Wellcome Centre for Integrative Neuroimaging, FMRIB, Nuffield Department of Clinical Neurosciences, University of Oxford, Oxford, UK. [5]National Institute for Health Research Bristol Biomedical Research Centre, University Hospitals Bristol NHS Foundation Trust and University of Bristol, Bristol, UK.

References

1. Cross M, Smith E, Hoy D, Nolte S, Ackerman I, Fransen M, Bridgett L, Williams S, Guillemin F, Hill CL: The global burden of hip and knee osteoarthritis: estimates from the global burden of disease 2010 study. Ann Rheum Dis 2014:annrheumdis-2013-204763.
2. Beswick AD, Wylde V, Gooberman-Hill R, Blom A, Dieppe P. What proportion of patients report long-term pain after total hip or knee replacement for osteoarthritis? A systematic review of prospective studies in unselected patients. BMJ Open. 2012;2(1):e000435.
3. Kurtz S, Ong K, Lau E, Mowat F, Halpern M. Projections of primary and revision hip and knee arthroplasty in the United States from 2005 to 2030. JBJS. 2007;89(4):780–5.
4. National Joint Registry for England W, Northern Ireland and the Isle or Man,: 14th Annual Report 2017. In.; 2017.
5. Jeffery AE, Wylde V, Blom AW, Horwood JP. "It's there and I'm stuck with it": patients' experiences of chronic pain following total knee replacement surgery. Arthritis Care Res (Hoboken). 2011;63(2):286–92.
6. Smith TO, Dainty JR, MacGregor AJ. Changes in social isolation and loneliness following total hip and knee arthroplasty: longitudinal analysis of the English longitudinal study of ageing (ELSA) cohort. Osteoarthritis Cartilage. 25(9):1414–9.
7. Jinks C, Ong BN, Richardson J. A mixed methods study to investigate needs assessment for knee pain and disability: population and individual perspectives. BMC Musculoskelet Disord. 2007;8(1):59.
8. Boonstra AM, Schiphorst Preuper HR, Balk GA, Stewart RE. Cut-off points for mild, moderate, and severe pain on the visual analogue scale for pain in patients with chronic musculoskeletal pain. Pain. 2014;155(12):2545–50.
9. Patient Reported Outcome Measures (PROMs) [https://digital.nhs.uk/data-and-information/publications/statistical/patient-reported-outcome-measures-proms]. Accessed 2 Aug 2016.
10. Dawson J, Fitzpatrick R, Murray D, Carr A. Questionnaire on the perceptions of patients about total knee replacement. J Bone Joint Surg Br. 1998; 80-B(1):63–9.
11. The EuroQol Group. EuroQol - a new facility for the measurement of health-related quality of life. Health Policy. 1990;16(3):199–208.
12. Macrae WA. Chronic pain after surgery. Br J Anaesth. 2001;87(1):88–98.
13. Werner MU, Kongsgaard UE. I. Defining persistent post-surgical pain: is an update required? Br J Anaesth. 2014;113(1):1–4.
14. Lenguerrand E, Wylde V, Gooberman-Hill R, Sayers A, Brunton L, Beswick AD, Dieppe P, Blom AW. Trajectories of pain and function after primary hip and knee arthroplasty: the ADAPT cohort study. PLoS One. 2016;11(2).
15. Halket A, Stratford PW, Kennedy DM, Woodhouse LJ. Using hierarchical linear modeling to explore predictors of pain after Total hip and knee arthroplasty as a consequence of osteoarthritis. J Arthroplast. 2010;25(2):254–62.
16. Scott CEH, Howie CR, MacDonald D, Biant LC. Predicting dissatisfaction following total knee replacement: a prospective study of 1217 patients. J Bone Joint Surg. 2010;92-B(9):1253–8.
17. Harris K, Dawson J, Doll H, Field RE, Murray DW, Fitzpatrick R, Jenkinson C, Price AJ, Beard DJ. Can pain and function be distinguished in the Oxford knee score in a meaningful way? An exploratory and confirmatory factor analysis. Qual Life Res. 2013;22(9):2561–8.
18. Cruz-Almeida Y, King CD, Goodin BR, Sibille KT, Glover TL, Riley JL, Sotolongo A, Herbert MS, Schmidt J, Fessler BJ. Psychological profiles and pain characteristics of older adults with knee osteoarthritis. Arthritis Care Res. 2013;65(11):1786–94.
19. Murphy SL, Lyden AK, Phillips K, Clauw DJ, Williams DA. Subgroups of older adults with osteoarthritis based upon differing comorbid symptom presentations and potential underlying pain mechanisms. Arthritis Res Ther. 2011;13(4):R135.
20. Egsgaard LL, Eskehave TN, Bay-Jensen AC, Hoeck HC, Arendt-Nielsen L. Identifying specific profiles in patients with different degrees of painful knee osteoarthritis based on serological biochemical and mechanistic pain biomarkers: a diagnostic approach based on cluster analysis. Pain. 2015; 156(1):96–107.
21. Frey-Law LA, Bohr NL, Sluka KA, Herr K, Clark CR, Noiseux NO, Callaghan JJ, Zimmerman MB, Rakel BA. Pain sensitivity profiles in patients with advanced knee osteoarthritis. Pain. 2016;157(9):1988–99.
22. Khalid S, Judge A, Pinedo-Villanueva R. An Unsupervised Learning Model for Pattern Recognition in Routinely Collected Healthcare Data. In Proceedings of the 11th International Joint Conference on Biomedical Engineering Systems and Technologies. HEALTHINF. 2018;5:266–73. ISBN 978-989-758-281-3. https://doi.org/10.5220/0006535602660273.
23. Dolan P. Modeling valuations for EuroQol health states. Med Care. 1997; 35(11):1095–108.
24. Judge A, Arden NK, Kiran A, Price A, Javaid MK, Beard D, Murray D, Field RE. Interpretation of patient-reported outcomes for hip and knee replacement surgery: identification of thresholds associated with satisfaction with surgery. J Bone Joint Surg Br. 2012;94-B(3):412–8.
25. Wylde V, Hewlett S, Learmonth ID, Dieppe P. Persistent pain after joint replacement: prevalence, sensory qualities, and postoperative determinants. Pain. 2011;152(3):566–72.
26. NHS Digital: Patient Reported Outcome Measures (PROMs) in England – Data Quality Note. Finalised data for April 2014 to March 2015. In.; 2016.
27. Open Government Licence for public sector information [http://www.nationalarchives.gov.uk/doc/open-government-licence/version/3/]. Accessed 22 Jan 2018.

Permissions

The contributors of this book come from diverse backgrounds, making this book a truly international effort. This book will bring forth new frontiers with its revolutionizing research information and detailed analysis of the nascent developments around the world.

We would like to thank all the contributing authors for lending their expertise to make the book truly unique. They have played a crucial role in the development of this book. Without their invaluable contributions this book wouldn't have been possible. They have made vital efforts to compile up to date information on the varied aspects of this subject to make this book a valuable addition to the collection of many professionals and students.

This book was conceptualized with the vision of imparting up-to-date information and advanced data in this field. To ensure the same, a matchless editorial board was set up. Every individual on the board went through rigorous rounds of assessment to prove their worth. After which they invested a large part of their time researching and compiling the most relevant data for our readers.

The editorial board has been involved in producing this book since its inception. They have spent rigorous hours researching and exploring the diverse topics which have resulted in the successful publishing of this book. They have passed on their knowledge of decades through this book. To expedite this challenging task, the publisher supported the team at every step. A small team of assistant editors was also appointed to further simplify the editing procedure and attain best results for the readers.

Apart from the editorial board, the designing team has also invested a significant amount of their time in understanding the subject and creating the most relevant covers. They scrutinized every image to scout for the most suitable representation of the subject and create an appropriate cover for the book.

The publishing team has been an ardent support to the editorial, designing and production team. Their endless efforts to recruit the best for this project, has resulted in the accomplishment of this book. They are a veteran in the field of academics and their pool of knowledge is as vast as their experience in printing. Their expertise and guidance has proved useful at every step. Their uncompromising quality standards have made this book an exceptional effort. Their encouragement from time to time has been an inspiration for everyone.

The publisher and the editorial board hope that this book will prove to be a valuable piece of knowledge for researchers, students, practitioners and scholars across the globe.

List of Contributors

Daniel Cury Ribeiro, Angus Belgrave, Ana Naden, Helen Fang, Patrick Matthews and Shayla Parshottam
Centre for Health, Activity and Rehabilitation Research (CHARR), School of Physiotherapy – University of Otago, Dunedin 9054, New Zealand

Klemens Trieb
Department of Orthopaedics, Klinikum Wels-Grieskirchen, Grieskirchnerstr 42, 4600 Wels, Austria

Andreas Meryk, Erin Naismith and Beatrix Grubeck-Loebenstein
Institute for Biomedical Aging Research, University of Innsbruck, 5020 Innsbruck, Austria

Sascha Senck
Computed Tomography Research Group, University of Applied Sciences Upper Austria, 4600 Wels, Austria

John D. Collins
School of Design, University of Limerick, Limerick, Ireland

Leonard O'Sullivan
School of Design and Health Research Institute, University of Limerick, Limerick, Ireland

Yong-Qing Yan and Qing-Jiang Pang
Department of Orthopaedics, Ningbo No.2 Hospital, Xibei Street No.41 Ningbo, 315010 Zhejiang, People's Republic of China

Ren-Jie Xu
Department of Orthopaedics, Suzhou Municipal Hospital/The Affiliated Hospital of Nanjing Medical University, No 26, Daoqian Street, Suzhou 215000, Jiangsu, People's Republic of China
Department of Orthopaedics, the First Affiliated Hospital, Orthopaedic Institute, Soochow University, Suzhou 215000, Jiangsu, People's Republic of China

Qi Cheng, Jin-long Tang, Jiang-jiang Gu, Kai-jin Guo and Feng-chao Zhao
Department of Orthopedic Surgery, The Affiliated Hospital of Xuzhou Medical University, No. 99 Huaihai West Road, Xuzhou, Jiangsu 221002, People's Republic of China

Wang-shou Guo and Bai-liang Wang
Department of Joint Surgery, China-Japan Friendship Hospital, Beijing 100029, People's Republic of China

Frederic Martens and Geoffrey Lesage
Department of Neurosurgery, OLV Ziekenhuis, Moorselbaan 164, 9300 Aalst, Belgium

Jeffrey M. Muir
Motion Research, 3-35 Stone Church Rd., Suite 215, Hamilton, ON L9K 1S4, Canada

Jonathan R. Stieber
Clinical Assistant Professor of Orthopaedic Surgery, New York University School of Medicine, 485 Madison Avenue, 8th Floor, New York, NY 10022, USA

Qiuke Wang, Yifei Liu, Ming Zhang, Yu Zhu, Lei Wang and Yunfeng Chen
Department of Orthopedic Surgery, Shanghai Jiao Tong University Affiliated Sixth People's Hospital, 600 Yishan Road, Shanghai 200233, People's Republic of China

Toru Akiyama
Department of Orthopaedic Surgery, Saitama Medical Center, Jichi Medical University, Saitama, Japan

Takashi Fukushima
Department of Orthopaedic Surgery, Saitama Medical Center, Jichi Medical University, Saitama, Japan
Department of Orthopaedic Surgery, Jichi Medical University, Tochigi, Japan

Katsushi Takeshita
Department of Orthopaedic Surgery, Jichi Medical University, Tochigi, Japan

Akira Kawai
Department of Musculoskeletal Oncology, National Cancer Center Hospital, Tokyo, Japan

Koichi Ogura
Department of Musculoskeletal Oncology, National Cancer Center Hospital, Tokyo, Japan
Department of Orthopaedic Surgery, Faculty of Medicine, The University of Tokyo, Tokyo, Japan

Nancy E. Lane
Department of Internal Medicine, University of California, Davis School of Medicine, Sacramento, CA, USA

Barton L. Wise
Department of Internal Medicine, University of California, Davis School of Medicine, Sacramento, CA, USA

Department of Orthopaedic Surgery, University of California, Davis School of Medicine, Sacramento, CA, USA
Center for Musculoskeletal Health, Departments of Orthopaedic Surgery and Internal Medicine, University of California, Davis School of Medicine, 4625 2nd Avenue, Suite 2002, Sacramento, CA 95817, USA

Jingbo Niu and Yuqing Zhang
Boston University School of Medicine, Boston, MA, USA

Felix Liu and John A. Lynch
Department of Epidemiology and Biostatistics, University of California, San Francisco, San Francisco, CA, USA

Joyce Pang
University of New Mexico School of Medicine, Albuquerque, NM, USA

Junfeng Zeng, Hao Liu, Xin Rong, Beiyu Wang, Yi Yang1, Xinlin Gao and Tingkui Wu
Department of Orthopedics, West China Hospital, Sichuan University, 37 Guoxue Lane, Chengdu 610041, Sichuan, China

Ying Hong
Department of Operation Room, West China Hospital, Sichuan University, Chengdu 610041, Sichuan, China

Fabienne Reynard
Department of Physiotherapy, Clinique romande de réadaptation Suva, Sion, Switzerland

Philippe Vuistiner and Bertrand Léger
Institute for Research in Rehabilitation, Clinique romande de réadaptation Suva, Sion, Switzerland

Michel Konzelmann
Department of Musculoskeletal Rehabilitation, Clinique romande de réadaptation Suva, Sion, Switzerland

Guanglei Zhao, Jin Wang, Jun Xia, Yibing Wei, Siqun Wang, Gangyong Huang, Feiyan Chen, Jie Chen, Jingsheng Shi and Yuanqing Yang
Division of orthopaedic surgery, Huashan Hospital, Fudan University, Shanghai 200040, China

Lars Helbig, Georg W. Omlor, Adriana Ivanova and Gerhard Schmidmaier
Clinic for Orthopedics and Trauma Surgery, Center for Orthopedics, Trauma Surgery and Spinal Cord Injury, Heidelberg University Hospital, Schlierbacher Landstrasse 200a, 69118 Heidelberg, Germany

Thorsten Guehring
Clinic for Trauma and Orthopaedic Surgery, BG Trauma Center Ludwigshafen at Heidelberg University Hospital, Ludwig-Guttmann-Strasse 13, 67071 Ludwigshafen on the Rhine, Germany

Robert Sonntag and J. Philippe Kretzer
Laboratory of Biomechanics and Implant Research, Clinic for Orthopedics and Trauma Surgery, Heidelberg University Hospital, Schlierbacher Landstrasse 200a, 69118 Heidelberg, Germany

Susann Minkwitz
Berlin-Brandenburg Center for Regenerative Therapies, Charité—Universitätsmedizin Berlin, 13353 Berlin, Germany

Britt Wildemann
Berlin-Brandenburg Center for Regenerative Therapies, Charité—Universitätsmedizin Berlin, 13353 Berlin, Germany
Experimental Trauma Surgery, Universitätsklinikum Jena, 07747 Jena, Germany

Tereza Kropáčková, Olga Šléglová, Olga Růžičková, Jiří Vencovský, Karel Pavelka and Ladislav Šenolt
Institute of Rheumatology, Prague, Czech Republic
Department of Rheumatology, 1st Faculty of Medicine, Charles University, Prague, Czech Republic

Junqi Huang
Department of Orthopaedics, Mianyang Central Hospital, Mianyang 621000, Sichuan, China

Wenzhi Bi, Gang Han, Jinpeng Jia, Meng Xu and Wei Wang
Department of Orthopaedics, PLA General Hospital, Beijing 100853, China

Yoon Yi Kim, Bo Mi Chung and Wan Tae Kim
Department of Radiology, Veterans Health Service Medical Center, 53, Jinhwangdo-ro 61-gil, Gangdong-gu, Seoul 05368, Republic of Korea

Charlotte M Mallon and Andrew J Moore
Bristol Medical School, University of Bristol, Bristol, UK

Rachael Gooberman-Hill
Bristol Medical School, University of Bristol, Bristol, UK
National Institute for Health Research Bristol Biomedical Research Centre, University of Bristol, Bristol, UK

Humaira Mahmood, Duncan E. T. Shepherd and Daniel M. Espino
Department of Mechanical Engineering, University of Birmingham, B15 2TT, Birmingham, UK

Haoda Yu, Haoyang Wang, Kai Zhou, Xiao Rong, Shunyu Yao, Fuxing Pei and Zongke Zhou
Department of Orthopedics, West China Hospital, Sichuan University, Chengdu 610041, China

Dominik Kaiser, Christian Gerber and Dominik C. Meyer
Department of Orthopaedics, University of Zurich, Balgrist University Hospital, Uniklinik Balgrist, Forch-strasse 340, 8008 Zürich, Switzerland

Elias Bachmann
Department of Orthopaedics, Biomechanical Research Laboratory, Balgrist Campus, University of Zürich, Zürich, Switzerland

Maliheh Ghaneei, Yong Li and Samer Adeeb
Department of Civil and Environmental Engineering, Donadeo-ICE, University of Alberta, 9203 116th St, Edmonton, AB T6G 1R1, Canada

Amin Komeili
Faculty of Kinesiology, University of Calgary, Calgary, Canada

Eric C. Parent
Department of Physical Therapy, Faculty of Rehabilitation Medicine, University of Alberta, Edmonton, Canada

L Finlayson
University of Edinburgh, Edinburgh, Scotland

T Czuba
Epidemiology and Register Center South, Lund, Sweden

M S Gaston
Department of Orthopaedic Surgery, Royal Hospital for Sick Children, Edinburgh, Scotland

G Hägglund
Lund University Department of Clinical Sciences, Orthopedics, Lund, Sweden

J E Robb
School of Medicine, University of St Andrews, St. Andrews, Scotland

Rienk Dekker, Juha M. Hijmans and Jan H. B. Geertzen
Department of Rehabilitation Medicine, University of Groningen, University Medical Center Groningen, CB41, 9700 RB Groningen, The Netherlands

Pieter U. Dijkstra
Department of Rehabilitation Medicine, University of Groningen, University Medical Center Groningen, CB41, 9700 RB Groningen, The Netherlands
Department of Oral and Maxillofacial Surgery, University of Groningen, University Medical Center Groningen, Groningen, The Netherlands

Jutamanee Poonsiri
Department of Rehabilitation Medicine, University of Groningen, University Medical Center Groningen, CB41, 9700 RB Groningen, The Netherlands
Sirindhorn School of Prosthetics and Orthotics, Faculty of Medicine Siriraj Hospital, Mahidol University, Bangkok, Thailand

Mira Park
Department of Preventive Medicine, School of Medicine, Eulji University, Deajeon, Republic of Korea

Hye-Young Shim
Department of Preventive Medicine, School of Medicine, Eulji University, Deajeon, Republic of Korea
Department of Rehabilitation Medicine, Seoul National University Bundang Hospital, Seoul National University College of Medicine, Seongnam, Republic of Korea

Hee-June Kim and Hee-Soo Kyung
Department of Orthopaedic Surgery, School of Medicine, Kyungpook National University, Kyungpook National University Hospital, Daegu, Republic of Korea

Ji-Yeon Shin
Department of Preventive Medicine, School of Medicine, Kyungpook National University, Daegu, Republic of Korea

Ming Guan, Yong Xu, Feng Li and Wei Xiong
Department of orthopedics, Tongji Hospital, Tongji Medical College, Huazhong University of Science and Technology, 1095#, Jiefang Ave, Wuhan, Hubei, China

Zi Li
Department of orthopedics, Tongji Hospital, Tongji Medical College, Huazhong University of Science and Technology, 1095#, Jiefang Ave, Wuhan, Hubei, China
Department of orthopedics, Taikang Tongji Hospital, Wuhan, Hubei, China

Dong Sun
Radiology department, Tongji Hospital, Tongji Medical College, Huazhong University of Science and Technology, 1095#, Jiefang Ave, Wuhan, Hubei, China

Mauro A. S. Melloni, Josiel De Almeida Ávila, Mauro Alexandre Páscoa, Camila Justino De Oliveira Barbeta, Vagner Xavier Cirolini, Ezequiel M. Gonçalves and Gil Guerra-Júnior
Departamento de Pediatria, Universidade Estadual de Campinas-Unicamp, Tessália Vieira de Camargo, 126, Cidade Universitária Zeferino Vaz, Campinas, SP Zip code: 13083-887, Brazil

Sara Khalid
Nuffield Department of Orthopaedics, Rheumatology and Musculoskeletal Sciences, University of Oxford, Botnar Research Centre, Windmill Road, Headington, Oxford OX3 7LD, UK

Rafael Pinedo-Villanueva
Nuffield Department of Orthopaedics, Rheumatology and Musculoskeletal Sciences, University of Oxford, Botnar Research Centre, Windmill Road, Headington, Oxford OX3 7LD, UK
MRC Lifecourse Epidemiology Unit, University of Southampton, Southampton, UK

Anushka Soni
Nuffield Department of Orthopaedics, Rheumatology and Musculoskeletal Sciences, University of Oxford, Botnar Research Centre, Windmill Road, Headington, Oxford OX3 7LD, UK
Wellcome Centre for Integrative Neuroimaging, FMRIB, Nuffield Department of Clinical Neurosciences, University of Oxford, Oxford, UK

Andrew Judge
Nuffield Department of Orthopaedics, Rheumatology and Musculoskeletal Sciences, University of Oxford, Botnar Research Centre, Windmill Road, Headington, Oxford OX3 7LD, UK
Musculoskeletal Research Unit, Translational Health Sciences, Bristol Medical School, University of Bristol, Learning and Research Building, Level 1, Southmead Hospital, Bristol BS10 5NB, UK
National Institute for Health Research Bristol Biomedical Research Centre, University Hospitals Bristol NHS Foundation Trust and University of Bristol, Bristol, UK

Vikki Wylde and Rachael Gooberman-Hill
Musculoskeletal Research Unit, Translational Health Sciences, Bristol Medical School, University of Bristol, Learning and Research Building, Level 1, Southmead Hospital, Bristol BS10 5NB, UK
National Institute for Health Research Bristol Biomedical Research Centre, University Hospitals Bristol NHS Foundation Trust and University of Bristol, Bristol, UK

Index

www.ingramcontent.com/pod-product-compliance
Lightning Source LLC
Chambersburg PA
CBHW080522200326
41458CB00012B/4305